T0249835

TECHNOLOGY for DIAGNOSTIC SONOGRAPHY

WAYNE R. HEDRICK, PH.D., FACR

Professor, Medical Radiation Biophysics,
Northeast Ohio Medical University, Rootstown, Ohio
Aultman Hospital, Canton, Ohio

PAUL R. WAGNER, BS, RDMS, RDCS, RVT

Program Director, Diagnostic Medical Sonography
South Hills School of Business and Technology
State College, Pennsylvania

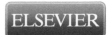

3251 Riverport Lane
St. Louis, Missouri 63043

Study Guide and Laboratory Exercise for Technology
for Diagnostic Sonography   ISBN: 978-0323081979

Library of Congress Cataloging-in-Publication Data
Study guide and laboratory exercises for technology for diagnostic sonography / Wayne R. Hedrick,
Paul R. Wagner. – 1st ed.
    p. cm.
    1. Diagnostic ultrasonic imaging–Problems, exercises, etc.   2. Diagnostic ultrasonic imaging–
Laboratory manuals. I. Hedrick, Wayne R. II. Wagner, Paul R.
    RC78.7.U4S78 2013
    616.07′543–dc23   2011044012

Publisher: Jeanne Olson
Managing Editor: Linda Woodward
Publishing Services Manager: Catherine Jackson
Project Manager: Sara Alsup
Design Direction: Paula Catalano

To Anne for your support and understanding... again.
(WRH)

To Leslie for your encouragement, support, and patience.
(PRW)

ACKNOWLEDGMENTS

The authors are indebted to the following diagnostic medical sonographers from our teaching institutions. They are a great resource of technical expertise, and create a challenging learning environment for residents and student sonographers:

James Allman, BS, RT, RDMS, RVT
Kelly Bourne, BA, BS
Rebecca Congon, RT, RDMS
Kathy Filicky, RT, RDMS
Valerie Hulett, RT(M), RDMS
Karen Karlen, RT, RDMS
Liz Ladrido, BS, RDMS, RVT
Beth Lampe, BS, RDMS, RDCS
Heather Massarelli, BS, RT, RDMS

Linda Metzger, RT, RDMS, RVT
Amy Mitan, BS, RT, RDMS
Robyn Nero, RT, RDMS
Michelle Neumeyer, RDMS
Angela Riker, RDMS
Susan Schmidt, RT, RDMS
Karry Smith, BS, RDMS
Sheri Tilton, RT, RDMS
Greg Tressler, RT(R), RDMS
Tricia Turner, BS, RDMS, RVT
Hannah Vickers, BS, RT, RDMS
Jessica Wheeler, BS, RDMS
Stephanie Wilson, BS, RVT, RDMS
Stephanie Yerian, RT, RDMS, RVT, RDC

TABLE OF CONTENTS

SECTION I
Sonography Principles

Chapter 1   Properties of Sound Waves, 2

Chapter 2   Interactions, 5

Chapter 3   Intensity and Power, 10

Chapter 4   Single-Element Transducers: Properties, 15

Chapter 5   Single-Element Transducers: Transmission and Echo Reception, 21

Chapter 6   Static Imaging, 26

Chapter 7   Image Formation in Real-Time Imaging, 29

Chapter 8   Real-Time Ultrasound Transducers, 33

Chapter 9   Real-Time Ultrasound Instrumentation, 41

Chapter 10   Digital Signal and Image Processing, 47

Chapter 11   Image Quality, 50

Chapter 12   Image Artifacts, 54

Chapter 13   Doppler Physics and Instrumentation, 59

Chapter 14   Doppler Spectral Analysis, 63

Chapter 15   Doppler Imaging, 67

Chapter 16   M-Mode Scanning, 70

Chapter 17   Clinical Safety, 73

Chapter 18   Performance Testing, 77

Answers to End of Chapter Questions, 85

APPENDICES

Appendix A   Computer Fundamentals, 91

Appendix B   Hemodynamics, 96

Appendix C   Contrast Agents, 101

SECTION II
Laboratory Exercises

Introduction to Laboratory Exercises, 104

Lab 1   Display Depth, Frame Rate, Freeze Frame, and Cine Loop, 105

Lab 2   Overall Gain and Output Power, 108

Lab 3   Time Gain Compensation, 110

Lab 4   Transmit Frequency: Resolution and Penetration, 113

Lab 5   Transmit Focus, 116

Lab 6   Magnification (Write Zoom), 119

Lab 7   Dynamic Range, 122

Lab 8   Persistence (Frame Averaging), 124

Lab 9   Gray-Scale Mapping, 126

Lab 10   Distance and Area Measurements, 128

Lab 11   Doppler Controls 1, 131

Lab 12   Doppler Controls 2, 135

Lab 13   Doppler Angle to Flow, 139

Lab 14   Nyquist Limit and Aliasing, 143

Lab 15   Color Doppler Controls: Part 1, 147

Lab 16   Color Doppler Controls: Part 2, 152

Lab 17   Application Presets, 155

Lab 18   Tissue-Mimicking Phantoms, 159

SECTION III
Review Questions

Review Questions, 162

Answers for Review Questions, 178

Glossary, 188

SECTION I

Sonography Principles

Properties of Sound Waves, 2

Interactions, 5

Intensity and Power, 10

Single-Element Transducers: Properties, 15

Single-Element Transducers: Transmission and Echo Reception, 21

Static Imaging, 26

Image Formation in Real-Time Imaging, 29

Real-Time Ultrasound Transducers, 33

Real-Time Ultrasound Instrumentation, 41

Digital Signal and Image Processing, 47

Image Quality, 50

Image Artifacts, 54

Doppler Physics and Instrumentation, 59

Doppler Spectral Analysis, 63

Doppler Imaging, 67

M-Mode Scanning, 70

Clinical Safety, 73

Performance Testing, 77

Answers to End of Chapter Questions, 85

Appendix A Computer Fundamentals, 91

Appendix B Hemodynamics, 96

Appendix C Contrast Agents, 101

Properties of Sound Waves

SOUND WAVES

- Sound is mechanical energy that is transmitted through a medium by forces acting on molecules.
  - Induced molecular motion is periodic whereby the molecules oscillate back and forth about their unperturbed positions.
  - Pressure fluctuations induce changes in molecular density (greater than and lower than the natural density).
    - Compression is a high-pressure (high-molecular-density) region in the medium created by the mechanical action of the sound wave.
    - Rarefaction is a low-pressure (low-molecular-density) region in the medium created by the mechanical action of the sound wave.
    - Acoustic pressure is expressed in units of pascal, megapascal, newton/m^2, or atmosphere.
- During linear propagation, molecular density exhibits sinusoidal behavior along the transmission path (plot of molecular density as a function of distance at an instant in time is a sine wave, as shown in Figure 1-1).

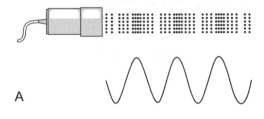

A

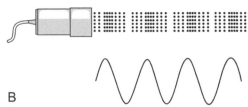

B

FIGURE 1-1 Particle density along the path of propagation varies with time, as shown by the sinusoidal curves. The high-density region denotes compression, and the low-density region denotes rarefaction. **A,** Initial observation. **B,** After a short time, the regions of high density and low density are displaced to the right along the direction of propagation and away from the sound source.

- Zones of rarefaction and compression alternate as sound is transmitted through the medium (see Figure 1-1).
  - Molecular density at a single location fluctuates with time ranging between compression and rarefaction.
  - Compression and rarefaction zones move away from the sound source and in the direction of sound propagation.
- Sound transmission cannot occur in a vacuum.
- The term *cycle* describes a sequence of amplitude changes (e.g., pressure or molecular density) that recur at regular intervals.
- *Frequency (f)* is the number of cycles per unit time.
  - The rate of density variation at a spatial location is the frequency.
  - The unit *hertz (Hz)* denotes one cycle per second.
  - The *period of the wave (T)* is the time for one complete cycle and equals the reciprocal of the frequency.
- *Ultrasound* is classified as sound waves with frequencies above the audible range of human hearing, and is generally considered >20 kilohertz (kHz).
- For longitudinal waves, the molecular (particle) motion is along the same direction as sound propagation (sound waves in liquids and tissue).
- For transverse waves, the molecular (particle) motion is perpendicular to the direction of sound propagation (sound waves in bone or metal).
- *Wavelength (λ)* is the distance for one complete cycle and is expressed in units of length—meter (m), centimeter (cm), or millimeter (mm).
  - Successive compression zones (or rarefaction zones) along the propagation path are separated by a distance equal to the wavelength.
- *Acoustic velocity (c)* is the speed at which the sound wave moves through a medium.
- The rate at which the wave transmits energy over a small area is the *intensity* (expressed in units of watts per centimeter squared [W/cm^2] or milliwatts per centimeter squared [mW/cm^2]).
- As sound intensity is increased, molecular density and acoustic pressure in the compression zone are also increased, accompanied by longer particle oscillation length and faster particle velocity.

- Intensity does not affect frequency, wavelength, and acoustic velocity during linear propagation.
- At high intensity, such as in tissue harmonic imaging, nonlinear propagation alters particle velocity and distorts the sinusoidal wave.

PROPERTIES OF SOUND-PROPAGATION MEDIA

- *Elasticity* is the ability of an object to return to its original shape and volume after a force has caused spatial distortion.
- *Density* (ρ) is the mass of the medium per unit volume (expressed in units of kilogram per cubic meter [kg/m^3] or gram per cubic centimeter [g/cm^3]).
- *Compressibility* indicates the fractional decrease in volume when pressure is applied to a medium.
- *Bulk modulus (B)* is the negative ratio of stress and strain.
  - *Stress* is the force per unit area applied to the medium.
  - *Strain* is the fractional change in volume of the medium.
- *Acoustic velocity* (c) depends on the density (ρ) and bulk modulus (B) of the medium:

$$c = \sqrt{\frac{B}{\rho}}$$

- Acoustic velocity is inversely proportional to the square root of the density.
- The density and bulk modulus of a material are interdependent.
  - A change in density is usually coupled with a larger and opposing change in bulk modulus.
  - Bulk modulus is the dominant factor in the determination of acoustic velocity.
- The average acoustic velocity in soft tissue is 1540 meters per second (m/s) or 1.54 millimeters per microsecond (mm/μs) and is compared with different media in Table 1-1.

- Acoustic velocity is considered to be independent of frequency in the sonography range of 2 to 20 megahertz (MHz).

TABLE 1-1	Acoustic Velocity of Different Media
Material	**Acoustic Velocity (m/s)**
Air	330
Soft tissue	1540
Bone	4080
Fat	1459
Blood	1575

m/s, meters per second.

FREQUENCY, WAVELENGTH, AND VELOCITY

- Frequency (f), wavelength (λ), and acoustic velocity (c) are interdependent, as shown by the following equation:

$$c = f\lambda$$

- Since acoustic velocity is constant for a particular medium, an increase in frequency results in a decrease in wavelength.
- Frequency remains constant as sound passes through media with different acoustic velocities (consequently, wavelength must change).
- As a rule of thumb, the wavelength (mm) in soft tissue is calculated by dividing 1.54 by the frequency expressed in MHz.

SOUND TRANSMISSION

- In sonography, the sound source as well as the detector of echoes is the *transducer*.
- The transducer may operate in continuous or pulsed ultrasound-generating mode, depending on the application.
- *Continuous-wave (CW) transmission* continuously emits a constant frequency and constant peak-pressure amplitude sound wave from the source.
- *Pulse-wave (PW) transmission* is a short-duration burst of sound (a few cycles in length) emitted from the sound source.

REVIEW QUESTIONS

1. What is the unit for frequency?
2. What are the two properties of a medium that affect the acoustic velocity in the medium?
3. For breast examination, the sonographer replaces a 5-MHz transducer with a 10-MHz transducer. Which of these two transducer frequencies generates the shortest wavelength in soft tissue?
4. What is the acoustic velocity of a 5-MHz ultrasound wave in soft tissue?
5. What is the acoustic velocity of a 10-MHz ultrasound wave in soft tissue?

PROBLEMS

1. What is the wavelength of ultrasound in a medium if the velocity is 1540 m/s and the frequency is 5 MHz?
2. What is the wavelength of ultrasound in a medium if the velocity is 4080 m/s and the frequency is 5 MHz?
3. What is the velocity of ultrasound in a medium if the wavelength is 0.04 cm and the frequency is 4 MHz?
4. What is the period of a wave whose frequency is 6 MHz?
5. Calculate the frequency of an ultrasound wave that has a wavelength of 0.45 mm in soft tissue.

MULTIPLE CHOICE QUESTIONS

1. Which of the following wave types is associated with ultrasound transmission in soft tissue?
   A. Longitudinal
   B. Transverse
   C. Electromagnetic
   D. Tidal

2. Which of the following terms describes the region of decreased molecular density induced by sound propagation in a medium?
   A. Compression
   B. Focal
   C. Fresnel
   D. Rarefaction

3. Which tissue type has the highest acoustic velocity?
   A. Bone
   B. Fat
   C. Muscle
   D. Soft tissue

4. Above what lower frequency limit are sound waves classified as ultrasound?
   A. 20 Hz
   B. 2000 Hz
   C. 20,000 Hz
   D. 200,000 Hz

5. Which quantity describes the energy transmission rate over a small area?
   A. Acoustic velocity
   B. Frequency
   C. Intensity
   D. Wavelength

Interactions

SPECULAR REFLECTION

- Reflection at a specular interface causes a fraction of the incident sound energy to be redirected into the medium from which it came (Figure 2-1).
  - Specular reflectors are larger than the wavelength of the sound beam.
  - The angle of incidence equals the angle of reflection.
  - At normal incidence, the reflected wave is directed back to the sound source along the same propagation path as that of the incident wave.
  - The intensity of the reflected wave depends on the composition of the interface.
  - The *acoustic impedance (Z)* of a medium is the resistance to the transmission of sound and equal to the product of density (ρ) and acoustic velocity (c):

$$Z = \rho c$$

  - The unit for acoustic impedance is the *rayl*, which equals to kg/m^2-s.
  - Acoustic impedances for different media are listed in Table 2-1.
  - Differences in acoustic impedance at an interface cause sound reflection.

TABLE 2-1	Acoustic Impedances for Different Media
Material	**Acoustic Impedance (Megarayls)**
Air	0.0004
Water	1.48
Soft tissue	1.63
Fat	1.38
Blood	1.62
Bone	7.8
Lung	0.26

TABLE 2-2	Percentage Reflections for Soft Tissue Interfaces
Interface	**Reflection Percentage**
Soft tissue—air	99.9
Soft tissue—lung	52
Soft tissue—bone	43
Soft tissue—fat	0.69
Soft tissue—muscle	0.04

- The *reflection coefficient for intensity (α_r)*, which equals the ratio of *reflected intensity (I_r)* to *incident intensity (I_i)*, is given by

$$\alpha_r = \frac{I_r}{I_i} = \left(\frac{Z_2 - Z_1}{Z_2 + Z_1} \right)^2$$

  for normal incidence, where Z_1 and Z_2 are the respective acoustic impedances of the media that compose the interface.
- Incident ultrasound intensity that is not reflected is transmitted through the interface.
- The reflection coefficient is independent of frequency for specular reflectors.
- The percentage reflection at different interfaces is shown in Table 2-2.

DIFFUSE REFLECTION

- *Diffuse reflection* occurs when a sound beam is incident on a large (greater than a wavelength), irregular surface and is reflected in multiple directions.
- The intensity of the reflected sound waves is typically much lower than that in specular reflection.

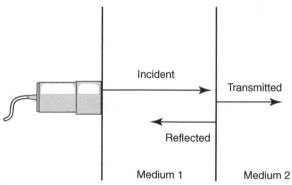

FIGURE 2-1 Specular reflection caused by a sound wave striking a large, smooth interface at normal incidence. The acoustic impedances of the media that compose the interface determine the relative intensities of the transmitted and reflected waves.

• Diffuse reflection is relatively independent of the orientation of the interface.

SCATTERING

• *Scattering* causes sound energy to radiate in all directions after a sound beam strikes a small interface with physical dimensions less than a wavelength (Figure 2-2).
  • Scatter intensity depends on the number of scatterers per volume.
  • Scattering is responsible for the internal texture of organs in the image but is weaker than specular reflection.
  • Scattering has strong frequency dependence.

REFLECTIVITY

• *Reflectivity* is the combination of factors (acoustic impedance mismatch, size, shape, surface evenness, and angle of incidence) that determine the intensity of an echo created at an interface.

REFRACTION

• For nonperpendicular beam incidence on a specular reflector, the reflector wave is not redirected back to the sound source, but reflected at an angle and refraction of the transmitted beam may occur.
• *Refraction* is the change in direction of a sound beam as it enters a medium (Figure 2-3).
  • Angular displacement is based on the ratio of the velocity of sound in the respective media and obeys Snell's law:

$$\frac{c_i}{c_t} = \frac{\sin \theta_i}{\sin \theta_t}$$

  where θ_i is the incident angle, θ_t the transmitted angle, c_i the velocity of sound in the incident medium, and c_t the velocity of sound in the transmitted medium.
  • Refraction does not depend on acoustic impedance mismatch at the interface.
  • At normal incidence or if velocity of sound is the same for two media, refraction does not occur.

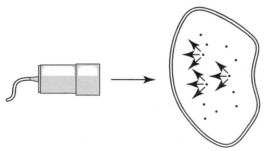

FIGURE 2-2 **Scattering**. Echoes are emitted in all directions from small reflectors (appropriately the size of the wavelength or smaller). The strength of the echoes is relatively independent of the incident beam direction.

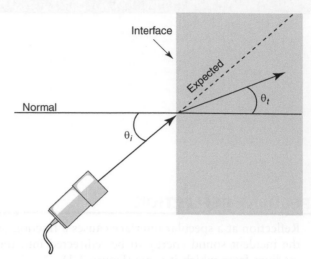

FIGURE 2-3 **Refraction**. The velocity of a sound beam in the incident medium is greater than that in the transmitted medium, causing the beam to be bent toward the normal ($\theta_i > \theta_t$).

DIVERGENCE AND DIFFRACTION

• *Divergence* causes a sound beam to radiate outward with a reduction in intensity as the beam moves away from a small source.
• The rate of divergence (and rate of intensity reduction) depends on the diameter of sound source (more pronounced as the source is made smaller).
• Diffraction causes a sound beam to diverge after passing through a small aperture.

INTERFERENCE

• Waves from more than one source combine by interference when they overlap.
• *Interference* is the point-by-point addition of waves (Figure 2-4), which depends on amplitude, frequency, and phase of the respective waves.
  • The resultant wave from the constructive interference has greater amplitude than do individual waves.
  • The resultant wave from the destructive interference has smaller amplitude than do individual waves.
  • Complex patterns are possible when the combined waves differ in amplitude, frequency, and phase.

ABSORPTION

• *Absorption* is the process whereby sound energy is converted into heat.
• Energy is transferred from ultrasound to the medium and cannot be recovered.
• The rate of absorption is directly proportional to the frequency.
• Ease of molecular motion (viscosity of medium) affects the absorption rate.
• In diagnostic sonography, the temperature rise is generally less than 1°C.

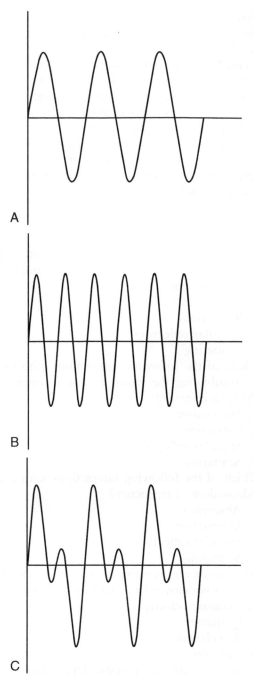

FIGURE 2-4 Wave Interference. Note that **B** has a different frequency from **A**. Thus **C** is the point-by-point amplitude summation of these two waves along the horizontal axis.

ATTENUATION

- *Attenuation* is the reduction in intensity from scattering and absorption as sound propagates through a medium (Figure 2-5).
- Intensity and peak pressure exhibit an exponential decrease as a function of distance.
- The rate of attenuation is directly proportional to frequency but also depends on the properties of a medium.

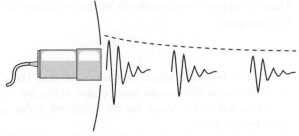

FIGURE 2-5 Attenuation. Decrease in acoustic pressure as a pulsed sound beam penetrates the medium. The dashed curve demonstrates an exponential loss in the peak acoustic pressure.

TABLE 2-3	Loss of Intensity by Attenuation in Different Media
Material	**Relative Intensity* (1 cm at 1 MHz)**
Blood	0.96
Fat	0.87
Soft tissue	0.83–0.89
Skull	0.01
Lung	0.0001
Water	0.9995

*Note: A value of 1 corresponds to no reduction in intensity.
cm, centimeter; *MHz*, megahertz.

- Values for the fractional intensity that remains after transmission through different media (1 cm in thickness) at a frequency of 1 MHz are listed in Table 2-3.

ECHO RANGING

- A transmitted pulsed wave is required to determine the depth of the reflector from the source.
- The time between transmitted pulse and detected echo is measured (Figure 2-6).
- Acoustic velocity (c) along a straight-line path is assumed to be a constant (1540 m/s).

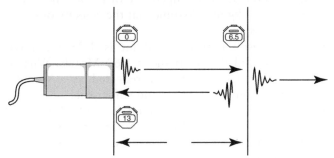

FIGURE 2-6 Principle of Echo Ranging. The distance to the interface is determined by measuring the time delay between the transmitted pulse and the received echo. A constant acoustic velocity must be assumed to convert time into depth.

- Time (t) is converted to depth of the reflector (z) by the equation:

$$z = \frac{ct}{2}$$

where the factor 2 takes into account that the distance between the sound source and reflector must be traversed twice, once by the transmit pulse and once by the echo.
- Time between transmitted pulse and detected echo is 13 μs for each centimeter in depth for soft tissue.

REVIEW QUESTIONS

1. For a breast examination, the sonographer replaces a 5-MHz transducer with a 10-MHz transducer. Which transducer frequency produces the strongest echo from a reflector at a depth of 5 cm? Assume that the transmitted intensity is the same for each frequency.
2. What is the change in frequency for a 5-MHz sound wave transmitted through an interface composed of fat and soft tissue?
3. What is the effect on wavelength when an ultrasound wave moves from a low–acoustic velocity medium to a high–acoustic velocity medium?
4. If an ultrasound beam is directed at an interface with a 10-degree angle of incidence and the acoustic velocity in the incident medium is greater than that in the transmitted medium, what is the change in direction of the transmitted beam (bends toward the normal, bends away from the normal, no change as it continues on straight line path)?
5. If an ultrasound beam is directed at an interface with a 10-degree angle of incidence and the acoustic velocity in the incident medium is equal to that in the transmitted medium, what is the change in direction of the transmitted beam (bends toward the normal, bends away from the normal, no change as it continues on straight line path)?

PROBLEMS

1. What is the acoustic impedance of tissue whose density is 1060 kg/m^3? Assume that the velocity of sound in tissue is 1540 m/s.
2. The acoustic impedance of fat is 1.38 megarayls (Mrayls) and that of tissue is 1.63 Mrayls. What is the percentage of intensity reflected at a specular interface composed of fat and soft tissue?
3. The acoustic impedance of fat is 1.38 Mrayls and that of tissue is 1.63 Mrayls. What is the percentage of transmission at a specular interface composed of fat and soft tissue?
4. What is the depth of an interface in soft tissue if the elapsed time between the transmitted pulse and the detected echo is 104 μs?

5. What is the elapsed time between the transmitted pulse and the detected echo if the interface is 5 cm from the transducer?
6. Calculate the transmitted angle if an ultrasound beam is directed at a large interface composed of soft tissue and bone. The angle of incidence is 10 degrees. Assume that the sound beam moves from soft tissue into bone.
7. Calculate the transmitted angle if an ultrasound beam is directed at a large interface composed of fat and soft tissue. The angle of incidence is 10 degrees. Assume that the sound beam moves from fat into soft tissue.

MULTIPLE CHOICE QUESTIONS

1. Which of the following interactions with matter is responsible for the internal texture of organs in the ultrasound image?
   A. Diffuse reflection
   B. Refraction
   C. Specular reflection
   D. Scattering
2. Which of the following interactions with matter is responsible for the major outline of organs in the ultrasound image?
   A. Diffraction
   B. Refraction
   C. Specular reflection
   D. Scattering
3. Which of the following interactions with matter is independent of frequency?
   A. Absorption
   B. Attenuation
   C. Specular reflection
   D. Scattering
4. What parameter remains unchanged when an ultrasound wave moves from fat to soft tissue?
   A. Acoustic velocity
   B. Frequency
   C. Wavelength
   D. Intensity
5. What is the unit for acoustic impedance?
   A. Rayl
   B. Decibel
   C. Hertz
   D. Curie
6. Which of the following interface compositions is most likely to generate the strongest echo?
   A. Soft tissue and muscle
   B. Soft tissue and fat
   C. Soft tissue and lung
   D. Soft tissue and water
7. Which tissue type has the highest rate of attenuation?
   A. Bone
   B. Fat
   C. Muscle
   D. Soft tissue

8. The depth of a reflector is 6 cm from the transducer. How long after the transmited pulse does the echo from this interface arrive at the transducer?
   A. 13 μs
   B. 39 μs
   C. 78 μs
   D. 156 μs

9. Which interaction is associated with the divergence of an ultrasound beam after it passes through a small aperture?
   A. Diffraction
   B. Interference
   C. Scattering
   D. Specular reflection

10. Which interaction produces a resultant wave from the summation of multiple waves?
    A. Diffraction
    B. Interference
    C. Scattering
    D. Specular reflection

11. Which interaction transfers energy from ultrasound to soft tissue?
    A. Refraction
    B. Absorption
    C. Scattering
    D. Specular reflection

Intensity and Power

MEASUREMENT OF INTENSITY

- Intensity is the rate of energy flow through an area expressed in units of watts per centimeter squared (W/cm^2) or milliwatts per centimeter squared (mW/cm^2).
- The instantaneous intensity (I) is determined from the measurement of acoustic pressure (p) in which the acoustic velocity (c) and the density (ρ) of the medium are known.

$$I = \frac{p^2}{\rho c}$$

- The term *free-field* describes conditions in which pressure (intensity) measurements are performed in water without reflectors or other disturbances to the ultrasonic field.
- Intensity determined in water is converted to the clinical situation (intensity in tissue) by applying correction (derating) factors.
- The hydrophone is a device that measures the time-varying pressure in the ultrasonic field.
- Ultrasound incident on the hydrophone induces a voltage that is directly proportional to pressure.
- By squaring the voltage signal, pressure is converted into instantaneous intensity.
- The physical size of the hydrophone is small (0.5 mm in diameter) to minimized spatial averaging.
- Spatial mapping is accomplished by moving the hydrophone to different locations within the ultrasonic field.

INTENSITY DESCRIPTORS

- Diagnostic medical ultrasound transducers produce complex, spatially and time-varying acoustic fields.
- Intensity descriptors are simplified characterizations of the intensity with respect to space and time.
- Temporal variations of pulsed-wave intensity are classified by temporal peak, pulse average, and temporal average (Figures 3-1 and 3-2).
    - Temporal peak (TP) intensity is the maximum intensity when accessed on the basis of time.
    - Pulse average (PA) intensity is time-varying intensity averaged over the duration of a single pulse.

- Temporal average (TA) intensity is time-varying intensity averaged over the pulse repetition period.
- For a given pulse sequence, temporal peak has the highest numerical value, followed by pulse average, and then by temporal average.
- Ultrasound intensity generated by continuous-wave devices usually refers to temporal-averaged intensity.
- Duty cycle is the fraction of time the transducer is actively generating ultrasound energy.
    - For imaging, the duty cycle is less than 1%.
    - For continuous-wave devices, the duty cycle is 100%.
- Temporal average intensity equals the product of the duty factor and pulse average intensity.

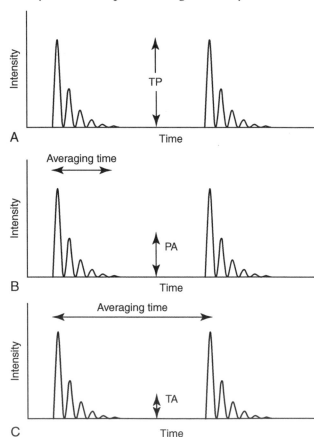

FIGURE 3-1 Temporal descriptors. Specification of intensity with respect to time measured at a point in the ultrasonic field. **A,** Temporal peak (TP). **B,** Pulse average (PA). **C,** Temporal average (TA).

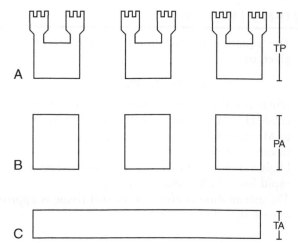

FIGURE 3-2 Temporal Averaging. A, The highest points on the sand castles (*turrets*) correspond to the temporal peak (TP). **B,** Sand making up the turrets has been stacked on the base of each castle. This corresponds to the pulse average (PA). **C,** The sand has been flattened to cover the area between the castles. This corresponds to the temporal average (TA).

- Spatial variations of pulsed-wave intensity are classified by spatial peak and spatial average.
  - The maximum intensity of all temporal intensity values within the ultrasonic field is the spatial peak (SP).
  - Averaging of the temporal intensity over the cross-sectional area of the beam is the spatial average (SA).
- Six combinations of spatial and temporal descriptors are possible:
  I(SPTP)—Spatial peak, temporal peak intensity
  I(SPPA)—Spatial peak, pulse average intensity
  I(SPTA)—Spatial peak, temporal average intensity
  I(SATP)—Spatial average, temporal peak intensity
  I(SAPA)—Spatial average, pulse average intensity
  I(SATA)—Spatial average, temporal average intensity

POWER

- *Power* is the energy radiated per unit time, usually expressed in milliwatts (mW), watts (W), or joules per second (J/s).
- Power equals the intensity integrated over the entire cross-section of the beam (or more simply, the product of intensity and area if the intensity is constant).
- The I(SATA) is approximated by the ratio of the power to the scan cross-sectional area (or power equals the product of the averaged intensity and duty factor).

ATTENUATION

- Scattering and absorption both contribute to the attenuation of ultrasound intensity as sound propagates through a medium.
- Fractional loss of peak amplitude pressure and intensity per unit distance depends on the medium and frequency (Figure 3-3).

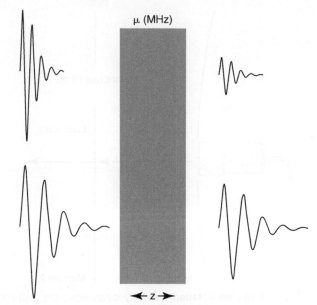

FIGURE 3-3 Attenuation. Intensity loss depends on the tissue via the attenuation coefficient (μ), the frequency of the sound wave, and the path length (z). High frequency sound waves undergo more rapid attenuation for the same medium and path length, as illustrated by the reduced amplitude on the right-hand side.

- The attenuation rate increases linearly with frequency.
- Attenuation by different media along the propagation path as well as specular reflection, diffuse reflection, and divergence contribute to the overall reduction in intensity.
- Specular reflection and diffuse reflection occur at the boundary between tissue types and redirect the beam.
- Divergence radiates the energy over a larger area thereby reducing the intensity (similar to distance from a hot stove).

DECIBEL

- Relative change in intensity is expressed in decibels (dB).
- Equation for decibels is given by:

$$\text{Level (dB)} = 10 \log\left(\frac{I}{I_{ref}}\right)$$

where I is the intensity at the point of interest, and I_{ref} is the initial or reference intensity.
- Since intensity is proportional to the square of the pressure amplitude, the decibel equation must be modified for pressure amplitude:

$$\text{Level (dB)} = 20 \log\left(\frac{p}{p_{ref}}\right)$$

where p is the peak pressure at the point of interest, and p_{ref} is the initial or reference peak pressure.
- A negative decibel result indicates a reduction in intensity compared with the reference value.
- Negative sign often replaced with the descriptor "loss" to indicate a decrease in intensity along the propagation path.

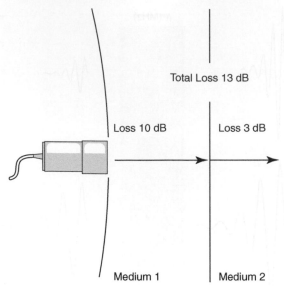

FIGURE 3-4 Decibel Notation. Intensity losses along the path are additive. Thus, the total intensity loss from the transducer to the point in medium 2 is 13 dB.

- Decibel losses along path segments are additive to yield the decibel loss for the entire path (Figure 3-4).
- Loss of 3 dB corresponds to a reduction in intensity by a factor of 2 or the equivalent of one half-value layer (HVL).
- The reduction factor from decibel loss is determined using the relationship 3 dB per HVL.
  - Divide the loss in decibel by 3 dB to yield number of HVLs (n).
  - 2^n equals the factor by which intensity was reduced.
  - As an example, a loss of 21 dB corresponds to 7 HVLs, or a reduction in intensity by a factor of 2^7 or 128.
- Attenuation rates for different media are shown in Table 3-1.
  - The attenuation rate for soft tissue is generally considered to be 0.7 decibel per centimeter-megahertz (dB/cm-MHz) but ranges from 0.5 to 0.8 dB/cm-MHz.
  - The attenuation rate for soft tissue at 5 MHz is 2.5 to 4 dB/cm.
  - The attenuation rate for soft tissue at 10 MHz is 5 to 8 dB/cm.

TABLE 3-1	Attenuation Rates for Different Media	
Material	**Attenuation Rate (dB/cm-MHz)**	
Blood	0.18	
Fat	0.6	
Soft tissue	0.5–0.8	
Skull	20	
Lung	40	
Water	0.0022	

dB/cm-MHz, decibel per centimeter-megahertz.

INTENSITY LOSS

- The equation to calculate loss from attenuation is given by:

$$\text{Intensity loss (dB)} = \mu\, f\, z$$

where μ is the intensity attenuation coefficient in dB/cm-MHz, f is the frequency of the ultrasound wave in MHz, and z is the distance traveled in the medium in centimeters.
- High values of the attenuation coefficient indicate rapid loss of ultrasound intensity.
- The attenuation coefficient for soft tissue is approximately 0.7 dB/cm-MHz.
- Compare the absolute reflected intensity from a specular reflector located at a distance of 2 cm and 4 cm: Attenuation for the longer path reduces the reflected intensity, even though the acoustic mismatch is unchanged.

ECHO INTENSITY

- Attenuation along the path and percent reflection from the interface affect the detected echo intensity.
- Percent reflection at the interface (%R) is converted into decibels by:

$$\text{Loss (dB)} = 10 \log\left(\frac{100}{\%R}\right)$$

- The bone–tissue interface at a depth of 5 cm in soft tissue shows a 24.7 dB intensity reduction for the detected echo with a frequency of 3 MHz:

$$\text{Loss (dB)} = \text{Loss (transmit)} + \text{Loss (return)} + \text{Loss (reflection)}$$

$$\text{Loss (dB)} = \mu\, f\, z\, \text{(transmit)} + \mu\, f\, z\, \text{(return)} + 10 \log\left(\frac{100}{\%R}\right)$$

$$\text{Loss (dB)} = (0.7 \text{ dB/cm-MHz})\,(3 \text{ MHz})\,(5 \text{ cm})$$
$$+ (0.7 \text{ dB/cm-MHz})\,(3 \text{ MHz})\,(5 \text{ cm}) + 10 \log\left(\frac{100}{43}\right)$$

$$\text{Loss (dB)} = 10.5 \text{ dB} + 10.5 \text{ dB} + 3.7 \text{ dB} = 24.7 \text{ dB}$$

- Structures with the same reflectivity are not necessarily depicted in an image with the same signal level because of differences in path length (effect of attenuation).
- A loss of 24.7 dB yields an echo intensity (I_e) of 6.8 mW/cm^2 for a transmitted intensity (I_t) of 2 W/cm^2:

$$\text{Loss (dB)} = 10 \log\left(\frac{I_e}{I_t}\right)$$

$$-24.7 = 10 \log\left(\frac{I_e}{2\text{W/cm}^2}\right)$$

$$-2.47 = \log\left(\frac{I_e}{2W/cm^2}\right)$$

$$0.0034 = \frac{I_e}{2W/cm^2}$$

$$I_e = 6.8 \text{ mW/cm}^2$$

REVIEW QUESTIONS

1. What is the rate of attenuation in decibel per centimeter-megahertz (dB/cm-MHz) for ultrasound propagating through soft tissue?
2. What property of the decibel notation allows the calculation of total loss from attenuation and reflection?
3. What are the units for intensity?
4. What is the unit for pressure?
5. What interactions contribute to loss of ultrasound intensity?
6. A comparison of the pulsed ultrasound output from two transducers shows 8 W/cm² at 6 MHz versus 10 W/cm² at 3.5 MHz. Which pulsed wave will undergo the fastest rate of intensity loss in soft tissue?
7. What fractional change in intensity is associated with a 3-dB loss?

PROBLEMS

1. If the rate of attenuation for fat is 1.8 dB/cm at 3 MHz, what is the rate of attenuation at 6 MHz?
2. What is the attenuation loss in decibels for an ultrasound wave that penetrates 1 cm of fat? Assume the frequency to be 3 MHz, the acoustic velocity to be 1460 m/s, and the attenuation coefficient to be 0.6 dB/cm-MHz.
3. If an ultrasound beam has a transmitted intensity of 2 W/cm² and the detected echo has an intensity of 0.005 W/cm², what is the intensity loss in decibels?
4. Calculate the relative intensity level in decibels for an echo generated at a soft tissue–bone interface that is at a depth of 4 cm. The ultrasound beam travels through soft tissue before being reflected at the interface. The transducer frequency is 5 MHz, and the rate of attenuation is 0.7 dB/cm-MHz.
5. Calculate the relative intensity in decibels for an echo generated at a soft tissue–lung interface that is at a depth of 3 cm. The ultrasound beam travels through soft tissue before being reflected at the interface. The transducer frequency is 5 MHz, and the rate of attenuation is 0.7 dB/cm-MHz.

6. Calculate the returning echo intensity as a fraction of the transmitted intensity if the intensity of the detected echo is described as 50 dB below the transmitted intensity.
7. What is the power for a transducer if the I(SATA) is 32 mW/cm² and the scanned area is 3 cm²?
8. If the I(SAPA) is 2 W/cm² and the duty cycle is 0.001, what is the I(SATA)?
9. If the intensity loss along the beam path is 30 dB, by what factor has the intensity been reduced?
10. If the intensity loss along the beam path from point A to point B is 5 dB and the intensity loss along the beam path from point B to point C is 2 dB, what is the intensity loss along the beam path from point A to point C?
11. If the rate of attenuation is 2.1 dB/cm at a frequency of 3 MHz, what would be the rate of attenuation at 10 MHz?
12. Calculate the loss in decibels if the intensity is reduced by a factor of 8.

MULTIPLE CHOICE QUESTIONS

1. Which material has the highest rate of attenuation?
   A. Blood
   B. Fat
   C. Lung
   D. Soft tissue
2. Which material has the lowest rate of attenuation?
   A. Blood
   B. Fat
   C. Lung
   D. Soft tissue
3. What factor primarily affects the absolute echo intensity detected by the transducer?
   A. Acoustic velocity
   B. Beam width
   C. Spatial pulse length
   D. Transmitted intensity
4. What factor affects the ratio of echo intensity compared with transmitted intensity?
   A. Pulse duration
   B. Path length
   C. Transmitted intensity
   D. Pulse repetition frequency
5. What wave property is changed by an increase in intensity (assume linear propagation)?
   A. Wavelength
   B. Frequency
   C. Acoustic velocity
   D. Acoustic pressure
6. What is the unit for power?
   A. Joule
   B. W/cm²
   C. mW
   D. Pascal

7. What medium is used for free-field intensity measurement?
   A. Soft tissue
   B. Water
   C. Tissue-mimicking material
   D. Acoustic gel

8. What is the effect on instantaneous intensity if the measured pressure increases by a factor of 2?
   A. No effect
   B. Intensity increases by a factor of 2
   C. Intensity increases by a factor of 4
   D. Intensity decreases by a factor of 1.4

9. Which temporal intensity descriptor will have the highest numerical value for a transducer?
   A. Temporal peak
   B. Pulse average
   C. Temporal average
   D. One cycle average

10. What is the duty cycle for continuous-wave Doppler transducer?
   A. 0.1 %
   B. 1%
   C. 10%
   D. 100%

11. What affects the rate of loss of beam intensity as the pulsed ultrasound wave propagates through tissue?
   A. Beam width
   B. Frequency
   C. Pulse duration
   D. Initial intensity

Single-Element Transducers: Properties

TRANSDUCER BASICS

- A *transducer* is a device that converts one form of energy into another (sound to electrical, and vice versa).
- In the transmission mode, the ultrasound transducer generates a sound beam when voltage is applied across the crystal.
- In the reception mode, pressure fluctuations caused by the incident sound wave on the transducer are converted into an electrical signal.
- *The piezoelectric effect* is a phenomenon exhibited by crystalline materials, in which an electrostatic voltage is produced across the crystal when the shape of the crystal is deformed.
- Design criteria for the transducer used in imaging include an ultrasound wave of the proper frequency in the megahertz (MHz) range, directional control, limited spatial extent (beam width and pulse length), and capability of pulsed-wave operation.
- Megahertz frequencies (2–20 MHz) are necessary to achieve <1-mm wavelengths for good spatial resolution.
- Applying of the echo ranging principle, pulsed-wave ultrasound enables the depth of the reflector to be measured.
- Limited beam width and limited pulse length restrict the region in which the returning echo could have been formed.

PIEZOELECTRIC PROPERTIES

- Alignment of dipolar molecules enables expansion and contraction of the crystal when a voltage is applied to the crystal (Figure 4-1).
- Natural vibrational frequency is established by the thickness of the crystal.
- The thickness of the crystal is equal to one-half the natural resonance wavelength.
- Lead zirconate titanate (PZT) is a common piezoelectric material used in ultrasonography.
- The alignment of dipoles in piezoelectric crystals is destroyed by high temperature.

TRANSDUCER CONSTRUCTION

- The simplest ultrasound transducer has a single piezoelectric crystal, which is in the form of a disc (Figure 4-2).
- The crystal has thin, silver electrodes plated on each side of a cylindrical disc.
- A matching layer is located on the patient side of the crystal.
- The matching layer improves energy transfer from crystal to patient, thus shortening pulse duration and increasing pulse intensity.
- The acoustic impedance of the matching layer is intermediate between those of the crystal and tissue.
- A quarter-wavelength transducer has a matching layer, which has a thickness of one-quarter wavelength.
- Multiple matching layers taper the acoustic impedance between the crystal and tissue and thereby improve the transmission of sound energy into the patient (less ringing).
- The backing material is located next to the crystal on the side opposite the matching layer.
- For continuous-wave ultrasound, the backing material has an acoustic impedance very different from that of the crystal.
- For pulsed-wave ultrasound, the backing material has an acoustic impedance similar to that of the crystal to reduce ringing and to produce a pulse of short duration.
- Radiofrequency shielding surrounds the crystal, the matching layer, and the backing material and is designed to reduce environmental electromagnetic radiation interference.
- Focusing reduces beam width at a specific distance from the transducer.
- Compared with a nonfocused beam, a focused beam causes the ultrasound energy to be concentrated in a smaller volume within the focal region, which results in improved spatial localization and stronger echo formation.

• The advantages of composite materials include low acoustic impedance (better matching with tissue), wide frequency bandwidth (broadband transducers), and improved sensitivity.

REVIEW QUESTIONS

1. What is the purpose of the transducer?
2. What is the frequency range for common diagnostic medical ultrasound transducers?
3. Why is a megahertz operating frequency important in ultrasound imaging?
4. What effect is associated with materials that have aligned dipolar molecules in which an incident sound wave induces an electrical signal in the material?
5. What crystal material is commonly used in diagnostic medical ultrasound transducers?
6. What physical property of the piezoelectric crystal determines the natural vibrational frequency?
7. What is the purpose of the matching layer placed between the crystal and the patient?
8. What components of the transducer are designed to suppress ringing?
9. Why is a pulsed sound wave necessary for imaging?
10. What is pulse repetition frequency?
11. What factors determine the spatial pulse length of the transmitted ultrasound wave?
12. What is the purpose of focusing the ultrasound beam?
13. What parameter is used to characterize the range of frequencies that compose the ultrasound pulse?
14. What is the relationship between pulse duration and bandwidth?
15. What is duty factor?
16. What is the approximate pulse duration for ultrasound imaging?
17. What is the relationship between pulse repetition period and pulse repetition frequency?
18. Why is the generation of a unidirectional beam a desirable feature in an ultrasound transducer?
19. Why is the generation of an ultrasound with a small beam width a desirable feature in a transducer?
20. Label the diagram of the single-element transducer (Figure 4-5) with the following components: crystal, insulating case, matching layer, and backing material.

PROBLEMS

1. What is the maximum pulse repetition frequency (PRF) if the depth of interest is 8 cm?
2. What is the pulse repetition period (PRP) corresponding to a PRF of 9625 pulses per second?
3. What is the spatial pulse length (SPL) for a 3.5-cycle pulse if the frequency is 5 MHz?

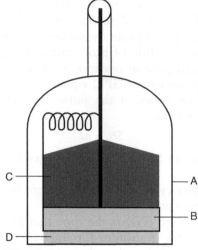

FIGURE 4-5 Single-element transducer.

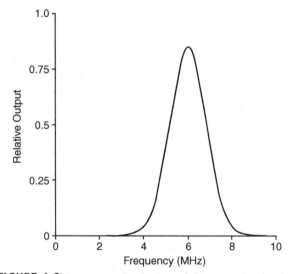

FIGURE 4-6 Frequency distribution of the transmitted pulse.

4. Determine the pulse duration (PD) for a 3.5-cycle transmitted pulse if the frequency is 5 MHz.
5. Calculate the duty factor for a 5-MHz transducer that produces 3.5 cycles per pulse. The pulse repetition frequency is 1500 pulses per second.
6. What is the fractional bandwidth for a 2.5-cycle, 5-MHz pulsed wave?
7. What is the pulse duration for a pulsed wave with a bandwidth of 2 MHz and a center frequency of 5 MHz?
8. Examine the graph of the frequency distribution for a transducer in Figure 4-6. What is the operating frequency?
9. Examine the graph of the frequency distribution for a transducer in Figure 4-6. What is the bandwidth?

MULTIPLE CHOICE QUESTIONS

1. What is a design feature of an ultrasound transducer used for B-mode imaging?
   A. Operating frequency in the megahertz (MHz) range
   B. Produces a directional beam
   C. Capability to turn sound beam on and off rapidly
   D. All of the above

2. For which application would the selected transducer operate at the highest frequency?
   A. Abdomen
   B. Breast
   C. Cardiac
   D. All applications use the same operating frequency

3. Why is an operating frequency of 200 kHz not appropriate for B-mode imaging?
   A. Wavelength is too long
   B. Attenuation is too rapid
   C. Power is too high
   D. Transducer footprint is too large

4. Which phenomenon is associated with materials that have aligned dipolar molecules in which an electrical impulse causes the bipolar material to expand and contract producing a sound wave?
   A. Quadrature phase principle
   B. Converse piezoelectric effect
   C. Doppler effect
   D. Huygens' principle

5. What component of the transducer contains lead zirconate titanate?
   A. Crystal
   B. Matching layer
   C. Backing material
   D. Electrodes

6. Which of the following transducer properties is most closely associated with crystal thickness?
   A. Center frequency
   B. Bandwidth
   C. Low Q-value
   D. Pulse duration

7. What is the primary purpose of the backing material placed next to the crystal?
   A. Suppress ringing in the transmitted pulse
   B. Reduce transducer footprint
   C. Reduce acoustic impedance mismatch between crystal and patient
   D. Insulate the patient from the high-temperature crystal

8. What component of the transducer is designed to shorten the transmitted ultrasound pulse and improve the energy transfer across the crystal–tissue interface?
   A. Electrodes
   B. Matching layer
   C. Backing material
   D. Radiofrequency (RF) shielding

9. What affects the maximum pulse repetition frequency?
   A. Attenuation of sound in tissue
   B. Crystal thickness in the transducer
   C. Distance to the point of interest
   D. Width of the field of view

10. Three transducers operating at a center frequency of 5 MHz produce a 2.5-cycle pulse, a 3-cycle pulse, or a 5-cycle pulse. Which transducer has the highest pulse repetition frequency for a scan range of 5 cm?
    A. 2.5-cycle
    B. 3-cycle
    C. 5-cycle
    D. Equal in pulse repetition frequency

11. Three transducers operating at a center frequency of 5 MHz produce a 2.5-cycle pulse, a 3-cycle pulse, or a 5-cycle pulse. Which transducer has the shortest pulse duration?
    A. 2.5-cycle
    B. 3-cycle
    C. 5-cycle
    D. Equal in pulse duration

12. What does the bandwidth indicate when applied to the transmitted ultrasound pulse?
    A. Mean of the frequencies present
    B. Median of the frequencies present
    C. Range of frequencies present
    D. Highest 10% of frequencies present

13. What can destroy the alignment of the dipolar molecules in a crystal?
    A. High temperature above 200°C
    B. Pulse repetition frequency above 1000 Hz
    C. Fast rotational movement of the transducer during scanning
    D. Application of a 300-volt electrical pulse across the crystal

14. Which transducer attribute results in a narrow bandwidth?
    A. Low Q-value
    B. Rapidly damped transmitted pulse
    C. Continuous wave
    D. Thin crystal thickness

15. What parameter characterizes the fraction of time that the transducer is actively generating ultrasound?
    A. Duty factor
    B. Crystal thickness
    C. Operating frequency
    D. Bandwidth

16. Compare the pulse duration with the interval of no transmission during a pulse–listen cycle in B-mode imaging.
    A. Pulse duration is 100 times greater than the listen cycle
    B. Pulse duration can be greater than or less than the listen cycle

C. The listen cycle is the same as pulse duration

D. The listen cycle is much greater than pulse duration

17. What is the purpose of focusing?

A. Increase the maximum pulse repetition frequency

B. Narrow the beam width at the depth of interest

C. Reduce the need for attenuation signal correction

D. Decrease the spatial pulse length

18. A transducer specification sheet states that the Q-value is 1000. Which application is most appropriate for this transducer?

A. B-mode imaging

B. Continuous-wave Doppler

C. Pulsed-wave Doppler

D. Any of the above

19. A transducer specification sheet states that the backing material is air. Which application is most appropriate for this transducer?

A. B-mode imaging

B. Continuous-wave Doppler

C. Pulsed-wave Doppler

D. Any of the above

20. What is the advantage of a tampered matching layer compared with a single matching layer?

A. Increased maximum pulse repetition frequency

B. Reduced spatial pulse length

C. Increased operating frequency

D. Reduced beam width

Single-Element Transducers: Transmission and Echo Reception

AXIAL RESOLUTION

- Axial resolution is the ability to resolve, as separate entities, two adjacent objects that lie along the beam axis.
- Axial resolution depends on spatial pulse length (SPL).
  - As operating frequency is increased, SPL is shortened (resolution is improved).
  - As ringing is decreased, pulse duration is shortened (resolution is improved).
- One-half of SPL is the smallest distance between reflectors that allows the reflectors to be resolved.
  - Echoes form reflectors located closer than one-half of SPL are processed as a single echo, and two scanned objects are presented as one structure in the display.
- SPL is not affected by attenuation along the beam path.
- Axial resolution is essentially constant throughout the scan range (independent of depth).
- Higher operating frequency, lower Q-value, increased damping, and shorter pulse duration reduce SPL and improve axial resolution.

LATERAL RESOLUTION

- Lateral resolution is the ability to resolve, as separate entities, two adjacent objects that lie perpendicular to the beam axis.
- A narrow beam width improves lateral resolution.
- A narrow beam width also enables a truer representation of single, small objects along the direction perpendicular to the beam axis.
- An object with physical dimensions smaller than the beam width is spatially depicted, with the lateral extent being equal to the beam width.

ULTRASONIC FIELD

- Huygens' principle states that a large sound source can be divided into a collection of small radiating sources.

- Each small individual source creates an ultrasonic field.
- Ultrasonic fields from all the small sources combine by interference to form a complex beam pattern.
- The near field, or the Fresnel zone, is the region extending from the transducer to the point of beam divergence (Figure 5-1).
  - The near field is associated with a narrow beam width.
  - A continuous wave produces axial pressure variations within the near field.
  - The pulsed wave with multiple frequency components diminishes axial pressure variations within the near field.
- The far field, or the Fraunhofer zone, is the region beyond the near field, in which the beam diverges rapidly and is associated with poor lateral resolution.
- The distance from the transducer that the near field extends into the patient is the near-field depth (NFD).
  - Larger diameter of the crystal (D) increases NFD.
  - Higher operating frequency of the transducer (f) extends NFD.
  - NFD is inversely proportional to the acoustic velocity of a medium (c).
  - NFD is inversely proportional to the wavelength in a medium (λ).

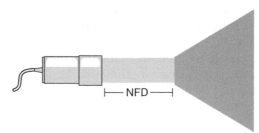

FIGURE 5-1 Beam pattern from a single-element transducer showing the near field (*light gray*) and far field (*dark gray*). Distance NFD indicates the depth of the near field.

- These relationships are summarized by the following equation to calculate NFD:

$$NFD = \frac{D^2 f}{4c} = \frac{D^2}{4\lambda}$$

- High frequency improves lateral resolution, but the increased rate of attenuation may cause unacceptable signal loss (lack of penetration).
- Increased crystal diameter extends NFD but broadens the beam width near the transducer.
  - For shallow depths, a small-diameter crystal with a narrow beam width improves lateral resolution.
  - As scan range is increased, a larger-diameter crystal is necessary to extend NFD and maintain lateral resolution.
- The angle of divergence of the beam in the far field (φ) indicates the changing beam width with depth.
  - Increasing the crystal diameter (D) decreases the angle of divergence.
  - Increasing the frequency of the transducer (f) decreases the angle of divergence.
  - Increasing the wavelength in the medium (λ) increases the angle of divergence.
  - The angle of divergence is proportional to the acoustic velocity of a medium (c).
  - These relationships are summarized in the following equation to calculate the angle of divergence (φ):

$$\sin \varphi = \frac{1.22\lambda}{D} = \frac{1.22c}{Df}$$

- The self-focusing effect narrows the beam width with in the near field (smaller than the diameter of the crystal).
- Side lobes are additional projections of ultrasound energy that radiate away from the main beam.

FOCUSING

- Focusing reduces the beam width and increases the intensity of the transmitted wave within the ultrasonic field.
- The focal zone is the region with the narrowest beam width and the highest intensity.
- The focal length is the distance from the transducer to the focal point (center of the focal zone).
- The depth of field is the length of the focal zone (Figure 5-2).
- Mechanical focusing methods include the use of an acoustic lens placed in front of the crystal and a curved crystal (Figures 5-3 and 5-4).
- In the manufacturing of the transducer, the radius of curvature of the lens or crystal controls the degree of focusing (Figure 5-5).
  - More curvature decreases the beam width, and the focal zone moves closer to the transducer.

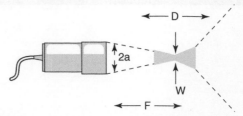

FIGURE 5-2 Focused Transducer. Parameters describing the ultrasonic field for a single-element focused transducer, aperture (*2a*), depth of field (*D*), focal length (*F*), and beam width (*w*).

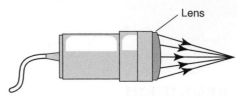

FIGURE 5-3 Mechanical Focusing. Focused single-element transducer with an acoustic lens.

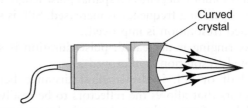

FIGURE 5-4 Mechanical Focusing. Focused single-element transducer with a curved piezoelectric crystal.

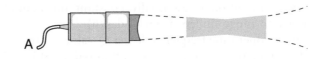

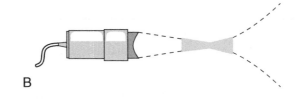

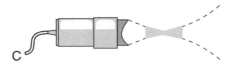

FIGURE 5-5 **The Radius of Curvature of the Piezoelectric Crystal Affects Beam Focusing.** For a higher degree of focusing, the beam width decreases, the focal zone moves closer to the face of the transducer, and the intensity increases in the focal zone. **A,** Weak or long focusing. **B,** Medium focusing. **C,** Strong or short focusing.

- The focal length is fixed for the transducer with mechanical focusing and cannot be adjusted by the sonographer.
  - Transducers with different fixed focal lengths are selected by application (obsolete technology).
- The f-number is the ratio of focal length to aperture.
  - A low f-number indicates strong focusing.
- Lateral resolution is not constant throughout the scan range.

TRANSMIT POWER

- Transmit power controls the intensity of the transmitted sound wave.
- Intensity is varied by changing the excitation voltage to the crystal.
- Operator control of power is usually specified in decibels of percent of maxium.
- High transmit power causes a proportionate rise in echo intensity and improves the detection of weak reflectors.
- High power levels increase patient exposure and should therefore be used with caution.

RECEPTION

- An echo striking the crystal induces a radiofrequency (RF) signal via the piezoelectric effect.
- RF waveform has the same shape as the echo pressure variations.

SIGNAL PROCESSING

- Amplification (receiver gain), which can be adjusted by the sonographer, increases the voltage of the RF signal.
- Time gain compensation (TGC) applies variable amplification as a function of depth.
  - Alternative names for time gain compensation include *depth gain compensation, swept gain control, depth-varied gain, distance-attenuation compensation,* and *sensitivity-time control.*
  - TGC corrects signals for attenuation along the beam path.
  - Amplification increases with time and follows a reverse exponential function.
  - TGC is automatically applied during signal processing, and fine control of gain versus depth can be adjusted by the sonographer.
- Rectification modifies the RF signal so that only positive variations are present.
- Enveloping connects peak-to-peak variations to form a contour of the overall RF signal.
- Integration determines the area under the enveloped signal.
- The induced RF signal with its fast oscillations and varying amplitude over time (pulse duration) is converted to a single metric (voltage representing the area of the enveloped signal) at the depth of echo generation.
- Reject control, which can be adjusted by the sonographer, eliminates from display low-amplitude signals and noise below a threshold value.

A-MODE DISPLAY

- A-mode display involves two-dimensional presentation of signal strength versus time (scan depth) on the monitor.
- Each detected interface is shown as a voltage spike (Figure 5-6).
  - A voltage spike occurs at a time sweep corresponding to the depth of the reflector.
  - The height of the voltage spike represents signal strength.

DYNAMIC RANGE

- Dynamic range, often expressed in decibels (dB), indicates the range of signal magnitudes that can be preserved as distinct values by a system component.
- Dynamic range is quantified as the ratio of the largest signal to the smallest signal.
- Echo amplitudes, detected by the transducer, vary from 100 dB to 150 dB.
- The dynamic range is reduced by logarithmic amplification, TGC, and reject control.
- Display and recording components have the lowest dynamic range.

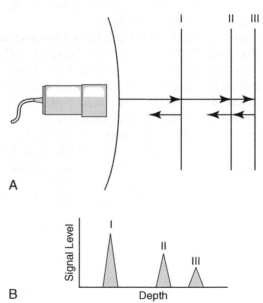

FIGURE 5-6 A-Mode Scan and Display. A, Three interfaces (I, II, and III). **B,** Display of the detected interfaces (relative signals and locations).

NOISE

- Noise is a variation in signal level, which is not correlated with echo intensity.
- Noise is random and inherent in the measurement process.
- Sources of noise include system electronics, RF interference, and power line fluctuations.
- Weak signals are difficult to detect in the presence of noise.
- The relative amplitude of a signal in the presence of noise is called the *signal-to-noise ratio (SNR)*.
- Signal averaging can reduce the noise component by making multiple measurements of the same entity.
  - Weak signals tend to reinforce.
  - Random noise variations tend to cancel one another.

REVIEW QUESTIONS

1. Why should the region of interest in the patient be within the near field of the transducer?
2. What is the effect on near-field depth if the operating frequency of a transducer is increased?
3. Which signal processing technique corrects for signal loss caused by attenuation?
4. What is represented by the horizontal axis in the A-mode display?
5. Name two methods to mechanically focus a single-element transducer.
6. What is the purpose of beam focusing?
7. What is noise?
8. What does noise affect?

PROBLEMS

1. Calculate the near-field depth for a 10-mm–diameter, nonfocused, 5-MHz transducer.
2. Calculate the near-field depth for a 12-mm–diameter, nonfocused, 5-MHz transducer. Note the effect of increased crystal diameter on near-field depth.
3. Calculate the near-field depth for a 10-mm–diameter, nonfocused, 3.5-MHz transducer. Note the effect of decreased frequency on near-field depth.
4. Calculate the far-field angle of divergence for a 10-mm–diameter, nonfocused, 5-MHz transducer.
5. Calculate the far-field angle of divergence for a 12-mm–diameter, nonfocused, 5-MHz transducer. Note the effect of increased crystal diameter on far-field divergence.
6. Calculate the far-field angle of divergence for a 10-mm–diameter, nonfocused, 3.5-MHz transducer. Note the effect of decreased frequency on far-field divergence.
7. What is the dynamic range if the largest echo-induced signal is 0.01 volts and the smallest echo-induced signal is 0.0001 volts?

MULTIPLE CHOICE QUESTIONS

1. During scanning with a single-element transducer, what adjustment is available to the sonographer to change the focal length from 8 cm to 5 cm?
   A. Replace the matching layer
   B. Apply electronic focusing
   C. Select a different the acoustic lens
   D. None of the above
2. Which type of resolution is affected by spatial pulse length?
   A. Axial
   B. Contrast
   C. Lateral
   D. Temporal
3. Which of the following statements regarding TGC applied during signal processing is true?
   A. Constant amplification for all depths
   B. Variable amplification depending on the depth
   C. Constant amplification for all signal levels above the reject threshold
   D. Variable amplification depending on signal level
4. How can lateral resolution be improved?
   A. Increase TGC
   B. Increase power
   C. Reduce beam width
   D. Reduce pulse duration
5. How many lines of sight are presented simultaneously in the A-mode display?
   A. One
   B. Two
   C. Depends on pulse repetition frequency (PRF)
   D. Depends on operating frequency
6. Which signal processing technique is designed to eliminate low-amplitude signals and noise below a certain threshold?
   A. Rectification
   B. Enveloping
   C. Integration
   D. Reject
7. Which signal processing technique is designed to eliminate the negative component of the RF signal?
   A. Rectification
   B. Enveloping
   C. Integration
   D. Reject
8. At which step in signal processing is dynamic range the highest?
   A. Reception
   B. TGC
   C. Integration
   D. Display

9. What is the orientation of two adjacent objects in the definition of axial resolution?
   A. Objects lie along the direction of propagation
   B. Objects lie perpendicular to the direction of propagation
   C. Objects lie within the focal zone
   D. Objects lie within the near field
10. What is the depth dependence of spatial pulse length?
    A. Increases with depth
    B. Decreases with depth
    C. No change with depth
    D. Depends on focusing
11. What is the depth dependence of lateral resolution?
    A. Increases with depth
    B. Decreases with depth
    C. No change with depth
    D. Depends on focusing

12. During scanning with a single-element transducer, what adjustment is available to the sonographer to improve the detection of echo-induced signals from weak reflectors?
    A. Increase gain
    B. Increase TGC
    C. Increase power
    D. Increase PRF
13. Which ultrasound interaction allows Huygens' principle to predict the spatial variation of the ultrasonic field from a large radiating source?
    A. Refraction
    B. Reflection
    C. Interference
    D. Diffraction

Static Imaging

A-MODE SCANNING

- Pulsed-wave ultrasound is directed into the patient along a particular sampling direction (scan line) according to transducer orientation.
- Reflectors interrogated by the ultrasound beam along the propagation path generate echoes.
- Echoes incident on the transducer are separated in time, depending on the depth at which they were created.
- The echo-ranging principle establishes the depth of origin for detected echo.
- Time gain compensation (TGC) is applied to correct signal loss caused by attenuation.
- Each detected reflector is depicted by the signal strength of the echo versus time (scan depth) on the monitor.
- Multiple reflectors along the scan line are displayed as multiple spikes.
- The display is refreshed at the same rate as pulse repetition frequency (PRF).
- Changing the orientation of the transducer provides a different sampling direction.

SUMMARY OF A-MODE SCANNING

Single line of sight
Graphic display of echo strength versus depth
Echo placement via echo ranging
Time gain compensation applied
Display updated at rate equal to pulse repetition frequency

STATIC B-MODE IMAGING

- A static B-mode image is a two-dimensional spatial presentation of detected echoes (tomographic slice).
- Compilation of multiple scan lines while maintaining spatial correlation creates a composite two-dimensional image.
  - Each location in a two-dimensional image correlates with the spatial counterpart of scanned subject.
  - Brightness level at each location in a two-dimensional image denotes corresponding signal strength.

- Reflectors along each scan line are displayed as corresponding dots with varying degrees of brightness (Figure 6-1).
- Multiple scan lines are obtained by changing the orientation of the transducer.
- The registration arm senses the position and orientation of the transducer for each scan line.
- The position generator determines the sampling direction based on transducer position and orientation.
- For each scan line, the depth of the reflector is determined by the echo-ranging principle.
- Spatial mapping of the echo-induced signals in a digital image matrix is a combination of sampling direction and echo ranging.

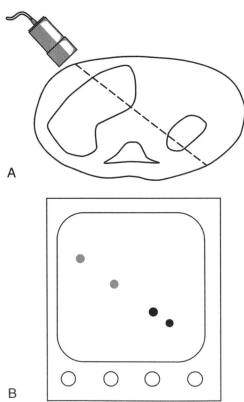

FIGURE 6-1 Single Scan Line in B-Mode. A, The transducer position defines the sampling direction. **B,** The interfaces encountered along the line of sight are represented as dots of varying degrees of brightness.

- The fidelity of geometric relationships must be maintained for all scan lines.
- The point of reference must be defined for each image acquisition.
- The digital scan converter stores signal levels associated with each reflector location throughout the field of view as the transducer is moved to new scanning directions.
- After image acquisition, the digital scan converter is read for display on the monitor.
    - The readout of signal strength is row by row (raster lines).
    - The scan data are converted to an analog video signal and routed to the monitor for display.
- Overwrite protect processing allows the highest signal from multiple scanning directions to be recorded for a detected interface.
- Moving interfaces are blurred in static B-mode images (poor temporal resolution).

SUMMARY OF STATIC B-MODE IMAGING

Large field of view
High signal-to-noise ratio
Multiple-angle sampling, which improves border definition of reflectors
Acquisition time of several seconds
Subject to motion artifacts
Restricted transducer movement
Single-depth focusing

REVIEW QUESTIONS

1. How many scan lines are shown simultaneously on an A-mode display?
2. At what rate is the A-mode display updated with the most recent scan data?
3. If two reflectors separated axially by 1 cm are encountered along the scan line, how many spikes are present in an A-mode display? Assume that the spatial pulse length is 0.9 mm.
4. If two reflectors separated axially by 0.04 cm are encountered along the scan line, how many spikes are present in an A-mode display? Assume that the spatial pulse length is 0.9 mm.
5. Assume that two reflectors with identical reflectivity are encountered along the scan line at a depth of 3 cm and 5 cm, respectively. Which one will most likely generate an echo with the highest intensity? Assume a nonfocused 5-MHz transducer.
6. Assume that two reflectors with identical reflectivity are encountered along the scan line at a depth of 3 cm and 5 cm, respectively. Which one will most likely generate an echo with the highest intensity?

Assume a 5-MHz transducer with a focal length of 5 cm and depth of field of 1 cm.

7. If two reflectors separated laterally by 0.1 cm are encountered at a depth of 3 cm, how many spikes will be present in the A-mode display?
8. If four received signals have relative amplitudes of 0.1, 0.2, 0.7, and 1.5, how many spikes will be present in the A-mode display for a reject control setting of 0.5?
9. What major modifications to the A-mode scanner are necessary to engineer the static B-mode scanner?
10. How many scan lines are shown simultaneously on a static B-mode display?
11. The matrix size for a static B-mode scanner is changed from 512×512 to 2000×2000. Would this improve the image quality with respect to spatial detail? Why, or why not?
12. How is the focal length for a static B-mode transducer changed?
13. Why is the border of a large, curved reflector well defined in a static B-mode image?
14. Why is the border of a large, moving reflector blurred in a static B-mode image?

PROBLEMS

1. What is the duration of a single horizontal A-mode trace if the scan range is 7 cm?
2. If the matrix size is 350×750 and the field of view is 5 cm $\times$ 11 cm, what is the pixel size?
3. If TGC were not applied, by what factor would the signal be reduced from a reflector located 5 cm from a 5-MHz transducer?

MULTIPLE CHOICE QUESTIONS

1. Which of the following is a function of the digital scan converter?
    - A. Storing echo-induced signals until readout
    - B. Controlling position and orientation of transducer
    - C. Applying time gain compensation (TGC) amplification
    - D. Calculating position of the reflector
2. In a static B-mode image, what characteristic of the reflector is represented by the brightness of the pixel displayed on the monitor?
    - A. Physical size
    - B. Signal level
    - C. Velocity
    - D. Depth
3. In static B-mode scanning, why must the orientation and position of the transducer be known?
    - A. To apply TGC properly
    - B. The magnetic field of Earth affects signal level
    - C. To determine the direction of sampling
    - D. Because it affects the focusing of the ultrasound beam

4. During static B-mode acquisition, a single, small reflector is interrogated by five different scan lines as the transducer is moved across the patient. How many echo-induced signals are ultimately stored for readout by the digital scan converter?
   A. One
   B. Two
   C. Five
   D. Ten

5. How is the digital scan converter read for display?
   A. In a scan line sequence
   B. In a row by row sequence of the matrix
   C. Highest to lowest signal level
   D. Largest to smallest reflector

6. What is the frame rate for static B-mode imaging?
   A. 1 fps
   B. 15 fps
   C. 100 fps
   D. None of the above

Image Formation in Real-Time Imaging

BASIC PRINCIPLES

- B-mode imaging compiles successive two-dimensional images of the sampled region, and these images are typically displayed in real-time at a frame rate of 15 or more frames per second.
- Varying brightness levels or shades of gray in the image depict the relative reflectivities of the structures within the sampled region.
- The field of view (FOV) is the physical region interrogated by the ultrasound scanning, in which the detected echoes are mapped in the two-dimensional image.
- The depth of the FOV is the scan range and is in the direction of propagation.
- The width of the FOV is the physical dimension over which the ultrasound beam is directed during image acquisition and is generally perpendicular to the direction of propagation.
- Spatial mapping of the echo-induced signals in the image is a combination of echo ranging and directional beam scanning.
- A pulsed sound beam with a narrow beam width is directed along a well-defined path.
- Only reflectors along the sampling path (scan line) generate echoes, which are received at the transducer in a linear time sequence governed by the depth of echo formation.
- The depth of echo formation is determined by the echo-ranging principle.
- The time interval between the transmitted pulse and the detected echo yields the distance along the direction of propagation to the reflector that created the echo.
  - A constant acoustic velocity for tissue is assumed.
  - A straight path for the transmitted pulse and the detected echo is assumed.
- After the data are collected for one scan line, the next transmitted pulse is directed along a different sampling direction.
- Each B-mode frame is composed of echoes received from multiple scan lines (Figure 7-1).

- In this scheme, at least one transmitted pulsed wave is required for each scan line.
- Beam direction is controlled automatically by mechanical or electronic means in a well-defined pattern without intervention by the sonographer (Figure 7-2).
- The scan converter retains the echo-induced signals from each scan line and then translates this information into the two-dimensional image format for readout.

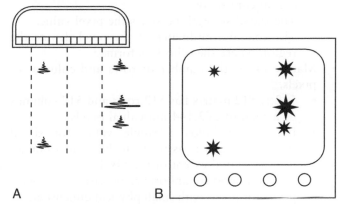

A   B

FIGURE 7-1 Image Formation in B-Mode Ultrasound. **A,** Echo-ranging data measured with three scan lines, which allows spatial mapping of detected echoes along the direction of sampling. The origin and amplitude of each echo along the respective beam paths (*dashed lines*) are shown. **B,** Image display on monitor. The brightness of the dot represents the strength of the detected echo.

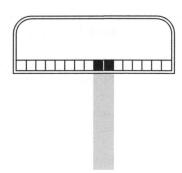

FIGURE 7-2 Beam Transmission. Independent electronic control of each crystal element allows selective excitation, which defines the sampling direction. The two excited elements are shown in black, and the sound beam originates at that location in the array.

ANALOG-TO-DIGITAL CONVERSION

- An analog signal such as the voltage induced by an echo is continuously variable (i.e., may assume any value between 0 and 1 millivolt).
- The digital signal is limited to discrete steps (only certain values are possible between 0 and 1 millivolt, such as 0.1, 0.2, 0.3, etc.).
- Analog signals must be translated into binary signals for processing by the computer.
- Some signal accuracy is sacrificed by digitalization.
  - A range of analog signal values are represented within each digital step.
  - Increase in the number of bits (bit depth) improves digital signal accuracy.

SPATIAL REPRESENTATION

- The FOV is divided into small, square (or rectangular) picture elements called *pixels*.
- Each pixel corresponds to a particular region in the patient and signifies the signal associated with that region.
  - The echo-induced signal must undergo analog-to-digital conversion.
  - The signal strength becomes the pixel value.
  - The spatial coordinates of the pixel denote the region where the echo was formed.
- Matrix size is the number of rows and columns of pixels.
  - 512 × 512 matrix has 512 rows and 512 columns or a total of 262,144 individual pixels.
  - Each pixel holds a single value for signal strength, which is assumed to be valid throughout the spatial extent of the pixel.
  - The assumption of uniform response is most appropriate for pixels with small physical dimensions.
  - Some spatial accuracy is lost by digital representation of pixel location.
  - Spatial accuracy is generally improved by using an image matrix with more pixels.

IMAGE DISPLAY

- The monitor is an output device that displays matrix data as an image.
  - The cathode ray tube uses a modulated, scanning electron beam to control brightness.
  - The liquid crystal display manipulates polarized light to regulate brightness for each monitor pixel.
- Monitor formats include television video and computer graphics.
  - Commercial television has 525 raster lines and 30 frames per second.
  - Computer graphics have fewer limitations with respect to number of pixels and frame rate (typically much higher than available with commercial television).

- The geometric relationship between pixels must be retained in the displayed image.
- The brightness level for a displayed pixel depends on pixel value and the lookup table that translates pixel value to brightness (gray scale map).
- Changes in gray scale map alter the brightness composition in the displayed image but not pixel values.

TIME CONSIDERATIONS

- Acoustic velocity of tissue is assumed to be 1540 meters per second (m/s).
- The echo-ranging principle requires a measurement time of 13 microseconds (μs) for every centimeter in distance from the transducer.
- Time for data collection for a single scan line depends on the scan range.
  - A time of 65 μs is required for a range of 5 cm.
  - A longer time of 195 μs is required for a range of 15 cm.
- The minimum time for data collection for a frame depends on the number of scan lines and range.
- Consider a frame composed of eight scan lines.
  - A time of 520 μs is required for a scan range of 5 cm.
  - A longer time of 1560 μs is required for a scan range of 15 cm.
- Time to collect data via beam steering and echo ranging imposes a limitation on frame rate.
- The maximum frame rate (FR_{max}) is a function of scan range (R), acoustic velocity (c), and the number of scan lines per frame (n).

$$FR_{max} = \frac{c}{2Rn} = \frac{PRF_{max}}{n}$$

- Reducing the number of scan lines, the scan range, or both increases the maximum frame rate.
- The time required for data collection for each frame equals the reciprocal of the maximum frame rate.
- The number of scan lines per frame (n) and pulse repetition frequency (PRF) determine the actual frame rate (FR), which is often less than the maximum frame rate.

$$FR = \frac{PRF}{n}$$

BEAM WIDTH

- An echo is created regardless of the lateral position of the object within the ultrasonic field.
- An object with physical dimensions smaller than the beam width is spatially mapped in the image with the lateral extent equal to the beam width.
  - Spatial location of small objects cannot be defined more accurately than the limitation imposed by measurement technique (in this case beam width).

- To depict small objects with corresponding small dimensions in the image, a narrow beam width is necessary.

LATERAL RESOLUTION

- Lateral resolution is the ability to resolve, as separate entities, two adjacent objects that lie perpendicular to the beam axis.
- Scan line density is the number of scan lines per distance across the width of the FOV.
- A narrow beam width and high scan line density improve lateral resolution (Figure 7-3).
- A narrow beam width and high scan line density also improve the border definition of small objects—a more accurate representation of object shape.
- A B-mode image is commonly composed of 120 to 200 scan lines.
- Expanding the width of the FOV can affect scan line density.

TEMPORAL RESOLUTION

- Accurate representation of moving objects depends on frame rate.
- High frame rates are required to depict fast-moving structures throughout the range of motion without jerkiness.
- Frame rate may be increased by reducing the scan lines or the scan range.
  - Fewer total scan lines in the frame degrades lateral resolution.
  - Decreased scan range restricts the FOV.

REVIEW QUESTIONS

1. What technique is employed to locate the depth of the reflector (distance from the transducer)?
2. Why is pulsed-wave ultrasound necessary for B-mode imaging?
3. Why is a narrow beam width necessary for B-mode imaging?
4. Why are multiple transmission pulses required to form a single B-mode image?
5. How is an echo-induced signal level represented in a B-mode image?
6. What is a scan line?
7. List the assumptions necessary for B-mode image formation.
8. How many echoes would be generated if three widely spaced (>>SPL), small reflectors were encountered along the scan line?
9. How many echoes would be detected if three small reflectors were encountered at the same depth along a single scan line?
10. When is slow frame rate desirable?

PROBLEMS

1. Calculate the maximum frame rate if the scan range is 10 cm and each frame is composed of 120 scan lines.
2. Calculate the time to form one frame if the image has 120 scan lines and a scan range of 10 cm.
3. Calculate the pulse repetition frequency for a 5-MHz transducer if the frame rate is 20 fps and each frame is composed of 120 scan lines.

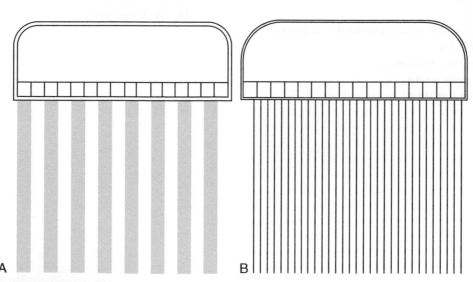

FIGURE 7-3 Effect of Line Density on Lateral Resolution. A, Low number of scan lines (total of 8 denoted by gray regions) results in poor lateral resolution. **B,** Lateral resolution is improved by increasing line density (total of 32).

4. Calculate the pulse repetition frequency for a 3.5-MHz transducer if the frame rate is 20 fps and each frame is composed of 120 scan lines.

5. If the scan range is 8 cm and the frame rate is 48 fps, how many scan lines are possible for each frame?

6. How much time is required to listen for echoes for a scan line, which is sampled to a depth of 10 cm?

7. If the frame rate is 15 fps and the PRF is 2100 pulses per second, how many scan lines are acquired for each frame?

8. If 200 scan lines compose each frame acquired at a rate of 20 fps, what is the maximum scan range?

9. If each frame is composed of 200 scan lines and is acquired at a rate of 30 fps, what is the maximum scan range?

10. If the pulse repetition frequency is 2100 pulses per second and each frame is composed of 150 scan lines, what is the frame rate?

MULTIPLE CHOICE QUESTIONS

1. Which parameter primarily affects lateral resolution?
   A. Spatial pulse length
   B. Scan line density
   C. Crystal thickness
   D. Power

2. Which parameter would you change to increase the frame rate?
   A. Operating frequency
   B. Pulse repetition frequency
   C. Beam width
   D. Power

3. If the width of the FOV is expanded, what must increase to maintain lateral resolution?
   A. Operating frequency
   B. Pulse repetition frequency
   C. Beam width
   D. Scan range

4. What is required for good temporal resolution?
   A. High frame rate
   B. High operating frequency
   C. Narrow beam width
   D. Short pulse duration

5. How many scan lines usually compose an image?
   A. 1
   B. 120
   C. 1000
   D. 5000

6. How is beam steering controlled during data acquisition?
   A. By the operator during scanning
   B. Preset selected by the operator
   C. Independent of the operator
   D. By random selection by the computer

7. Which device translates echo data, scan line by scan line, into a two-dimensional image format?
   A. Transducer
   B. Analog-to-digital converter
   C. Monitor
   D. Scan converter

8. For which B-mode imaging application is a continuous wave transducer the most appropriate choice?
   A. Scan range less than 5 cm
   B. Frame rate above 50 fps
   C. Extremely narrow beam width
   D. None of the above

9. What is the consequence in B-mode imaging if the acoustic velocity in tissue is less than 1540 meters per second (m/s)?
   A. The object is shifted laterally in the image
   B. The object is represented with increased lateral extent
   C. The object is shifted along the beam axis in the image
   D. All of the above

10. The shape of a 2-cm diameter stationary object in a B-mode image is not well defined. What adjustment may improve the presentation of the object?
    A. Decrease frame rate
    B. Decrease PRF
    C. Decrease operating frequency
    D. Decrease power

Real-Time Ultrasound Transducers

MECHANICAL SECTORS

- One or more piezoelectric crystals mounted on the mechanical arm are moved to different locations during frame acquisition.
  - Mechanical steering limits frame rate.
  - Fixed mechanical focusing is done to a single, specific depth.
- The mechanical sector transducer is considered an antiquated technology and has largely been replaced by multiple-element array transducers.

FEATURES OF MECHANICAL SECTORS

Pie-shaped field of view (FOV)
Mechanical beam steering
Fixed mechanical focus
Increased sector angle enlarges the FOV
Width of the FOV increases with depth
Small footprint
High scan line density can be achieved with high pulse repetition frequency (PRF)
Scan line density is not uniform throughout the FOV (decreases with depth)
Relatively low cost

LINEAR ARRAYS

- Multiple, small, rectangular piezoelectric crystals are configured in a straight row along the face of the transducer.
  - Independent electronic control of each element during transmission and reception enables directional beam formation and electronic focusing.
  - The physical length of the array equals the width of the field of vision (FOV).
- Selected elements are activated during transmission to control sampling direction.
  - Since a small crystal size produces a short near field, a group of crystals are excited to enlarge the beam aperture.

- To achieve high scan line density, crystal groups are overlapped.
  - For example, a group of four crystals is shifted by one element for each successive transmission (e.g., crystals 1–4, then crystals 2–5, followed by crystals 3–6).
- Electronic sequencing by element selection enables the ultrasound beam to be directed across the FOV along different lines of sight.
  - Frame acquisition is completely automated with no intervention by the sonographer.
  - The number of crystal elements ultimately limits the maximum number of scan lines in an image.
- Electronic transmit focusing enables the focal length to be prescribed for each transmitted pulse.
  - The purpose of transmit focusing is to reduce beam width and improve lateral resolution within the scan plane.
  - Interference of the wave patterns from individual elements creates the net overall ultrasonic field.
  - The crystal elements in the group are not excited simultaneously but, rather, are offset in time to cause constructive interference at the depth of interest (producing the desired effect of reduced beam width as shown in Figure 8-1).
  - The timing sequence depends on the position of the crystal element in the excited group and the desired focal zone depth.
  - Only a single transmit focal zone at a specified depth can be formed with the transmitted pulse.
  - Each scan line can be focused to the same depth of interest, but the sonographer can change the depth of interest.
  - Multiple-zone transmit focusing (also called *confocal imaging*) requires each scan line to be sampled with as many transmit pulses as focal zones selected by the sonographer.
    - Lateral resolution is improved throughout the scan range.
    - Multiple transmit focal zones typically slow the frame rate.

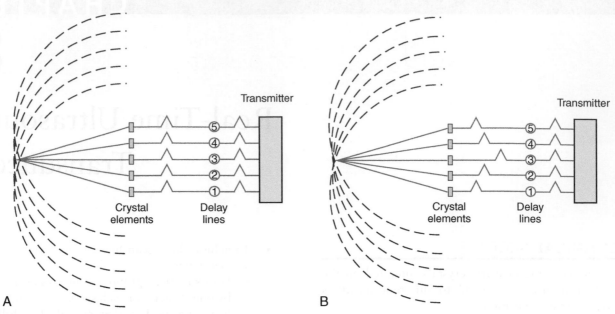

A **B**

FIGURE 8-1 Electronic Focusing. A, If five crystals are stimulated simultaneously, the wavefronts do not arrive simultaneously at the target because the distance of travel for each wavefront is not the same. **B,** Transmit delay lines are used to excite the crystals at slightly different times (nanosecond delays between firings). The wavefronts arrive exactly simultaneously at the target point, and the result is a focused beam. Crystals 1 and 5 are stimulated first, followed by 2, 4, and then 3. Changing the time delays allows other points to become the center of focus.

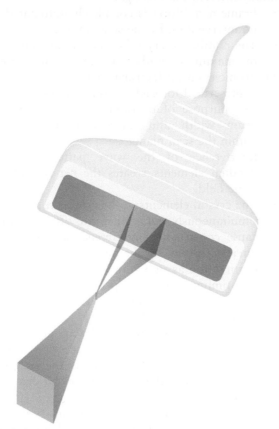

FIGURE 8-2 Beam pattern from both mechanical focusing and electronic focusing for one scan line in a linear array.

- Mechanical focusing in the elevation direction is fixed (Figure 8-2).
  - All elements are focused to the same depth.
  - Fixed focusing results in nonuniform slice thickness throughout the FOV.

- Aperture focusing is a form of electronic transmit focusing in which the number of crystals fired in a group depends on the depth of focus (Figures 8-3 and 8-4).
  - A large aperture extends the depth of focus.
  - The ratio of focal length to aperture size denotes focusing characteristics (given by f-number).
- Apodization varies the excitation voltage to each element to control that element's contribution to the overall transmit beam pattern.
- Dynamic receive focusing uses beam formation to improve lateral resolution and signal-to-noise ratio.
  - The echo wavefront from a reflector does not arrive simultaneously at all the elements in the array (Figure 8-5).
  - By delaying the individual echo signal at each crystal until the wavefront has arrived at all crystals in the receiver group, synchronization reinforces the summed output and restricts the sampled region (focusing during reception).
  - The delay time for a particular crystal element depends on the position of that crystal element in the group and the depth of sampling, which is known by echo ranging.
  - Delay times are adjusted during the acquisition to focus all depths along the scan line.
  - A dynamic aperture adjusts the number of receiving crystals contributing to beam formation as a function of depth.
  - Dynamic receive processing incurs no loss in frame rate or line density.
  - Each element with independent control of transmission and reception is a channel.
  - Increased channel number improves lateral resolution.

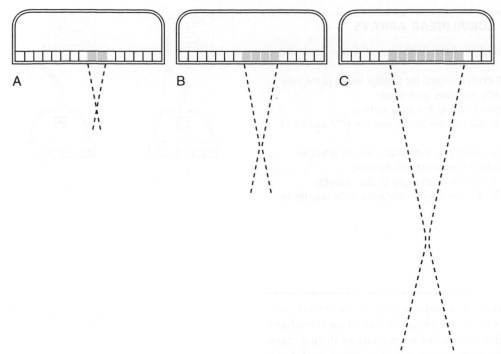

FIGURE 8-3 Aperture Focusing. A, Two crystals are fired for a short focus. **B,** Four crystals are fired for a medium focus. **C,** Eight crystals are fired for a long focus.

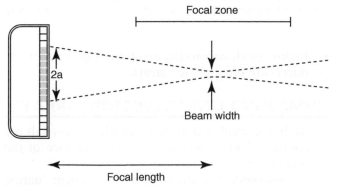

FIGURE 8-4 Depth of Field. The beam width is narrowest within the focal zone, which is affected by aperture size (2a), focal length, and frequency.

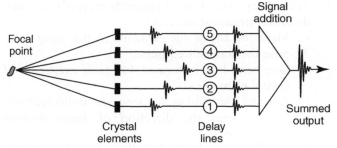

FIGURE 8-5 Dynamic Receive Focusing. The echo wavefront from the object arrives at crystal 3 first, then at 2 and 4, and finally at 1 and 5. By delaying the individual echo signal at each crystal until the wavefront has arrived at all five crystals, focusing is applied to the received signals to produce a summed output.

FEATURES OF LINEAR ARRAYS

Rectangular field of view (FOV)
In-plane FOV width equals the physical length of the array
Scan lines are parallel
Constant scan line density within the FOV
Electronic directional control by sequential element activation
Transmit and dynamic receive electronic focusing
Depth of transmit focus can be changed by the operator
Multiple transmit focal zones are possible and can be selected by the operator
Mechanical focusing in the elevation direction (fixed depth)

CURVILINEAR ARRAYS

- Multiple, small, rectangular piezoelectric crystals are configured in an arc along the face of the transducer.
  - Independent control of each element during transmission and reception enables directional beam formation and electronic focusing.
  - The width of the FOV extends beyond the physical length of the array.
  - The radius of the curvature determines the width of the FOV.
- Sequential activation of selected elements sweeps the respective scan lines across the FOV.
- Electronic directional control, electronic transmit focusing, aperture focusing, apodization, dynamic receive focusing, and mechanical focusing in the elevation direction, as described for linear arrays, also apply to curvilinear arrays.

FEATURES OF CURVILINEAR ARRAYS

Trapezoid field of view (FOV) with curved border near the transducer

In-plane FOV width extends beyond the physical length of the array

The width of the FOV increases with depth

Scan lines are perpendicular to the array surface

Scan line density is not uniform throughout the FOV (decreases with depth)

Electronic directional control by sequential element activation

Transmit and dynamic receive electronic focusing

Depth of transmit focus can be changed by the operator

Multiple transmit focal zones are possible and can be selected by the operator

Mechanical focusing in the elevation direction (fixed depth)

PHASED ARRAYS

- Multiple, small, rectangular piezoelectric crystals configured in a straight row along the face of the transducer.
  - Independent control of each element during transmission and reception enables directional beam formation and electronic focusing.
  - The width of the FOV extends beyond the physical length of the array.
- Time delay activation of elements controls scan line direction (transmit steering).
  - Most (or all) of the elements in the array compose the transmitted pulse.
  - One scan line is formed for each excitation of crystal elements.
  - Altering the timing sequence to individual elements varies the direction of beam steering (Figure 8-6).
  - The sector angle can be adjusted by the sonographer to alter the width of the FOV.
- Electronic transmit focusing, aperture focusing, apodization, dynamic receive focusing, and mechanical focusing in the elevation direction, as described for linear arrays, also apply to phased arrays.

FEATURES OF PHASED ARRAYS

Sector format for field of view (FOV)

Width of the FOV increases with depth

Small footprint

Scan line density is not uniform throughout the FOV (decreases with depth)

Electronic transmit steering by time delay activation of elements

Large-angle beam steering degrades spatial resolution

Transmit and dynamic receive electronic focusing

Depth of transmit focus can be changed by the operator

Multiple transmit focal zones are possible and can be selected by the operator

Mechanical focusing in the elevation direction (fixed depth)

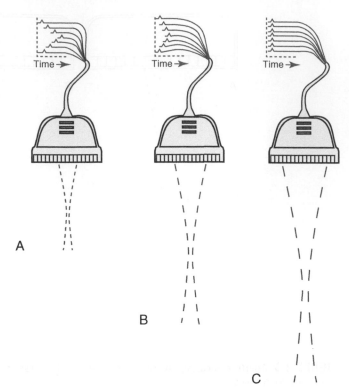

FIGURE 8-6 Beam Steering with a Phased Array. By altering the time delay sequences, the direction of propagation can be varied from one transmitted pulse to the next. Three scan lines are shown.

- Endovaginal, endorectal, and transesophageal transducers are often phased arrays.

COMPOUND LINEAR (VECTOR) ARRAYS

- Multiple, small, rectangular piezoelectric crystals are configured in a straight row along the face of the transducer.
  - Independent control of each element during transmission and reception enables directional beam formation and electronic focusing.
  - The width of the FOV extends beyond the physical length of the array.
- Central scan lines are acquired by element selection (as with linear array).
- Scan lines at the periphery are acquired by transmit steering (as with phased array).
- Electronic transmit focusing, aperture focusing, apodization, dynamic receive focusing, and mechanical focusing in the elevation direction, as described for linear arrays, also apply to vector arrays.

ANNULAR PHASED ARRAYS

- Concentric rings of piezoelectric crystals surround a single, central, circular piezoelectric element (4 to 16 total elements).
  - Independent control of each element during transmission and reception enables electronic focusing.

FEATURES OF VECTOR ARRAYS

> Trapezoid field of view (FOV) with a flat border near the transducer
> The width of the FOV increases with depth
> Generally has a smaller footprint than linear arrays and can be manufactured with a very small footprint for endosonographic probes
> Scan line density is uniform in the central FOV
> Scan line density decreases with depth outside the central FOV
> Electronic directional control is a combination of element selection and time delay activation of elements
> Large-angle beam steering degrades spatial resolution
> Transmit and dynamic receive electronic focusing
> Depth of transmit focus can be changed by the operator
> Multiple transmit focal zones are possible and can be selected by the operator
> Mechanical focusing in the elevation direction (fixed depth)

- Time delays focus the beam at a particular depth in both the in-plane direction and the elevation direction.
- Beam widths for both the in-plane direction and the elevation direction are symmetrical.
- Annular array must be mechanically steered to collect different scan lines.

FEATURES OF ANNULAR PHASED ARRAYS

> Sector format for the field of view (FOV)
> The width of the FOV increases with depth
> Small footprint
> Scan line density is not uniform throughout the FOV (decreases with depth)
> Mechanical steering
> Large-angle mechanical beam steering does not degrade spatial resolution
> Transmit and dynamic receive electronic focusing
> Transmit focusing reduces in-plane and elevation beam widths
> Depth of transmit focus can be changed by the operator
> Multiple transmit focal zones are possible and can be selected by the operator

1.5D LINEAR ARRAYS

- Multiple, small, rectangular piezoelectric crystals are configured in multiple straight rows (~6 rows) along the face of the transducer.
  - Inter-row spacing is 10 times the wavelength.
  - Independent control of each element during transmission and reception enables directional beam formation and electronic focusing.
  - The physical length of the array equals the width of the FOV.

- Time delays for elements in different rows focus the beam at a particular depth in both the in-plane direction and the elevation direction.
- Dynamic focusing replaces fixed mechanical focusing in the elevation direction.
- During transmission, selected elements are activated to control the scan line direction.
- Aperture focusing, apodization, and dynamic receive focusing, as described for linear arrays, also apply to 1.5D arrays.

FEATURES OF 1.5D LINEAR ARRAYS

> Rectangular field of view (FOV)
> In-plane width equals the physical length of the array
> Scan lines are parallel
> Electronic directional control by element activation
> Transmit and dynamic receive electronic focusing
> Transmit focusing reduces in-plane and elevation beam widths
> The depth of transmit focus can be changed by the operator
> Multiple transmit focal zones are possible and can be selected by the operator
> No mechanical focusing in the elevation direction

HANAFY LENS

- Multiple, small, rectangular, variable-thickness piezoelectric crystals are configured in a straight row along the face of the transducer.
  - Each crystal is thinnest at the center, with the thickness increasing toward the outer edge along the elevation direction.
  - Multiple resonant frequencies are transmitted simultaneously (broad bandwidth).
- Broadband frequency components narrow the beam width in the elevation direction.
- This focusing technique provides an alternative to the 1.5D array.

TWO-DIMENSIONAL (2D) ARRAYS

- Multiple, small, rectangular piezoelectric crystals are configured in a two-dimensional matrix across the face of the transducer.
  - A large number of elements (>9000) is required.
  - Independent control of each element during transmission and reception enables directional beam formation and electronic focusing.
  - Time delays for elements in different matrix locations focus the beam at a particular depth in both the in-plane direction and the elevation direction.

- Electronic steering in all directions without moving the transducer permits volumetric acquisitions.

TRANSDUCER DESIGN

- Side lobes are secondary lobes that originate at the transducer and radiate outward at various angles to the main beam.
  - Crystal vibrations in the direction(s) perpendicular to the thickness direction cause side lobes.
  - Side lobes contribute to clutter and may introduce artifacts from off-axis structures.
  - Side lobes are reduced by apodization, large aperture, and high frequency.
- Grating lobes are secondary lobes caused by the regular periodic spacing of elements in linear and phased arrays.
  - Grating lobes are eliminated if the element-to-element distance is less than one wavelength.
  - Subdicing reduces the occurrence of grating lobes by dividing an element into many subelements that electronically act in concert.
  - At large steering angles in phased arrays, the number and intensity of grating lobes are increased.
- Crystal element isolation attempts to decouple each element mechanically and electronically from its neighbors.
  - Each element is assembled with separate ground wires and signal wires.
  - Elements are mechanically linked by matching layers, backing layers, focusing lenses, and housing.
  - The crystal dimensions in the direction(s) perpendicular to the thickness direction are designed to be dissimilar from the thickness dimension and, therefore, have different resonant frequencies.

REVIEW QUESTIONS

1. What is the advantage of the annular phased array compared with the linear array?
2. What is the disadvantage of the annular phased array compared with the linear array?
3. What transmit focusing method is used for mechanical sector scanners?
4. Why have curvilinear arrays essentially replaced linear arrays for abdominal imaging?
5. What is the purpose of the Hanafy lens?

PROBLEMS

1. Calculate the f-number for a focal length of 6 cm using an aperture 3 cm in length.
2. How much time is required to form a 150-line image using a linear array, if the scan range is 10 cm?
3. How much time is required to form a 150-line image using a phased array, if the scan range is 10 cm?

MULTIPLE CHOICE QUESTIONS

1. Which condition is most likely to entail a large aperture for transmission in a multiple-element transducer?
   A. High frequency above 10 MHz
   B. Wide field of view beyond the physical size of the array
   C. Fast frame rate above 15 fps
   D. Scan range beyond 15 cm
2. What transmit focusing method for the elevation direction (slice thickness) is used in linear array transducers?
   A. Use of acoustic lens
   B. Decreasing the element spacing to less than one wavelength
   C. Time delay to excite crystal elements
   D. Apodization

TRANSDUCER CHARACTERISTICS

Type	Scanning Mechanism	In-Plane Focusing	Slice Thickness Focusing	Image Format	Footprint
Mechanical sector	Mechanical	Mechanical	Mechanical	Sector	Pointed
Linear array	Electronic sequencing	Electronic	Mechanical	Rectangular	Flat
Curvilinear array	Electronic sequencing	Electronic	Mechanical	Trapezoidal, curved near transducer	Curved
Phased array	Electronic steering	Electronic	Mechanical	Sector, straight near transducer	Small, flat
Vector array	Electronic steering	Electronic	Mechanical	Trapezoidal, straight near transducer	Flat
Annular phased array	Mechanical	Electronic	Electronic	Sector	Pointed

3. What transmit focusing method for the elevation direction (slice thickness) is used in phased array transducers?
   A. Use of acoustic lens
   B. Decreasing the element spacing to less than one wavelength
   C. Time delay to excite crystal elements
   D. Apodization

4. What transmit focusing method is used in linear array transducers to narrow the in-plane beam width at a specified depth?
   A. Use of acoustic lens
   B. Use of curved crystal elements
   C. Time delay to excite crystal elements
   D. Subdicing of the crystal elements

5. What transmit focusing method is used in phased array transducers to narrow the in-plane beam width at a specified depth?
   A. Use of acoustic lens
   B. Use of curved crystal elements
   C. Time delay to excite crystal elements
   D. Subdicing of the crystal elements

6. For a linear array, what method defines the sampling direction (scan line) within the field of view for the transmitted pulse?
   A. Crystal elements selection
   B. Time delay to excite the crystal elements
   C. Mechanical movement of the crystal elements
   D. Frequency response of the crystal elements

7. For an annular phased array, what method defines the sampling direction (scan line) within the field of view for the transmitted pulse?
   A. Crystal element selection
   B. Time delay to excite the crystal elements
   C. Mechanical movement of the crystal elements
   D. Frequency response of the crystal elements

8. For a phased array, what method defines the sampling direction (scan line) within the field of view for the transmitted pulse?
   A. Crystal element selection
   B. Time delay to excite the crystal elements
   C. Mechanical movement of the crystal elements
   D. Frequency response of the crystal elements

9. For a curvilinear array, what method defines the sampling direction (scan line) within the field of view for the transmitted pulse?
   A. Crystal element selection
   B. Time delay to excite the crystal elements
   C. Mechanical movement of the crystal elements
   D. Frequency response of the crystal elements

10. For a mechanical sector scanner, what method defines the sampling direction (scan line) within the field of view for the transmitted pulse?
    A. Crystal element selection
    B. Time delay to excite the crystal elements
    C. Mechanical movement of the crystal elements
    D. Frequency response of the crystal elements

11. What is a characteristic of dynamic receive focusing?
    A. Signals from multiple crystals are summed
    B. Induced signals at multiple elements undergo time delays
    C. Focusing is applied to all depths along the scan line
    D. All of the above

12. How can the sonographer improve lateral resolution throughout the scan range for a linear array?
    A. Use multiple transmit focal zones
    B. Lower the operating frequency
    C. Widen the field of view
    D. Increase the power

13. Which transducer limits the width of the field of view to the physical width of the crystal array?
    A. Linear array
    B. Phased array
    C. Curvilinear array
    D. Vector array

14. What is the image format for a linear array?
    A. Rectangular
    B. Sector
    C. Trapezoid with straight edge at transducer
    D. Trapezoid with curved edge at transducer

15. What is a likely result if transmit focusing is changed from one focal zone to three focal zones?
    A. Improved axial resolution
    B. Reduced frame rate
    C. Increased image brightness
    D. Degraded lateral resolution

16. What is apodization with respect to elements that form the transmitted pulse?
    A. Changing the number of elements for each pulse
    B. Varying the excitation voltage across the element group
    C. Increasing the time for voltage excitation across the element group
    D. Regulating the delay time for voltage excitation across the element group

17. For a linear array, what parameter is most dependent on depth?
    A. Scan line density
    B. Width of the field of view
    C. Slice thickness
    D. Axial resolution

18. Which type of transducer enables electronic focusing in the elevation direction?
    A. Linear array
    B. Phased array
    C. Curvilinear array
    D. 1.5D linear array

19. Which type of transducer enables electronic steering and focusing for a volume acquisition without moving the transducer?
A. Annular phased array
B. Curvilinear array
C. 1.5D linear array
D. Two-dimensional rectangular array

20. Which design feature reduces the occurrence of grating lobes in linear arrays by dividing each crystal element into multiple, small, electrically connected elements?
A. Apodization
B. Adding additional rows of crystals
C. Subdicing
D. Variable crystal element thickness

Real-Time Ultrasound Instrumentation

B-MODE ACQUISITION

- B-mode image formation is a multiple-step process, executed in real-time, but dependent on operator input.
- Table 9-1 lists the associated components and operator controls or processing options during image acquisition with multiple-element arrays.
- A pulser generates a short voltage pulse that stimulates a crystal to emit ultrasound.
- The transmitted ultrasound beam is a compilation of ultrasound waves from multiple crystals stimulated at nearly the same time.
  - Crystal elements in the group define the beam aperture.
  - The beam aperture affects transmit focusing (wider aperture for longer focal lengths).
- The timed sequence of crystal excitations directed by the transmit beam former enables electronic focusing and electronic sequencing or steering.
- High voltage necessary for crystal excitation is isolated from the receiver circuit by the transmit and receive switches.
- The communication pathway between the crystal and the pulser (or the crystal and the signal reception) is a channel.
- During reception, echo-induced radiofrequency (RF) signals from multiple channels are amplified (gain and time gain compensation [TGC]) prior to dynamic receive focusing by the receive beam former.
- In the receive beam former, the RF signal for each channel undergoes analog-to-digital conversion before interpolation, time delay, apodization, and summing (Figure 9-1).
- Signal processing refers to the manipulation of time-varying scan line data to enhance the information content.
  - Envelope detection simplifies the RF signal so that a single metric represents the echo strength.
  - Logarithmic amplification compresses signal amplitudes ranging over several orders of magnitude to 256 values (1 byte).

TABLE 9-1	Real-Time Image Formation	
Function	**Components**	**Controls/ Processing**
Transmission	Pulsers Transmit beam former Piezoelectric elements Transmit and receive switches	Power Transmit focal zone(s) Aperture Apodization Scan range Frame rate Pulse repetition frequency (PRF) Scan line density Write zoom
Reception	Piezoelectric elements Transmit and receive switches	Active channels
Amplification	Amplifier Timing circuits	Receiver gain Time gain compensation (TGC) Selective enhancement
Dynamic receive focusing	Receive beam former	Analog-to-digital converter (ADC) Interpolation (ADC sampling rate) Time delay Apodization Summing
Signal processing	Computer algorithms	Envelope detection Compression Edge enhancement/ smoothing Reject control
Scan data to image format	Scan converter	Matrix size Bilinear interpolation
Image processing	Computer algorithms Buffer	Edge enhancement/ smoothing Compression Persistence Gray-scale mapping
Display	Monitor	Real-time Freeze frame Cine

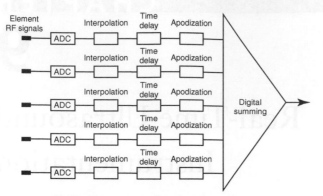

FIGURE 9-1 Digital receive beam former.

- Logarithmic amplification emphasizes the differences between weaker signals because a proportionally larger fraction of the compressed signal range is assigned to low signal values.
- Edge enhancement (or smoothing) is a digital filtering technique that emphasizes (or de-emphasizes) abrupt changes in signal levels (boundaries of reflectors).
- Reject control accepts only signals greater than a prescribed amplitude for further processing or display.
- The scan converter transforms the line-by-line scan data into the matrix format for image composition (Figure 9-2).
- Matrix size is the number of addressable pixels in the matrix (product of the number of rows and the number of columns).
- Bilinear interpolation assigns values to pixels not interrogated by a scan line.
- Image processing pertains to the manipulation of data in a matrix format to enhance the information content.

- Real-time, freeze frame, and cine are the three most common modes for display.

OPERATOR CONTROLS

- Power control (typically denoted in decibel [dB] difference from maximum output or percentage of maximum output) adjusts the intensity of the transmitted ultrasound beam.
  - Alternative labels for the power control are *transmitter, transmit power, output, acoustic power,* and *energy output.*
- High intensity levels increase the signal-to-noise ratio and improve sensitivity.
- A change in power setting is often accompanied by an automatic commensurate adjustment in receiver gain to maintain overall image brightness.
- The depth control sets the scan range for the field of view (FOV).
- Write zoom improves spatial detail by reducing the size of the displayed FOV.
- Frame rate, scan range, pulse repetition frequency (PRF), and line density are interdependent and not necessarily under direct operator control.
- The operator selects the number and respective depths of transmit focal zones.
- The receiver gain sets overall brightness of the image but cannot improve the signal-to-noise ratio.
- TGC is a variable gain applied to compensate for attenuation.
- Fine adjustment of variable gain according to depth is manually applied by the operator.
- Edge enhancement (or smoothing) alters the spatial definition of reflector boundaries.

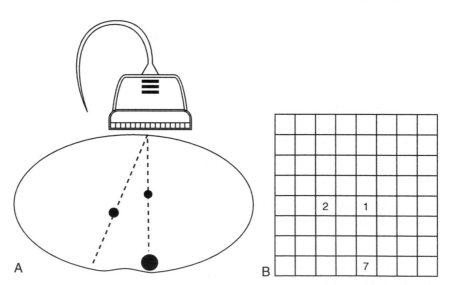

FIGURE 9-2 Scan Conversion. A, Sampling of the field of view along two lines of sight. Note that the two interfaces are detected along the central line of sight. The size of the black dot denotes the intensity of the reflected echo. **B,** An 8 × 8 matrix depicting the three structures observed in A. Note that the pixels corresponding to the various interfaces are assigned different values on the basis of the intensity of the reflected echoes.

- Persistence is a frame averaging technique to increase signal-to-noise ratio.
- Compression (or dynamic range) control alters image contrast by restricting signal levels that are shown with varying gray levels.
- Reject control eliminates low-amplitude signals and noise.
- Gray-scale mapping translates pixel value to brightness level for image display on the monitor.

COHERENT IMAGE FORMATION

- Outputs from multiple receive beam formers are processed simultaneously to improve the spatial mapping of the reflectors.
- The time-varying summed signals from each beam former (nonparallel adjacent scan lines) contain both axial and lateral spatial information.
- The final image is composed of synthetic scan lines derived from two-dimensional data sets.

MULTIPLE-FREQUENCY IMAGING

- A broad bandwidth transducer operates at two or more center frequencies.
- The operator-selectable center frequency allows an examination to be conducted with the appropriate tissue penetration at the highest possible frequency without changing transducers.

CONFOCAL IMAGING

- The center frequency for transmit-zone focusing is depth dependent.
- Focusing at shallow depths is accomplished with high center frequency, which is then lowered as the depth of the transmit focal zone is increased.
- Each scan line is composed of multiple transmit pulses.
- High pulse repetition frequency or parallel processing is necessary to maintain frame rate.

DYNAMIC FREQUENCY FILTERING

- A short pulse with a broad bandwidth is used for transmission.
- The receiver center frequency and bandwidth are automatically adjusted to lower frequencies as sampling progresses to deeper depths.
- Since noise is proportional to receiver bandwidth, progressively narrowing the bandwidth reduces image noise.
- In high definition imaging, the bandwidth of the transmitted pulse is altered to extend the depth of penetration (shifts to low-frequency components) or to improve lateral resolution at shallow depths (shifts to high-frequency components).

FREQUENCY COMPOUNDING (FREQUENCY FUSION)

- A short pulse with a broad bandwidth is used for transmission.
- During reception, echo pressure variations are faithfully converted into RF signals with a matched broad bandwidth.
- The echo frequency spectrum is subdivided into frequency bands by filters, processed separately, and then recombined to form a frequency-averaged image.
- The summing of frequency images can be adjusted to emphasize penetration, resolution, or tissue texture.
- A common application is reduction of speckle and noise to improve contrast resolution.

SPATIAL COMPOUNDING

- Frames acquired with different steered beam angles are combined to reduce speckle, clutter, and noise while improving border definition of specular reflectors.
- Multiple frames, each with parallel scan lines oriented at a unique angle, are held in a buffer.
- Averaging of the frames in the buffer is performed in real-time with no loss in frame rate.
- Each reflector is sampled from multiple directions, which increases the likelihood of a favorable incident angle for high reflectivity.
- The composite image is subject to motion blurring, since the sampling interval extends over several frames.
- Increasing the number of steering angles (and thus frames) enhances the compounding effect.

EXTENDED FIELD OF VIEW

- Automated scan line sequencing in B-mode restricts the size of the FOV.
  - The physical width of the linear array defines the width of the FOV.
  - Electronic steering of phased arrays limits the lateral extent of the FOV.
- Extended field of view imaging expands the FOV by forming a panoramic image composed of multiple frames as the transducer is moved across the patient.
- Since scanned anatomy is nearly the same, sequential frames acquired at high frame rate contain many common image features.
- Computer matching of image features in successive frames allows the superposition of shared anatomy while expanding the FOV.
- The fidelity of the registration is corrupted by tissue motion and off-plane rotation.

CODED EXCITATION

- Long coded waveforms during transmission improve signal-to-noise ratio, increase scan range, or both.
- Binary encoding and frequency modulation (chirp) are two methods to regulate the transmitted waveform.
- Echo intensity variation from a single reflector has the same pattern as the transmitted waveform.
- Signal processing with the known coded waveform isolates each reflector signal with a short axial extent from the echo wavetrain.
- A long spatial pulse length may hinder the imaging of superficial structures.
- Coded waveforms compared with conventional B-mode have lower peak intensity, but more total transmitted energy per pulse/receive cycle.

ZONE SONOGRAPHY

- The serial format of the line-by-line acquisition for conventional B-mode imaging imposes time constraints on image formation.
  - Acoustic velocity and path length fix the transit time for a scan line.
  - An image with 200 scan lines requires 200 pulse/receive cycles.
- In zone sonography, the acquisition time for a frame is greatly reduced by sampling a large region with a broad transmit beam (e.g., 20 pulse/receive cycles across the FOV).
- Echo wavetrain data for each channel following each transmitted pulse are stored in a buffer.
- Computer processing of the channel data by iterative reconstruction generates the ultrasound image within a few milliseconds (~5 ms).
- Speed of data acquisition allows extremely rapid frame rates (10 times faster than conventional B-mode imaging).
- Transmit focusing is not applied in zone sonography.

TISSUE HARMONIC IMAGING

- At high intensity, nonlinear propagation distorts the ultrasound waveform from its normal sinusoidal shape.
- The altered shape is caused by differing acoustic velocities during compression and rarefaction.
- The distorted waveform gives rise to additional frequency components called harmonics.
- Harmonic frequencies are integral multiples of the fundamental frequency.
- As the sound wave propagates through the medium, the waveform becomes more distorted, and harmonic components become more pronounced.
- Loss of intensity by attenuation ultimately reestablishes linear propagation and prevents further formation of harmonics.

- Harmonics are present in the central portion of the transmitted beam but are offset from the face of the transducer.
- The intensity of the second harmonic is lower than the intensity of the fundamental frequency but higher than that from all other harmonics.
- A reflector interrogated by fundamental and harmonic frequencies will generate an echo with these same frequency components.
- Two methods of tissue harmonic imaging—harmonic band filtering and pulse phase inversion—detect the second harmonic frequency in the presence of the fundamental frequency.
- Harmonic band filtering applies a filter to the echo-induced signal to remove the contributions at the fundamental frequency.
  - Only the isolated tissue harmonic signal is processed for image formation.
  - The purity of the harmonic filter band depends on the overlap between fundamental and harmonic components in the frequency spectrum.
  - A long spatial pulse length improves the separation of harmonics from the fundamental band.
- Pulse phase inversion sums signals from two transmitted pulses along the same scan line to eliminate the fundamental frequency (Figure 9-3).
  - Consecutive transmitted pulses are shifted in phase by 180 degrees.
  - If propagation is linear, then the summed signals are canceled completely.
  - For nonlinear propagation, the summed signals yield only the harmonic component.
  - Two successive measurements of echo-induced signals increase the signal-to-noise ratio but are subject to motion artifacts.

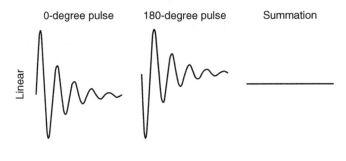
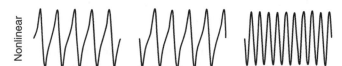

FIGURE 9-3 Pulse Phase Inversion to Isolate the Second Harmonic Signal. Two transmit pulses with opposite phases sample each scan line. For linear propagation, the echoes consist of the fundamental frequency only but are opposite in phase. The summed signal is zero. In the case of nonlinear propagation, the echoes each have a harmonic component, which does not cancel when summed. Note that the summed signal is twice the fundamental frequency.

- A short spatial pulse length preserves the axial resolution.
- Contributions from clutter, grating lobes, and side lobes at the fundamental frequency are suppressed in tissue harmonic imaging.
- Higher relative attenuation rates for harmonics decrease overall penetration.
- At the same transmitted frequency, the effective beam width is narrower than that from B-mode imaging because harmonic production occurs near the main beam axis and within the focal zone.

ELASTOGRAPHY

- The displacement of tissue (strain) following the application of a compression force (stress) measures elasticity.
- Strain elastography uses manual compression by the transducer to apply stress.
  - Precompression and compression A-line echo signal patterns are compared to determine relative tissue displacement.
  - Multiple A-lines with short time-division segments enable two-dimensional image formation.
  - B-mode and elasticity images are displayed side-by-side on the monitor in real-time.
- In shear wave elastography, manual compression is replaced by acoustic radiation force.
  - Acoustic radiation force is generated by a series of closely spaced pulses, similar to those used for color Doppler.
  - A conical shear wave radiates outward from the force line.
  - The velocity of the shear wave is proportional to the elasticity of tissue.
  - Measurements of shear wave velocity are overlaid on the simultaneously acquired B-mode image.
- Fluids, which are not compressible, yield signal voids in the elasticity image.
- Cancerous lesions may affect the elasticity of surrounding tissue more strongly than do noncancerous lesions; thus, the relative lesion size in B-mode imaging versus elastography may be used to characterize tissue.

3D ULTRASOUND

- The spatial relationships within a scanned tissue volume are represented as a three-dimensional image or set of images.
- A series of two-dimensional data sets (analogous to B-mode images) are acquired throughout the tissue volume.
- The plane data sets are assembled in parallel, in a wedge, in a cone, or in an arbitrary orientation, depending on the acquisition method.
- Reconstruction of the three-dimensional volume fills in the regions not sampled during acquisition by interpolation between known voxel values (two-dimensional data sets whose geometric relationship to the scanned volume is well defined).
- Selected information extracted from the three-dimensional volume is viewed interactively using computer graphics.
  - Multiplanar reformatting typically displays three orthogonal planes simultaneously.
  - The face of a polyhedron is positioned within the reconstructed volume to depict a two-dimensional image.
  - Surface rendering connects all similar voxels along a boundary to visualize surface morphology.
  - Volume rendering, such as maximum intensity projection, forms a two-dimensional image based on voxels encountered along each sampling ray (viewing line of sight through the three-dimensional volume).

4D ULTRASOUND

- The fourth dimension, time, is combined with volumetric sampling to depict the dynamic behavior of structures.
- Surface-rendered planes or multiple planes are displayed in real-time.
- Mechanically steered multiple-element arrays or two-dimensional rectangular arrays acquire the volume data set.
- Rectangular arrays contain thousands of elements, each controlled independently.
  - Electronic focusing and steering are applied to obtain scan lines throughout the scanned volume.
- Time constraints limit the number of scan lines that compose the volume data set.
- Slow frame rates, long computation times, and transducer cost restrict the use of 4D ultrasound.

MULTIPLE CHOICE QUESTIONS

1. What is the advantage of spatial compounding?
   A. Improved definition of curved structures
   B. Faster frame rates
   C. Increased field of view
   D. Reduced mechanical index
2. What is the advantage of tissue harmonic imaging?
   A. Faster frame rates
   B. Improved contrast
   C. Improved axial resolution
   D. Greater depth penetration
3. What limitation of conventional B-mode scanning is improved with zone sonography?
   A. Penetration
   B. Spatial resolution
   C. Frame rate
   D. Slice thickness

4. What is the reason for higher transmit intensity for tissue harmonic imaging compared with B-mode imaging?
   A. To eliminate aliasing
   B. To match the piezoelectric crystal response
   C. To induce nonlinear propagation
   D. To create a large beam aperture

5. Which imaging technique measures the displacement of tissue when a force is applied?
   A. Frequency fusion
   B. Elastography
   C. Zone sonography
   D. Spatial compounding

6. What is the communication pathway between the crystal and the receiver?
   A. Analog-to-digital converter
   B. Channel
   C. Pulser
   D. Universal serial bus

7. What operator control averages frames in a buffer to improve signal-to-noise ratio?
   A. Edge enhancement
   B. Persistence
   C. Gain
   D. Beam former

8. What is apodization applied during ultrasound transmission?
   A. Variation of excitation voltage to the crystal elements in the group
   B. Selection of the crystal elements in the transducer for excitation
   C. Timing of voltage excitation to the crystal elements in the group
   D. Isolation of the crystal elements from the receiver during transmission

9. What is the characteristic of the formation of harmonics during tissue harmonic imaging?
   A. Intensity is twice the fundamental intensity
   B. Frequency is twice the fundamental frequency
   C. Wavelength is twice the fundamental wavelength
   D. Acoustic velocity is twice the fundamental acoustic velocity

10. Which imaging technique employs long transmitted waveforms to improve signal-to-noise ratio?
    A. Spatial compounding
    B. Extended field of view
    C. Zone sonography
    D. Coded excitation

11. Which imaging technique employs feature matching in subsequent frames to expand spatial mapping in the horizontal direction?
    A. Spatial compounding
    B. Extended field of view
    C. Zone sonography
    D. Write zoom

12. What type of transducer is designed to acquire a volume data set?
    A. Annular array
    B. Stationary linear array
    C. Mechanical movement of a multiple-element array
    D. Mechanical movement of a mechanical sector

13. What is the problem encountered with two-dimensional rectangular arrays in 4D imaging?
    A. High electronic noise
    B. High channel number
    C. Steering only in planes parallel to the matrix rows
    D. Mechanical focusing in the elevation direction

14. In tissue harmonic imaging, where are harmonics most likely to be formed?
    A. Uniformly throughout the ultrasonic field
    B. Near the transducer–tissue interface
    C. Near the beam axis
    D. At the focal zone and beyond

15. Which of the following probably would *not* increase the signal-to-noise ratio?
    A. Persistence
    B. Spatial compounding
    C. Increased transmit power
    D. Increased receiver gain

16. Which component places the received signals in an image format?
    A. Beam former
    B. Scan converter
    C. Analog-to-digital converter
    D. Gray scale map

17. Where does dynamic beam focusing occur?
    A. Beam former
    B. Scan converter
    C. Analog-to-digital converter
    D. Gray-scale map

18. Which is *not* a transmit focusing method?
    A. Apodization
    B. Aperture
    C. Excitation delay times
    D. Element subdicing

19. What is the basis for the adjustment of transmit frequency in confocal imaging?
    A. Echo-induced signal strength
    B. Depth of transmit focal zone
    C. Frame rate
    D. Scan line density

20. Which imaging technique employs pulse phase inversion?
    A. Coded excitation
    B. Frequency compounding
    C. Tissue harmonic imaging
    D. Elastography

Digital Signal and Image Processing

SIGNAL AMPLIFICATION

- Time gain compensation (TGC) is the exponential amplification of signals as a function of elapsed time following the transmitted pulse.
- TGC is used to compensate for attenuation along the beam path so that reflectors with equal reflectivity at different depths are assigned the same signal level.
- For every scan line throughout the field of view (FOV), TGC is applied in the same manner.
- TGC assumes that all tissues along the beam path have the same rate of attenuation.
- Adaptive TGC applies a unique gain function for each scan line on the basis of an analysis of the depth-dependent gain settings for other scan lines.
- Adaptive TGC is performed in real-time without operator input and produces variable amplification throughout the image.
- Selective enhancement (also called time gain compensation) enables the sonographer to amplify signals from a particular depth of interest.
- Operator control of TGC is in the form of a series of slide keys, each key corresponding to a particular depth and whose displacement denotes the amount of amplification.
- Receiver gain increases the amplitude of all signals (and consequently, noise) by the same factor.
- Receiver gain is the primary control for overall brightness of the image.

REJECT CONTROL

- Reject control, which can be adjusted by the sonographer, eliminates low signals and noise below a threshold value from the image.
- Operator adjustment of reject control can reduce the dynamic range by removing low signals.

COMPRESSION

- Operator control of compression (also called *dynamic range and logarithmic compression*) reduces the dynamic range by removing low signals.

- A reduction in dynamic range provides contrast enhancement for the remaining displayed signals.
- Low dynamic range produces high image contrast (whites and blacks).
- High dynamic range produces low image contrast (intermediate grays).

EDGE ENHANCEMENT

- Edge enhancement is a filtering technique that is applied to scan line data to accentuate a change in signal level.
- The effect of edge enhancement is to emphasize the boundary between different tissue types.

SCAN CONVERSION

- Line-by-line signal acquisition is converted into a matrix format for image display.
- The sound beam cannot sample every pixel in the matrix.
- The value assigned to unsampled pixels is calculated by averaging the signal amplitudes in neighboring pixels.
- The most widely used scan conversion method is bilinear interpolation.

MATRIX FORMAT

- Write zoom (also called *regional expansion*, *reduced field of view*, *FOV size*, *res*, *scale*, *mag*, and *zoom*) is a magnification technique to distribute the pixels in an image matrix over a smaller FOV.
- Improved spatial resolution is possible because the physical dimensions of the zoomed region are smaller than the original FOV and the displayed matrix size is unchanged.
- Panning allows the operator to move the FOV to a new anatomic location during scanning.
- During panning, a subdivision of the maximum FOV for a particular transducer is displayed.
- Persistence or frame averaging adds successive frames to reduce noise.

- The most recently acquired frame is combined with previous frames held in a buffer.
- Frame rate can be maintained at 15 to 20 fps, but each displayed image is an average of multiple preceding frames.
- Since the effective time of sampling for a displayed frame is increased, blurring of fast moving structures is more pronounced.
- Adaptive frame averaging improves the signal-to-noise ratio without lag by the addition of buffer data to selective regions of the image associated with slow-moving structures (based on the frame-to-frame variation of pixel values).
- Edge enhancement is a filtering technique that can be applied to the matrix format data to accentuate the signal change at a boundary.
  - The visibility of small, high-contrast structures is improved but is accompanied by increased noise.
  - Changing the magnitude or the number of filter-weighting factors varies the amount of edge enhancement.
- Smoothing is a filtering technique that can be applied to the matrix format data to reduce noise.
  - The visibility of large, uniform structures is improved but is accompanied by increased blur.
  - Changing the magnitude or the number of filter-weighting factors varies the amount of smoothing.

DISPLAY

- Freeze frame suspends data collection and displays the last frame acquired.
  - Annotation, region of interest definition, and distance measurements can be performed on the freeze-frame image.
  - A freeze-frame image may be sent to a Picture Arching and Communication System (PACS) or recorded as a hard copy.
- Gray-scale mapping establishes the relationship between pixel value and brightness displayed on the monitor.
  - Each pixel is displayed uniformly as a particular shade of gray, depending on the pixel value.
  - High pixel values are typically displayed as white or near-white.
  - Multiple pixel values may be displayed with the same shade of gray because a range of pixel values is normally associated with one brightness level.
  - The gray-scale map (linear, logarithmic, exponential) can be selected by the operator.
  - Contrast enhancement redistributes the gray scale over a narrower range of pixel values so that pixels with similar values are displayed with different shades of gray.
    - The logarithmic map improves the contrast of weak signals.
    - The inverse log (exponential) map emphasizes variations in high-amplitude signals.

- The selection of a gray-scale map does not alter the pixel values in an image.
- Equalization is a method to enhance contrast by automatically adjusting the translation of pixel value to brightness level.
  - The distribution of pixel values is analyzed so that each brightness level displays the same number of pixels in the image.
  - For a linear gray-scale map, if no pixels have values associated with a particular brightness level, then that shade of gray is absent in the image.
  - The advantage of equalization is that all brightness levels are used in the display of the image and contrast is improved.
- Black-and-white inversion changes the gray-scale map so that high pixel values are displayed as black or near-black.
- Read zoom (also called *zoom*, *mag*, and *size*) is a magnification technique that displays pixels in a larger format on the monitor.
  - Pixel-to-pixel variations are seen more easily.
  - Image data are not changed, and spatial detail is not improved.

MULTIPLE CHOICE QUESTIONS

1. Which technique reduces the dynamic range during signal processing?
   A. Receiver gain
   B. Gray-scale map
   C. Time gain compensation
   D. Edge enhancement
2. Which technique reduces the dynamic range during signal processing?
   A. Reject
   B. Scan conversion
   C. Bilinear interpolation
   D. Read zoom
3. Which adjustment by the operator will likely improve spatial resolution?
   A. Receiver gain
   B. Gray-scale map
   C. Time gain compensation
   D. Write zoom
4. Which signal processing technique lowers image noise?
   A. Write zoom
   B. Edge enhancement
   C. Persistence
   D. Receiver gain
5. What is scan conversion?
   A. Translation of the pixel value to a shade of gray
   B. Conversion of analog echo-induced signals into the digital format
   C. Mapping of scan lines to the matrix format
   D. Altering the autoscan sequence of scan lines

6. Which signal processing technique will most likely improve the low contrast resolution of a 2-cm diameter lesion?
   A. Frame averaging
   B. Edge enhancement
   C. Receiver gain
   D. Read zoom

7. Which signal processing technique increases the blurring of fast-moving reflectors?
   A. Frame averaging
   B. Edge enhancement
   C. Receiver gain
   D. Write zoom

8. Which signal processing technique compensates for attenuation along the beam path?
   A. Receiver gain
   B. Gray-scale map
   C. Time gain compensation
   D. Write zoom

9. What is the result of signal processing technique of logarithmic compression?
   A. Reduces the dynamic range of signals
   B. Enhances the edges across tissue boundaries
   C. Improves spatial resolution by reducing pixel size
   D. Increases the B-mode frame rate by reducing the number of scan lines

10. How is time gain compensation applied?
    A. Constant amplification independent of time
    B. Variable amplification based on time
    C. Variable amplification based on signal level
    D. Variable amplification based on steered direction

11. How is receiver gain applied?
    A. Constant amplification independent of time
    B. Variable amplification based on time
    C. Variable amplification based on signal level
    D. Variable amplification based on steered direction

12. What is reject control?
    A. Constant amplification independent of time
    B. Low-strength signals below a reference value are not stored in the scan converter
    C. Variable amplification based on signal level
    D. High-strength signals above a reference value are not stored in the scan converter

Image Quality

IMAGE TEXTURE

- The pattern of signals that form the image is a combination of reflected and scattered ultrasound from structures within the field of view (FOV).
  - Specular reflectors such as organ boundaries produce bright lines with little modulation.
  - Scattering from organ parenchyma create a granular pattern with bright and dark dots.
- Speckle is a composite interference pattern from numerous scattering events (Figure 11-1).
  - Individual scatterers are randomly distributed and too small to be resolved as unique entities in the image.
  - Dots fluctuate between bright and dark as the beam is swept through the region, hence the name *speckle*.
  - The interference pattern of size and brightness of the dots depends on frequency (Figure 11-2).

DESCRIPTORS OF IMAGE QUALITY

- The components of image quality include axial resolution, lateral resolution, contrast resolution, geometric distortion, noise, artifacts, and temporal resolution.

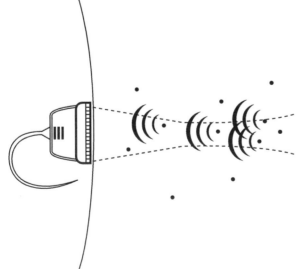

FIGURE 11-1 Speckle. Small reflectors in the beam (*black dots*) scatter the ultrasonic energy. The interference pattern produced at the transducer from numerous scatterers is called *speckle*.

- The components of image quality are interdependent.
- Improvement in one component is often coupled with deterioration of another.
- Power can affect image quality, particularly in the presentation of weak echo-induced signals.

AXIAL RESOLUTION

- Axial resolution is the ability to resolve, as separate entities, reflectors located near each other along the axis of propagation.
- Alternative names for axial resolution are *longitudinal*, *range*, *depth*, and *azimuthal resolution*.
- Axial resolution is primarily determined by spatial pulse length (SPL), which is a function of frequency and ringing.
- Axial resolution is fairly constant throughout the scan range.
  - Typical axial resolution at an operating frequency of 5 MHz is 0.5 to 2 mm.
  - Typical axial resolution at an operating frequency of 12 MHz is <0.5 mm.

LATERAL RESOLUTION

- Lateral resolution is the ability to resolve, as separate entities, reflectors located near each other along the direction perpendicular to the axis of propagation.
- Lateral resolution is primarily determined by beam width and scan line density.
- Factors that affect in-plane beam width include focusing (transmit focusing, dynamic receive focusing, aperture, apodization, and number of focal zones) and frequency.
- Factors that affect scan line density include number of lines per frame (often related to frame rate), width of the field of view, scan format, and number of elements in the array.
- For linear arrays, phased arrays, and curvilinear arrays, in-plane lateral resolution is not constant throughout the FOV.
- Typical lateral resolution for a B-mode imaging is 1 to 3 mm.

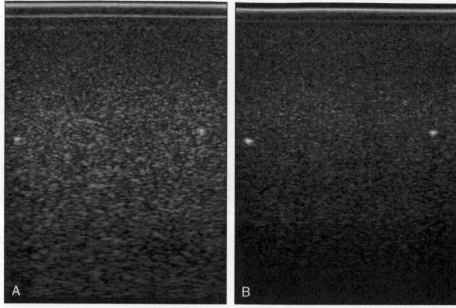

FIGURE 11-2 Frequency dependence of speckle. The speckle pattern varies with frequency. Sonograms of a tissue-mimicking phantom obtained with a transmit frequency of 5 MHz (**A**) and 11 MHz (**B**).

SLICE THICKNESS

- Slice thickness (out-of-plane beam width) is generally not constant throughout the FOV.
  - Fixed-focal-length, mechanical focusing for linear arrays, phased arrays, and curvilinear arrays establishes beam width in the elevation direction.
  - The smallest out-of-plane beam width is within the fixed focal zone.
  - The variability of slice thickness contributes to partial volume effects.

CONTRAST RESOLUTION

- Contrast resolution is the ability to discern reflectors that have different acoustic properties and depends on the magnitude of the signal difference as well as the size of the object.
  - Small reflectors with high signal levels are easily seen.
  - A large reflector with a weak signal level may be visible, whereas a small reflector at the same signal level is obscured by noise.
- Image contrast is the difference in brightness level for objects in the displayed image (monitor) or the difference in the optical density of objects in the printed image (film).
- Image contrast is composed of two components: intrinsic contrast and recording contrast.
  - Intrinsic contrast is the generation of pixel values in the scan converter from echo-induced signals.
    - Reflectivity, scan acquisition parameters, and signal processing techniques influence the pixel value stored for a reflector.
    - The difference in stored pixel values limits the displayed image contrast.

- Recording contrast is the translation of each pixel value to brightness level (monitor) or optical density (film).
  - The gray-scale map, which can be selected by the sonographer, establishes the relationship between pixel value and brightness level (or optical density).
  - Signal processing (e.g., dynamic range) can alter the displayed contrast.
- Interline interference and partial volume degrade contrast.

NOISE

- Noise is the random variation in signal level, which is not related to reflectivity.
  - Electronic sources (amplifiers, cabling, radiofrequency [RF] interference, and power line fluctuations) and acoustic sources (clutter) contribute to noise.
  - Clutter is spurious signals arising from echoes induced by ultrasound transmission unrelated to the main beam (multiple-path scattering as shown in Figure 11-3).
  - Speckle is often considered a form of acoustic noise.
  - Speckle, clutter, and noise cause homogeneous tissue to be displayed with non-uniform brightness level throughout its physical extent.
  - The presence of noise inhibits the ability to discern weak echo-induced signals.
- Methods to reduce noise include reject control, frame averaging, spatial compounding, frequency compounding, and spatial smoothing.

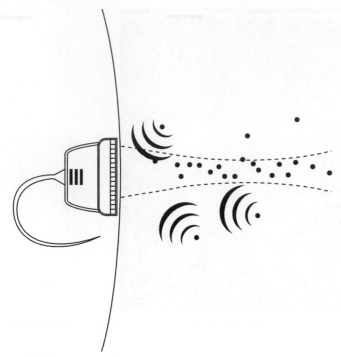

FIGURE 11-3 Clutter. Scatterers within the beam redirect sound energy to structures outside the beam, where additional scattering events enable the scattered sound energy to reach the transducer. The interference pattern produced by multiple path reflections is called *clutter*. Clutter suppresses contrast.

GEOMETRIC DISTORTION

- Geometric distortion is the inaccurate presentation of spatial relationships.
  - Size, shape, and relative positions of structures in the image should faithfully correspond to the reflectors within the scan plane.
  - Spatial mapping of echo-induced signals depends on scan line density, beam width, number of pixels, interpolation, and acoustic velocity.
  - Improperly calibrated image recording devices may introduce geometric distortion.
- Methods to improve spatial mapping include high scan line density, narrow beam width (good focusing characteristics along scan line), and spatial compounding.

ARTIFACTS

- An artifact is a structure in the image that does not correlate directly with actual tissue.
- Examples include reflectors missing in the image, structures in the image that are not representative of tissue, and reflectors geometrically displaced from their true locations.
- Artifacts are caused by acoustic properties of tissue, technical limitations, and equipment malfunction (see next chapter).

TEMPORAL RESOLUTION

- Temporal resolution is accurate depiction of the motion of reflectors and depends on frame rate and the rate of movement of the reflector.
- Methods to improve temporal resolution by operator controls include decreased scan line density, reduced scan range, lower persistence, and decreased sector angle.

MULTIPLE CHOICE QUESTIONS

1. Which operator control when adjusted would cause a change in frame rate?
   A. Transmit power
   B. Time gain compensation (TGC)
   C. Sector angle
   D. Center frequency
2. Which of the following is a type of acoustic noise?
   A. Clutter
   B. Partial volume
   C. Radiofrequency interference
   D. Amplifier voltage variations
3. Which image parameter primarily affects low contrast resolution?
   A. Axial resolution
   B. Lateral resolution
   C. Frame rate
   D. Noise
4. Which of the following when increased would improve lateral resolution?
   A. Number of transmit focal zones
   B. Transmit power
   C. TGC
   D. Frame rate
5. Which of the following when increased would improve axial resolution?
   A. Number of transmit focal zones
   B. Pulse repetition frequency (PRF)
   C. Center frequency
   D. Frame rate
6. Which of the following when increased would reduce image noise?
   A. Frame rate
   B. Persistence
   C. Receiver gain
   D. Scan range
7. How can the sonographer alter the contrast of the displayed image?
   A. Apply the read zoom
   B. Select a different gray-scale map
   C. Change the video display rate
   D. Increase the digital matrix size
8. Which of the following when increased would improve the detection of weak echoes?
   A. Reject control

B. Transmit power

C. Receiver gain

D. Frame rate

9. What affects image contrast represented by pixel values?

A. Receiver gain

B. Acoustic velocity along scan line

C. Reflectivity of interfaces

D. Frame rate

10. What is partial volume effect?

A. Multiple tissue types contained within the region corresponding to a pixel

B. Homogeneous object displayed with brightness variations caused by noise

C. Spatial misregistration of a large reflector

D. Loss of axial resolution outside the focal zone

11. In the case of linear arrays, phased arrays, and curvilinear arrays, why does slice thickness vary throughout the field of view?

A. Scan line density is not constant

B. Number of scan lines is limited by frame rate

C. Ultrasound intensity is reduced by attenuation

D. Electronic focusing is not applied in the elevation direction

Image Artifacts

DESCRIPTION

- An artifact is a structure in the image that does not correlate directly with actual tissue.
- Missing reflectors, structures not representative of tissue, and spatial misregistration of reflectors are forms of image artifacts.
- Artifacts are caused by the acoustic properties of tissue, technical limitations, and equipment malfunction.

SPATIAL MAPPING OF ECHOES

- The assignment of spatial origin of the detected echo is based on numerous assumptions.
- The transmitted wave travels along a straight-line path from the transducer to the object and back to the transducer.
- The attenuation of sound in tissue is uniform along the path.
- Beam dimensions are small in both section thickness and lateral directions.
- All detected echoes originate only from the axis of the main beam.
- All received echoes are derived from the most recently transmitted pulse.
- The ultrasound wave travels at the rate of 1540 meters per second (m/s) in tissue; thus the distance to the interface is determined from the time of flight (1 cm corresponds to 13 microseconds [μs]).
- Each reflector contributes a single echo when interrogated along a single scan line.
- The amplitude of the echo is derived from the object scanned and is correlated to the reflective properties of the object.

PARTIAL VOLUME

- Simultaneous sampling of tissues with different acoustic properties yields an intermediate result.
- The three-dimensional sampling volume of the ultrasound beam at a fixed point in time depends on the beam width in the lateral and elevation directions as well as spatial pulse length (SPL).
- Partial volume artifacts are more pronounced when the sampling volume is increased (Figure 12-1).

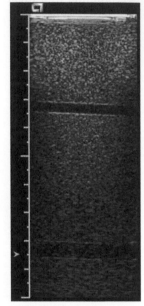

FIGURE 12-1 Partial Volume Artifact. Identical anechoic tubes located at 3 cm and 8 cm in a phantom. Even though transmit focal zone is set at 8 cm, fill-in is more predominant at 8 cm because slice thickness is increased at this depth by fixed mechanical focusing.

- When imaging a cyst, if the sampling volume extends beyond the cyst boundry, then echoes from the surrounding tissue cause fill-in near the border of the cyst.

ENHANCEMENT

- Regions distal to a low-attenuating structure are depicted with stronger signals compared with adjacent similar tissues, which are interrogated by beam paths that do not include the low-attenuating structure.
- Enhancement often occurs distal to cysts and liquid-filled structures, which normally have low attenuation (Figure 12-2).

SHADOWING

- Regions distal to a high-attenuating structure are depicted with weaker signals compared with adjacent similar tissues, which are interrogated by beam paths that do not include the high-attenuating structure.

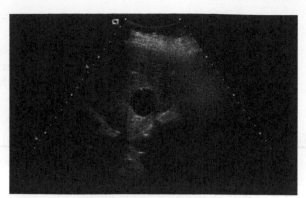

FIGURE 12-2 Attenuation Artifact. Enhancement distal to a liver cyst.

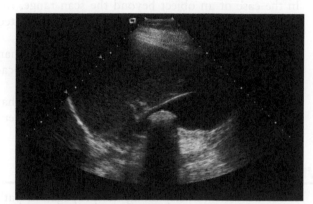

FIGURE 12-3 Attenuation Artifact. Shadowing distal to stones in the gallbladder.

- Shadowing often occurs distal to gallstones, bone, calcified plaque, bowel gas, and metal foreign bodies, which normally have high attenuation (Figure 12-3).

BANDING

- Transmit focusing creates regions of high intensity, which may lead to high echo-induced signals that are mismatched in amplitude compared with those arising from nearby depths.
- Multiple transmit focal zones are subject to banding when objects with identical reflectivity are not presented with the same brightness levels in adjacent focal zones.

REVERBERATION

- A reverberation artifact is manifested as a series of bright bands of decreasing intensity and equidistance from each other.
- An assumption of spatial mapping is violated in that multiple reflections from a single interface are recorded in the image.
- Reverberations often occur between an interface with a high acoustic impedance mismatch (soft tissue–gas, fat–muscle, or fluid–gas) and the transducer.
- Multiple reflections can also occur between two high-reflectivity structures along the beam path.

- The spacing between bands is equal to the separation of the reflectors.
- Reverberation artifacts are often observed in the bladder.

COMET TAIL

- Multiple internal reflections within a small but highly reflective object create multiple echoes, which are recorded in the image as a series of short bands distal to the object (Figure 12-4).
- The object has high or low acoustic impedance compared with surrounding tissue.
- The acoustic impedance mismatch at the boundary of the object forms two opposing interfaces that produce short-path reverberations.
- The physical extent of the comet tail is usually short, <2 cm in length.
- Comet tail artifacts typically arise from the lumen of the gallbladder when crystalline deposits are present.

RING DOWN

- A ring-down artifact occurs when a gas bubble resonates, resulting in a continuous emission of ultrasound.
- The track of the ring-down artifact may be extensive, extending from the point of origin to the limit of the depth of scanning.

MIRROR IMAGE

- The mirror image artifact occurs when a single object is depicted at two different locations in the image.

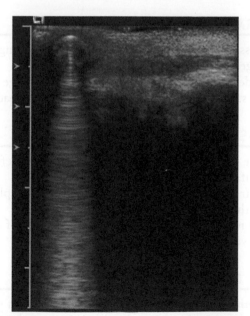

FIGURE 12-4 Comet Tail Artifact. The artifact is distal to a high acoustic impedance reflector (*BB near the eye*).

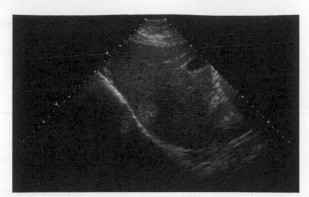

FIGURE 12-5 Mirror Image Artifact. The mass in the liver is replicated to form a second image distal to the diaphragm during tissue harmonic imaging at 3 MHz.

- The duplication of the object is symmetrical about a strong reflector.
- A mirror image artifact is formed when an object is located proximal to a highly reflective surface at which a strong reflection occurs (Figure 12-5).
- A mirror image artifact may also occur if the object is offset from a curved strong reflector or if the object and strong reflector are oriented at an angle.

REFRACTION (MISREGISTRATION)

- Refraction along the beam path causes an object to be misregistered in the image (the assigned location differs from the true position of the object).
- An assumption of spatial mapping is violated in that the ultrasound beam does not travel in a straight line through tissue.
- According to Snell's law, the amount of deviation from the expected straight-line path depends on the angle of incidence and the velocity of the media.

REFRACTION (DEFOCUSING)

- Loss of scan line coherence causes shadowing at the edges of a large, curved structure.
- A defocusing artifact often occurs at the edge of cystic structures and at the edge of the fetal head.

GHOST IMAGE

- The ghost image is a special case of a refraction artifact.
- Refraction by the rectus muscles causes duplication of the gestational sac.
- An indication of ghosting is the movement of the displayed structures in unison.

SIDE LOBE

- A highly reflective object along the path of a secondary lobe produces an echo that is incorrectly assigned a location along the direction of the main beam.

- An assumption of spatial mapping is violated in that the echo does not originate from the main beam.
- Since the intensity of the side lobe is much lower than that of the main beam, highly reflective objects such as gas and metal are usually responsible for this type of artifact.

RANGE AMBIGUITY

- At high pulse repetition frequency (PRF) and short scan range structures distal to the field of view (FOV) may be depicted in the image.
- The sampling time interval between transmitted pulses at high PRF is short.
- In the case of an object beyond the scan range, the echo is detected following the succeeding transmitted pulse.
- Since the measured time for the echo is shorter than the actual time, the object is misregistered at a location near the transducer.
- An assumption of spatial mapping is violated in that the echo does not originate from the most recent transmitted pulse.

VELOCITY ERROR

- If the acoustic velocity along the propagation path deviates from the assumed 1540 m/s, then the reflector is displaced in the image (Figure 12-6).
- If low acoustic velocity media are encountered along the scan line path to an object, then the measured time for an echo is delayed, and the object is mispositioned at increased depth.

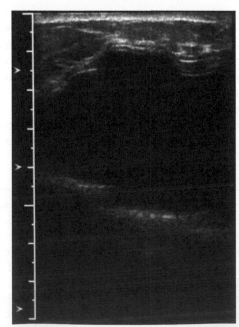

FIGURE 12-6 Velocity Error Artifact. Sonogram of the breast with a silicone implant, which has caused a disjointed image of the fibrous capsule surrounding the implant.

- If high acoustic velocity media are encountered along the scan line path to an object, then the measured time for an echo is shortened, and the object is mispositioned at a shallower depth.
- Velocity error causes measurements of distances, areas, and volumes to be incorrect.

CLASSIFICATION OF ARTIFACTS

Type	Effect	Cause
Partial volume	Fill-in	Beam width extending over different tissue types
Attenuation	Shadowing	Absorption greater than adjacent paths
Attenuation	Enhancement	Absorption less than adjacent paths
Reverberation	Equally spaced banding	Multiple echoes from a single reflector
Comet tail	Closely spaced bands of relatively high signal level	Multiple internal echoes from a single reflector
Ring down	Continuous band extending through field of view (FOV)	Gas bubble resonance
Mirror image	Duplication of structures	Presence of strong reflector near the object
Side lobe	Misregistration	Strong reflector interrogated by a secondary lobe
Refraction	Misregistration	Bending of sound waves along beam path
Refraction (defocusing)	Shadowing	Bending of sound waves by a curved surface
Range ambiguity	Misregistration	Echo not generated by most recent transmitted pulse
Velocity error	Misregistration	Velocity not constant along beam path

REVIEW QUESTIONS

1. Which artifact is associated with different tissue types within the sampled volume?
2. Which assumption for echo mapping is violated by refraction along the beam path?
3. If a deep-lying reflector is depicted near the transducer, what operating parameter may have been set incorrectly?
4. What must be present within the scanned field of view if a structure is duplicated in the image (mirror image artifact)?

5. Why are multiple internal echoes generated within a small object that produces the comet tail artifact?
6. Which artifact is associated with multiple reflections between the transducer and a strong reflector?

MULTIPLE CHOICE QUESTIONS

1. If the acoustic velocity of a lesion is 1450 meters per second (m/s), which spatial representation is not correct?
   A. The depth of the first detected interface of the lesion
   B. The axial length of the lesion
   C. The lateral extent of the lesion
   D. All of the above
2. Which substance is most likely to produce a side lobe artifact?
   A. Soft tissue
   B. Bowel gas
   C. Fluid
   D. Red blood cells (RBCs)
3. If signal enhancement occurs distal to a lesion in the breast, what is the likely composition of the lesion?
   A. Carcinoma
   B. Fluid
   C. Fat
   D. Calcium
4. What causes an error in distance measurement in the axial direction?
   A. Low scan line density
   B. Frame rate above 25 film photograph sequence frames per second (fps)
   C. Instrument calibration of 1600 m/s for acoustic velocity
   D. High pulse repetition frequency (PRF) above 2000 hertz (Hz)
5. Identify the artifact that would have occurred if a lesion is depicted in two locations, which are symmetrical with respect to the diaphragm.
   A. Reverberation
   B. Comet tail
   C. Mirror image
   D. Propagation error
6. Identify the artifact that would have occurred if the diaphragm shows a discontinuity distal to a lesion.
   A. Reverberation
   B. Comet tail
   C. Mirror image
   D. Velocity error
7. Identify the artifact that would have occurred if small bands of high signal extend from the near wall of the gallbladder.
   A. Reverberation
   B. Comet tail
   C. Mirror image
   D. Velocity error

8. Which artifact is commonly observed in the urinary bladder?
   A. Reverberation
   B. Comet tail
   C. Mirror image
   D. Velocity error

9. Which artifact is caused by multiple reflections along the propagation path?
   A. Attenuation
   B. Fill-in

   C. Mirror image
   D. Velocity error

10. Which artifact does *not* cause a spatial misregistration in the image?
    A. Attenuation
    B. Range ambiguity
    C. Mirror image
    D. Velocity error

Doppler Physics and Instrumentation

DOPPLER EFFECT

- A change in the frequency of sound is observed if there is relative motion between the source of the sound and the receiver of the sound.
- If the direction of movement of the source and the receiver is toward each other, then the observed frequency is higher than the transmitted frequency.
- If the direction of movement of the source and the receiver is away from each other, then the observed frequency is lower than the transmitted frequency.
- The change in frequency between the transmitted frequency and the received frequency is the *Doppler shift frequency* (or, simply, *Doppler shift*).
- The angle between the direction of motion and the direction of wave propagation is called the *Doppler angle* (Figure 13-1).
- The Doppler shift (f_D) depends on the relative velocity between source and receiver (v), the transmitted frequency (f), the acoustic velocity of the medium (c), and the Doppler angle (θ) as given by the Doppler shift equation:

$$f_D = \frac{2\, vf\, \cos\theta}{c}$$

- The combination of relative velocity and cosine of the Doppler angle gives the component of velocity along the direction of propagation.
- For a constant reflector velocity, the detected Doppler shift decreases as the Doppler angle is increased.
- If the Doppler angle is 90 degrees, the Doppler shift is zero.
- In the case of a stationary transducer, the Doppler shift equation predicts that an increase in reflector velocity causes a higher Doppler shift.
- If the Doppler shift and Doppler angle are measured, then the velocity of the moving interfaces (e.g., red blood cells in vessels) can be determined.
- If the Doppler angle is not included in the calculation of reflector velocity, then the result underestimates the true velocity.
- Uncertainty in the measurement of the Doppler angle, particularly at large angles, introduces error in the velocity computation.
- To avoid errors from large Doppler angles, Doppler signals from superficial blood vessels should be acquired at angles no greater than 60 degrees.
- Most Doppler units allow the operator to specify the direction of flow on the image and then automatically calculate the Doppler angle with respect to the transmitted beam direction.
- The Doppler shift frequency derived from flowing blood is typically in the audible range, which enables the use of speakers as output devices.
- Doppler shifts expressed in kilohertz (kHz) are not readily comparable between different instruments and facilities.
- The optimal transmitted frequency for Doppler is usually lower than that for B-mode imaging.

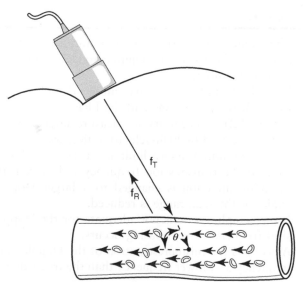

FIGURE 13-1 Doppler angle. Motion of red blood cells (RBCs) through the vessel, which is not parallel to the direction of travel of the sound beam. The observed frequency (f_R) differs from the transmit frequency (f_T). The angle θ is the Doppler angle.

CONTINUOUS-WAVE DOPPLER

- The continuous-wave (CW) Doppler transducer is configured with two crystals: one to transmit sound waves of constant frequency continuously and one to receive the returning echoes continuously.
- The CW transducer has a narrow bandwidth and a high Q-value.
- The sampling volume is defined by the geometric arrangement of the crystals.
- The measurement of the Doppler shift is based on wave interference.
  - The reflected sound wave from a moving interface varies slightly in frequency from the transmitted sound wave.
  - The echo-induced radiofrequency signal is combined with the reference signal from the oscillator to yield a complex waveform by wave interference.
  - Variation of the complex waveform is characterized by the beat frequency.
  - The isolation of the beat frequency by a processing technique called *demodulation* forms the Doppler signal.
  - The beat frequency is the difference in frequency between the transmitted wave and the received wave and, thus, equal to the Doppler shift frequency.
- Reflectors moving at a single, constant velocity produce a single beat frequency.
- Reflectors moving with a range of velocities produce multiple beat frequencies.
- Multiple beat frequencies representing all the detected motion comprise the complex Doppler signal.
- The CW Doppler signal is sent to the audio amplifier, filtered to remove unwanted components, and routed to a speaker for display.
- The wall filter removes low-frequency Doppler shifts associated with large, slow-moving reflectors (e.g., vessel walls) that can produce intense signals.
- A low-pass filter eliminates high-frequency noise, but its application imposes an upper limit on velocity measurement.
- The CW Doppler has high sensitivity to detect slow flow with small Doppler shift frequencies.
- Small differences in flow velocity can be detected with CW Doppler techniques.
- CW Doppler cannot use the echo ranging principle to ascertain the depth of moving reflectors.
- Time gain compensation (TGC) cannot be applied to correct signal loss by attenuation.

PULSED-WAVE DOPPLER

- By pulsing the transmitted wave, the echo-ranging principle is applied to obtain depth information about the origin of the Doppler signal.
- A long transmit pulse duration is necessary to detect slow flow.

- The received signals are electronically gated with respect to time to isolate the region that contributes to the Doppler signal.
  - The delay time before the gate is turned on determines the axial location of the sensitive volume.
  - The amount of time the gate is activated establishes the axial length of the sampling volume.
  - Other dimensions of the sampling volume are dictated by the beam width in the in-plane direction and beam width in the elevation direction.
- Multiple echoes from a moving reflector, separated in time, must be accrued to detect motion.
  - Transmitted pulses must be repeatedly directed along the scan line to interrogate the sampling volume.
  - Doppler signal acquisition requires longer time than does the assignment of echo strength in B-mode imaging.
- The pulsed-wave (PW) Doppler instrument modifies the basic CW design to include gating and a sample-and-hold circuit.
- Each transmitted pulse contributes one point to the complex Doppler signal (sum of beat frequencies associated with the movement of reflectors within the sampling volume).
- The sample-and-hold circuit is a buffer that assembles these point-by-point measurements to form the complex Doppler signal.
- Because the complex Doppler signal is sampled intermittently, beat frequencies must be inferred from the limited data available.
- The definition of the complex Doppler signal is improved by increasing the rate of sampling, which is the pulse repetition frequency (PRF).

ALIASING

- The Nyquist limit states that a minimum of two pulses per beat cycle is required to define beat frequency unambiguously.
- In PW Doppler, the maximum Doppler shift, $f_D(max)$, is equal to one-half the PRF.
- A high PRF is necessary to measure large Doppler shifts produced by high-velocity reflectors.
- The maximum velocity limit is raised to a higher value if the transmission frequency is lowered, the sampling direction is changed to a larger Doppler angle, or the scan range is reduced.
- If the sampling rate is not adequate for the Doppler shift frequency, then aliasing occurs.
- Aliasing is the misrepresentation of the Doppler shift frequency as a lower frequency than the true value.

DIRECTIONAL METHODS

- Demodulation yields the Doppler shift, but it cannot indicate if the motion was toward or away from the transducer.

- Single-sideband, heterodyne, or quadrature phase detection are additional signal processing techniques that can identify the direction of motion.
- Quadrature phase detection divides the received signal into two components, and then each component is mixed with a reference signal (one channel is 90 degrees out of phase with the other).
- Frequency domain processing is applied after quadrature phase detection to generate two output signals, each associated with a particular direction of flow.

DUPLEX SCANNERS

- Duplex Doppler scanners combine real-time B-mode imaging with CW or PW Doppler detection.
- B-mode imaging depicts stationary reflectors and aids in the placement of CW sampling direction or PW sampling volume.
- The cursor must be placed parallel to the vessel wall to properly define the Doppler angle for an accurate calculation of velocity.
- Real-time imaging is interrupted when the Doppler signal is collected, usually over a period of several milliseconds (ms).
- The flow information is acquired for a small region within the B-mode field of view and displayed in real-time.
- The global pattern of flow must be ascertained by sampling multiple regions, one after another, throughout the field of view (FOV).

CHARACTERISTICS OF DOPPLER INSTRUMENTS

Continuous-Wave Doppler	Pulsed-Wave Doppler
No range resolution	Depth information
Narrow bandwidth	Wide bandwidth
No velocity limit	Maximum velocity limit
High sensitivity to slow flow	Low sensitivity to slow flow
No aliasing	Aliasing

PROBLEMS

1. Assuming that a 2 MHz transducer is directed at an interface moving with a velocity of 15 centimeters per second (cm/s), what is the Doppler shift frequency? The Doppler angle is 30 degrees.
2. Assuming that a 2 MHz transducer is directed at an interface moving with a velocity of 15 cm/s, what is the Doppler shift frequency? The Doppler angle is 45 degrees.
3. Assuming that a 2 MHz transducer is directed at an interface moving with a velocity of 45 cm/s, what is the Doppler shift frequency? The Doppler angle is 30 degrees.

4. Assuming that a 4 MHz transducer is directed at an interface moving with a velocity of 15 cm/s, what is the Doppler shift frequency? The Doppler angle is 30 degrees.
5. Calculate the velocity of the moving reflector if a Doppler shift of 800 hertz (Hz) is observed. The Doppler angle is 30 degrees, and the operating frequency is 3 MHz.
6. Calculate the velocity of the moving reflector if a Doppler shift of 1200 Hz is observed. The Doppler angle is 30 degrees and the operating frequency is 3 MHz.
7. Calculate the velocity of the moving reflector if a Doppler shift of 800 Hz is observed. The Doppler angle is 30 degrees, and the operating frequency is 1.5 MHz.
8. Calculate the velocity of the moving reflector if a Doppler shift of 800 Hz is observed. The Doppler angle is 45 degrees, and the operating frequency is 3 MHz.
9. Calculate the minimum pulse repetition frequency to prevent aliasing if the velocity of the moving reflector is 25 cm/s. The Doppler angle is 30 degrees, and the operating frequency is 3 MHz.
10. Calculate the minimum pulse repetition frequency to prevent aliasing if the velocity of the moving reflector is 50 cm/s. The Doppler angle is 30 degrees, and the operating frequency is 3 MHz.
11. Calculate the minimum pulse repetition frequency to prevent aliasing if the velocity of the moving reflector is 25 cm/s. The Doppler angle is 45 degrees, and the operating frequency is 3 MHz.
12. Calculate the minimum pulse repetition frequency to prevent aliasing if the velocity of the moving reflector is 25 cm/s. The Doppler angle is 30 degrees, and the operating frequency is 1.5 MHz.

MULTIPLE CHOICE QUESTIONS

1. What is the beat frequency obtained with a continuous-wave (CW) Doppler instrument?
   A. One-half the rate of sampling along the scan direction
   B. Difference between transmitted frequency and received frequency
   C. Echo-induced signal from stationary reflectors
   D. Frequency of the received echo from moving reflector
2. What is the purpose of the wall filter applied during CW Doppler signal processing?
   A. Correct for attenuation along beam path
   B. Remove high-frequency noise
   C. Prevent aliasing of high-frequency Doppler shifts
   D. Eliminate signals from slow-moving reflectors
3. How is the sampling volume delineated in PW Doppler?
   A. Transmit focal zone
   B. Timing gates for received signals
   C. High-pass filters
   D. Dynamic receive focusing

4. What is aliasing?

A. The observed Doppler shift frequency lower than the true Doppler shift frequency

B. Poor detection of the Doppler shift frequency caused by low signal-to-noise ratio

C. Improper application of a low-pass filter to remove fast-velocity components

D. Doppler signal obtained with a Doppler angle greater than 80 degrees

5. What is a characteristic of CW Doppler ultrasound?

A. Aliasing can occur

B. Sensitive to slow flow

C. Excellent depth resolution

D. Wide transmitted bandwidth

6. What is a characteristic of PW Doppler ultrasound?

A. Aliasing cannot occur

B. Sensitive to slow flow

C. Maximum velocity limit

D. Narrow transmitted bandwidth

7. Which of the following is a feature of a duplex scanner?

A. Depicts global flow throughout the field of view

B. Sampling volume selected without operator input

C. Nearly simultaneous B-mode and Doppler acquisitions

D. Nearly simultaneous PW and CW Doppler acquisitions

Doppler Spectral Analysis

COMPLEX DOPPLER SIGNAL

- Red blood cells (RBCs) throughout the cross-section of a vessel move at different velocities.
- Velocity variations within the pulsed-wave (PW) Doppler sampling volume give rise to a complex Doppler signal, which is a combination of all the Doppler shift frequencies present.
- Spectral analysis is the determination of the individual Doppler shift frequencies that compose the complex Doppler signal.
- Spectral analysis, when repeated rapidly in time, characterizes the flow in vessels.

FAST FOURIER TRANSFORM

- Fast Fourier transform (FFT) is a mathematical algorithm that converts the complex Doppler signal into a series of single-frequency sine wave components.
- The algebraic summation of the series of sine waves yields the original complex Doppler waveform.
- Each single-frequency sine wave corresponds to a Doppler shift frequency and denotes RBCs moving at a specific velocity.
- The Doppler shift equation converts the Doppler shift frequency into velocity.
- The amplitude of each sine wave is the signal strength of RBCs moving at the velocity indicated by the Doppler shift frequency.
- The FFT determination of the Doppler shift frequency present in the complex Doppler signal is performed without prior knowledge of these frequency components.
  - All frequency components present are identified by spectral analysis.
  - In the absence of noise, the fidelity of the FFT is independent of the Doppler shift frequency distribution (whatever frequency components that are present are identified).

POWER SPECTRUM

- Sine wave is often depicted as the change in amplitude as a function of time.
- Frequency is derived from the time-dependent plot by measuring the number of cycles per unit time.

- Power spectrum is an alternative graphic display of the results of spectral analysis.
  - The amplitude (or magnitude) of individual frequency components is plotted as a function of frequency or velocity via the Doppler shift equation.
  - Each point on the horizontal axis corresponds to a specific velocity.
  - The displacement along the vertical axis indicates the relative number of RBCs moving with that velocity in the sampled volume.
- Flow velocities not present are depicted with zero magnitude in the power spectrum.
- The distribution of Doppler shift frequency is readily illustrated by the power spectrum.

DOPPLER SPECTRAL WAVEFORM

- The power spectrum shows the velocity distribution at the time of sampling.
- The velocity distribution of RBCs in a vessel is not constant with time.
- In order to display the changing velocity distributions, the power spectrum for the vessel must be obtained repeatedly over time.
- FFT processing analyzes the series of power spectra in real-time.
- A graphic plot of the power spectrum as a function of time is called the *Doppler spectral waveform*.
- Three variables (frequency or velocity, magnitude, and time) are shown in a two-dimensional display of the Doppler spectral waveform (Figure 14-1).
  - The vertical axis depicts for frequency or velocity as well as magnitude.
  - The displacement along the vertical axis represents increased frequency or velocity.
  - The brightness of the dot at a frequency point indicates magnitude.
  - The horizontal axis scrolls with time.
- Each analysis of a short time segment of the complex Doppler signal is presented as a single vertical line.
- Succeeding frequency spectral analyses are placed side by side, a fixed distance apart, and the vertical lines scroll left to right to build up a pattern.

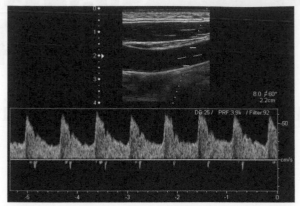

FIGURE 14-1 Doppler spectral waveform. The sample volume was positioned to encompass the full width of the vessel.

- The velocity scale of the Doppler spectral waveform is adjusted by changing the pulse repetition frequency.
- Time-varying physiologic signals (e.g., electrocardiogram) can be displayed in conjunction with brightness-modulated power spectra.
- A wall filter, applied to the Doppler signal to eliminate vessel wall thump, may also remove low-velocity blood flow components in the power spectra.

ALIASING

- Aliasing is characterized by wrap-around, whereby the high-velocity components above the Nyquist limit are misrepresented at lower velocity in the direction opposite to flow (Figure 14-2).
- The most common technique to remove aliasing is to increase the velocity scale, which is accomplished by raising the pulse repetition frequency (Figure 14-3).
- According to the Nyquist criterion, a higher pulse repetition frequency extends the maximum velocity limit.
- Other techniques to eliminate aliasing include baseline adjustment, increased angle of insonation, decreased depth to sample volume, and lower transmitted frequency.

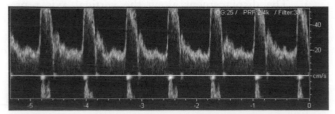

FIGURE 14-2 Aliasing artifact. High-velocity components demonstrate wrap-around (depicted at lower velocity in the opposite direction). The velocity range on the vertical scale is −20 to 50 centimeters per second (cm/s).

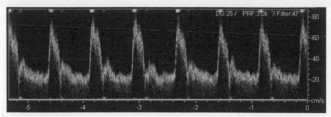

FIGURE 14-3 Velocity scale adjustment. The aliasing artifact in Figure 14-2 is removed by increasing the velocity range on the vertical scale from 0 to 85 centimeters per second (cm/s).

LIMITATIONS OF SPECTRAL ANALYSIS

- In the presence of noise, the complex Doppler signal is inexact, and FFT yields variations in the calculated frequency components.
- Each brightness-modulated dot in the Doppler spectral waveform represents a range of Doppler shift frequencies.
- Short sampling times (~10 milliseconds [ms]) are necessary to depict rapid changes in the velocity distribution.
- Sampling time imposes a limit on the frequency resolution of the Doppler spectral waveform.
- The frequency range for each dot equals the inverse of the sampling time (5 ms yields 200 hertz [Hz]).
- The movement of RBCs in and out of the sampling volume causes a fluctuation of the Doppler signal, which introduces additional frequency components above and below the idealized Doppler shift frequency (called *transit time broadening*).
- By the narrowing of the beam width or shortening of the receiver gate, transit time broadening becomes more pronounced.
- PW Doppler has a broad bandwidth, which gives rise to multiple Doppler shifts from a reflector moving at constant velocity.
- The physical size of the beam aperture creates a range of angles that intercept the vessel, which gives rise to multiple Doppler shifts from a reflector moving at constant velocity.

POWER SPECTRUM DESCRIPTORS

- FFT processing yields a frequency or velocity distribution with high information content.
- The information content of brightness-modulated power spectra is simplified by displaying a time-varying trace of a power spectrum descriptor (maximum frequency, mean frequency, median frequency, and mode frequency).
  - Maximum frequency is the calculated maximum frequency in the power spectrum with an upper cut-off limit applied.
  - Mean frequency is the average of all Doppler shifts in the power spectrum.

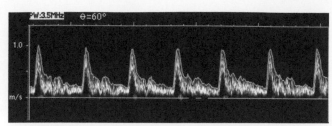

FIGURE 14-4 Maximum velocity waveform (*solid line*).

- Doppler shifts are equally divided above and below the median frequency.
- Mode frequency is the most prevalent Doppler shift in the power spectrum.
- Each FFT time segment is analyzed for the power spectrum descriptor.
- The time-varying trace of the highest Doppler shift converted to velocity is the maximum velocity waveform, the most commonly displayed descriptor (Figure 14-4).

DISTURBED FLOW

- A partial blockage of a vessel causes flow disturbance, which induces changes in the Doppler spectral waveform.
- Severe stenosis creates high-speed jets at the point of blockage.
- Peak velocity, in particular, increases as luminal size decreases and is used as an indicator of the severity of the stenosis.
- Eddy currents—that is, rotating elements—are present immediately distal to severe stenosis.
- Turbulence—that is, loss of flow coherence including reversal of flow components—may occur distal to severe stenosis (Figure 14-5).

REVIEW QUESTIONS

1. What method is used to determine the Doppler shift frequencies present in the complex Doppler signal?
2. What parameter is represented by the horizontal axis of the Doppler spectral waveform?

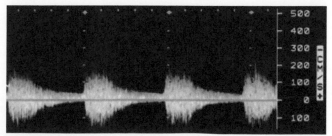

FIGURE 14-5 Disturbed flow. Doppler spectral waveform demonstrating turbulence.

3. What parameter is represented by the vertical axis of the Doppler spectral waveform?
4. How is time-dependent flow information acquired to form the Doppler spectral waveform?
5. At the time of measurement, no red blood cells (RBCs) are moving with a velocity of 30 to 50 centimeters per second (cm/s). How is this depicted in the Doppler spectral waveform?
6. If the sampled volume at the time of measurement contains RBCs moving at a constant velocity, how many Doppler shift frequencies should ideally be present?
7. What is aliasing with respect to the Doppler spectral waveform?
8. What is maximum velocity waveform?
9. What is the major advantage of the Doppler spectral waveform?
10. What is the major disadvantage of the Doppler spectral waveform?
11. Examine the Doppler spectral waveform in Figure 14-1. What is the highest velocity recorded throughout the cardiac cycle?

MULTIPLE CHOICE QUESTIONS

1. If the peak velocity increases from 50 centimeters per second (cm/s) to 90 cm/s, what change occurs in the Doppler spectral waveform?
   A. The displacement along the vertical axis becomes elongated
   B. The displacement along the horizontal axis becomes elongated
   C. Overall brightness is increased
   D. No change
2. If twice as many red blood cells (RBCs) flow at the peak velocity of 50 cm/s, what change occurs in the Doppler spectral waveform?
   A. The displacement along the vertical axis becomes elongated
   B. The displacement along the horizontal axis becomes elongated
   C. The brightness at the velocity peak is increased
   D. No change
3. Which technique cannot eliminate aliasing?
   A. Increasing the pulse repetition frequency (PRF)
   B. Increasing the velocity scale
   C. Increasing the angle of insonation
   D. Increasing the transducer frequency
4. What is the feature of flow at the site of 90% stenosis? Assume that the laminar flow has occurred prior to the stenosis.
   A. Laminar flow
   B. High-speed jets
   C. Flow reversal
   D. Turbulent flow

5. What is the feature of a disturbed flow immediately distal to 90% stenosis? Assume that the laminar flow occurred prior to the stenosis.
   A. Laminar flow
   B. Plug flow
   C. Eddy flow
   D. Uniform velocity

6. What is the feature of flow very distal to 90% stenosis? Assume that the laminar flow occurred prior to the stenosis.
   A. Laminar flow
   B. High-speed jets
   C. Eddy flow
   D. Uniform velocity

Doppler Imaging

IMAGE FORMATION

- Doppler imaging combines, in real-time, two-dimensional flow information depicted in color with gray-scale B-mode imaging.
- Stationary reflectors are assigned a gray level based on signal strength.
- Moving reflectors are assigned a color based on velocity or quantity of blood flow.
- Doppler imaging is more sensitive than B-mode imaging for the detection of flow in vessels.
- Doppler imaging enables global visualization of flow by displaying the two-dimensional spatial distribution of velocities and the temporal changes in velocity patterns.

COLOR DOPPLER IMAGING

- The mean velocity at each sampling site where motion is detected is color encoded by hue and superimposed on the B-mode image.
- The velocity color map, which can be selected by the operator, assigns shades of color to represent velocity range and direction of flow.
- Flow toward and flow away from the transducer are depicted simultaneously.
- Moving reflectors cause a phase shift in received echo signals, which indicates the presence and direction of motion.
- To assess motion, multiple echoes from the same reflector must be collected using a sequence of transmitted pulses, separated in time by the pulse repetition period.
- Packet size, or ensemble length, is the number of transmit pulses that interrogate a color scan line.
- The rapid acquisition and analysis of flow data are accomplished with autocorrelation detection.
  - The echoes received along the entire scan line are segmented by depth and then compared with the echo wavetrain obtained from the immediately preceding transmitted pulse.
  - Processing for all depth segments is done concurrently.
  - Autocorrelation for each depth segment yields a mean frequency estimate but does not provide spectral analysis of the Doppler signal.

- The dwell time for a color line is relatively long because multiple transmitted pulses (set by packet size) are required for the measurement of mean velocity.
- A large packet size improves the accuracy of the mean frequency estimate but increases the time required for data collection.
- The fixed echo canceller removes strong echoes from stationary reflectors before signal transfer to the autocorrelation detector (stationary reflectors are not a concern in color assignment).
- An asynchronous scanner acquires the B-mode image and flow data separately; these are later superimposed to form the color Doppler image.
  - The transmitted power, frequency, and steering can be optimized for both Doppler and B-mode scanning.
  - The width of the color field of view can be made smaller than the field of view (FOV) of the B-mode image.
  - Scan line density in color mode is usually lower than that of the B-mode image.
  - The spatial resolution for color and B-mode image components is not matched, since the axial sampling interval for the Doppler scan line is usually greater than that for the B-mode scan line.
- A synchronous scanner acquires echo and flow data simultaneously by dividing the signal into separate processing pathways for Doppler and B-mode components.
  - The transmitted power, frequency, and steering for the transmitted pulse cannot be optimized for both Doppler and B-mode scanning.
  - The FOV and spatial resolution are identical for the color and gray-scale components of the Doppler image.
- The combined Doppler mode displays the Doppler spectrum analysis with the color Doppler image.
  - Pulsed-wave (PW) Doppler spectral analysis is performed on a single selected region of interest.
  - The rate of image update for color Doppler is dramatically reduced.

COLOR DOPPLER OPERATOR CONTROLS

- The color map assigns flow velocities to various shades of color.
- The velocity scale specifies the direction and range of velocities in the color display.

- The baseline control shifts the center of the velocity scale to increase the velocity range in one direction.
- Color gain is the amplification applied to the Doppler component during processing.
- The color gate adjusts the axial length of the Doppler sampling volume.
- The color reject sets a signal strength threshold below which weak signals are not included in the color display.
- The color filter is a high-pass filter, which is applied to eliminate color encoding of tissue associated with vessel wall movement.
  - The color filter may eliminate low-velocity blood flow from the color display.
- The frame rate depends on the width of the color FOV, color line density, and packet size.
- Color persistence is a frame averaging technique to reduce noise and enhance regions with low-volume flow.
- The direction of sampling for the color FOV can be changed to improve the angle of insonation for the vessel of interest.
- The variance map assigns the spread of the velocity distribution in the sampled volume to various color shades.

POWER DOPPLER IMAGING

- Alternative terms for power Doppler imaging are *power flow Doppler, Doppler energy, color energy, color amplitude, color angio, ultrasound angio,* and *color power angio.*
- The amplitude of the Doppler signal at each sampling site where motion is detected is color encoded by hue and superimposed on the B-mode image.
- Autocorrelation detection measures the Doppler signal strength as well as mean velocity.
- The Doppler signal strength depends on the number of red blood cells (RBCs) within the sampling volume.
- The major advantage of power Doppler imaging is the visualization of flow in small vessels.
- The power Doppler image contains no flow direction or flow velocity information.
- Since all Doppler frequency shifts contribute to the Doppler signal strength, power Doppler imaging is relatively independent of angle of insonation.
- Power Doppler imaging is not subject to aliasing.
- Three-dimensional power Doppler imaging of organ vasculature is now possible.

IMAGE QUALITY

- Motion discrimination is a signal-processing technique designed to distinguish flowing blood from moving tissue.
- A high-pass filter is applied to remove low-frequency Doppler shifts associated with vessel wall movement;

however, it causes a corresponding loss of low-velocity flow components.
- A high frame rate enables rapidly changing flow patterns to be portrayed accurately.
- An increased frame rate is achieved by reducing the color line density, the width of the color FOV, the packet size, or all of these.
- Spatial mapping of Doppler signals depends on color gate, in-plane beam width, elevation beam width, and color line density.
- As the sampling volume is reduced, weak Doppler signals are less likely to be encoded in color.
- Vessel size and color pattern should be unaffected by scan depth (i.e., vessels with identical low characteristics should appear the same regardless of scan depth).

COLOR DOPPLER IMAGING ARTIFACTS

- Shadowing from enhanced attenuation by overlying structures may cause an absence of color in the vessel.
- At a high pulse repetition frequency (PRF), a deeply-lying vessel may be depicted in a more superficial location.
- Steering to improve the angle of insonation can cause misregistration of reflectors from grating lobes.
- Aliasing occurs if the velocity of flow exceeds the velocity limit of the color map.
- Aliasing is readily identified when adjoining regions show contrasting colors that represent maximum flow in opposite directions.
- A vessel interrogated along its length with different insonation angles will depict the flow incorrectly with varying colors.
- A nonuniform angle of insonation across a tortuous vessel will register the direction of the flow incorrectly.
- A mirror image of color flow is formed when a vessel is located proximal to a highly reflective surface at which near-total reflection occurs.
  - The spectral analysis of a mirror image is identical to that derived from a properly registered image of color flow.
- Color flash is a sudden burst of color that encompasses a wide region within the frame.
  - Movement of the transducer or tissue causes improper assignment of color.
  - Increasing the color filter, decreasing the persistence, or reducing the width of the color FOV suppresses the occurrence of a color flash artifact.
- Color bleed is the extension of color beyond the region of flow to adjacent tissue.
- Color noise is the color fill-in of hypoechoic regions caused by random variations in Doppler signal measurements.

- Color noise is most often attributed to high color gain or low color reject settings.
- The spectral analysis of color noise does not correspond to correlated flow profiles.
- Color bruit is the color encoding of tissue near the region of severe stenosis of a vessel.

MULTIPLE CHOICE QUESTIONS

1. What signal processing technique is applied in Doppler imaging to detect moving reflectors?
   A. Autocorrelation
   B. Fast Fourier transform
   C. Fixed echo canceller
   D. Harmonic filtering
2. What is packet size?
   A. Number of color lines in a Doppler image
   B. Number of transmit pulses for a color line
   C. Number of the gray-scale lines in a Doppler image
   D. Number of transmit pulses for a gray-scale line
3. What parameter of flow is color encoded in power Doppler imaging?
   A. Velocity
   B. Direction
   C. Flow velocity range
   D. Quantity of red blood cells (RBCs)
4. What adjustment can remove aliasing in color Doppler imaging?
   A. Increasing packet size
   B. Increasing number of color lines
   C. Decreasing width of color field of view
   D. Decreasing color gain
5. What parameter of flow is color encoded in color Doppler imaging?
   A. Mean velocity
   B. Maximum velocity
   C. Velocity spectral analysis
   D. Rate of velocity change
6. How can the accuracy of the velocity measurement in color Doppler imaging be improved?
   A. Increase packet size
   B. Increase the number of color lines
   C. Reduce width of the color field of view
   D. Reduce operating frequency
7. Which Doppler mode is *not* subject to aliasing?
   A. Color Doppler imaging
   B. Power Doppler imaging
   C. Pulsed-wave spectral analysis
   D. Duplex scanning with depth-defined sampling volume
8. If a cyst without flow is depicted in color, which color Doppler control is improperly set?
   A. Color persistence
   B. Color gain
   C. B-mode gain
   D. Packet size
9. If the tissue next to the vessel wall is shown in color, which color Doppler control is improperly set?
   A. Frame rate
   B. Color filter
   C. Packet size
   D. Color persistence
10. What adjustment can increase the frame rate in color Doppler imaging?
    A. Increasing the packet size
    B. Increasing the color line density
    C. Reducing the width of the color field of view
    D. Reducing the operating frequency

M-Mode Scanning

SCAN FORMAT

- The depth of the reflectors as a function of time is presented in a two-dimensional graphic display.
- M-mode sampling is done along one line of sight.
- Repeated measurements during the time of observation show the change in the position of each reflector along the line of sight.
  - Pulse repetition frequency (PRF) is generally less than 500 hertz (Hz).
- Quantitative analysis of the movement of reflectors, including velocity, amplitude, and pattern of motion, is accomplished with M-mode scanning.
- Stationary interfaces produce straight-line plots, whereas moving interfaces produce oscillating waveforms (Figure 16-1).
- Echo intensity is depicted in the graphic display by shades of gray, color brightness, or color hue.
- The information content of the M-mode trace contains reflector depth, signal level for each reflector, relative positions of the reflectors at each sampling time, and change in the axial position of each reflector with time.
- Motion in the lateral direction is not portrayed because sampling is limited to one line of sight.

M-MODE WITH B-MODE IMAGING

- The M-mode trace is combined with B-mode imaging on the display monitor.
- A line cursor placed on the B-mode image denotes the line of sight for the acquisition of the M-mode scan data (Figure 16-2).
- The visualized anatomy facilitates the placement of the line cursor so that the desired structures are depicted in the M-mode trace.

COLOR M-MODE IMAGING

- The M-mode trace is combined with color Doppler imaging on the display monitor.
- A line cursor placed on the color Doppler image denotes the M-mode sampling direction with respect to flow.
- Interface motion and blood flow along the line of sight are correlated.

OPERATOR CONTROLS

- Gain, independent of B-mode receiver gain, amplifies signals along the sampling direction.
- Log compression is applied to suppress low signals and noise.

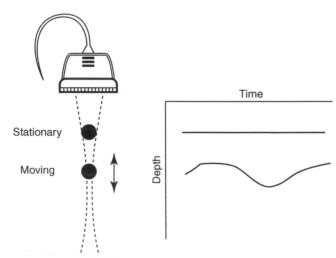

FIGURE 16-1 Principle of M-Mode Scanning. The depth of each interface encountered along the line of sight is monitored by repeated measurements during the time of observation. The M-mode display shows stationary and moving interfaces within the pulsed sound beam.

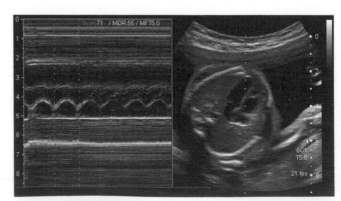

FIGURE 16-2 Combined M-mode with B-mode. M-mode trace of aortic valve at a depth between 4 and 5 cm.

- Filtering sharpens or smoothes boundaries of moving structures.
- Signal strength is encoded in gray levels or color according to the gray-scale map or the color map.
- Freeze function suspends M-mode data collection and displays the most recently acquired trace for prolonged viewing.
- The spatial dimension of the M-mode trace is magnified by time-gating the received signals so that a more narrow range of depths is displayed.
- The sweep rate adjusts the displayed temporal dimension of the M-mode trace.

MULTIPLE CHOICE QUESTIONS

1. How many lines of sight compose the M-mode trace?
   A. One
   B. One hundred
   C. Operator selectable
   D. Automatically set on the basis of reflector displacement
2. How many moving reflectors are depicted in the M-mode graphic display?
   A. One
   B. Depends on the sampling direction
   C. Depends on the number of lines of sight
   D. Depends on pulse repetition frequency
3. What information is contained in the two-dimensional M-mode trace?
   A. Two-dimensional spatial relationships similar to those in B-mode imaging
   B. Axial and lateral movements of reflectors along the sampling direction
   C. Only axial movement of reflectors along the sampling direction
   D. Only moving reflectors, with the exclusion of stationary reflectors
4. How is signal strength encoded in the two-dimensional M-mode trace?
   A. Gray level
   B. Deflection in the axial direction
   C. Deflection in the lateral direction
   D. Slope of the M-mode trace
5. How is reflector displacement portrayed in the two-dimensional M-mode trace?
   A. Gray level
   B. Deflection in the axial direction
   C. Slope of the M-mode trace
   D. Horizontal width of the M-mode trace
6. What is the advantage of combining M-mode scanning with B-mode imaging?
   A. Display of two-dimensional movement of reflectors on M-mode trace
   B. Ease of placement of M-mode sampling direction
   C. Extension of the velocity limit for accurate M-mode recording
   D. Improving B-mode temporal resolution
7. How is a stationary reflector portrayed in the two-dimensional M-mode trace?
   A. Circle
   B. Straight line
   C. Sine wave
   D. Saw tooth
8. Which M-mode pattern corresponds to the largest displacement?

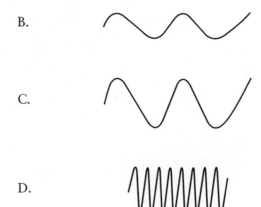

9. Which M-mode pattern corresponds to the reflector with the highest velocity?

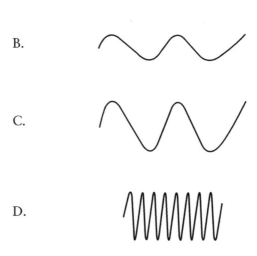

10. How is reflector velocity portrayed in the two-dimensional M-mode trace?
    A. Gray level
    B. Deflection in the axial direction
    C. Horizontal width of the M-mode trace
    D. Slope of the M-mode trace

11. Which of the following operator controls reduces the dynamic range of M-mode signals?
    A. Log compression
    B. Smoothing filter
    C. Sweep rate
    D. Freeze

12. Which of the following operator controls suspends the acquisition of M-mode signals?
    A. Log compression
    B. Smoothing filter
    C. Sweep rate
    D. Freeze

Clinical Safety

SYNOPSIS

- Ultrasound is *not* a form of ionizing radiation.
- No *acute* harmful effects of diagnostic medical sonography have been reported.

MECHANISMS OF BIOLOGIC DAMAGE

- The term *radiation force* describes the damage induced by mechanical motion.
  - During propagation, particles undergo extreme changes in velocity and acceleration, which gives rise to acoustic pressure applied to a surface.
  - The rapid movement of fluid near solid boundaries (microstreaming) can cause fragmentation of macromolecules.
- The absorption of sound causes heating of tissue (thermal effects).
  - Irreversible tissue damage can be induced by a period of increased temperature (depending on duration of elevated temperature).
  - The rate of temperature rise depends on the absorption coefficient of tissue, temporal averaged intensity, cross-sectional area of the beam, exposure time, and heat-transport processes.
  - Throughout the frequency range of diagnostic ultrasonography, the absorption coefficient of tissue increases with frequency.
- The dynamic behavior of microbubbles subjected to pressure fluctuations is called *cavitation*.
- Cavitation is subdivided into two forms: stable cavitation and transient cavitation.
- Stable cavitation involves pre-existing microbubbles in the medium, which are not destroyed by the action of the sound wave.
  - A microbubble expands and contracts in size during a wave cycle of rarefaction and compression.
  - Dissolved gas may leave the solution and contribute to the expansion of microbubbles.
  - At the resonant frequency (depending on bubble size), the vibration amplitude of surrounding liquid particles is maximized.
  - Stable cavitation may produce high shearing forces and microstreaming in localized areas near the microbubbles.

- Short-lived expansion and collapse of microbubbles is called *transient cavitation*.
  - During the rarefaction phase, microbubbles form and grow in size when dissolved gases leave the solution.
  - A large rate of growth can be sustained for a few acoustic cycles before complete collapse of the microbubble.
  - A rarefaction phase of long duration (low frequency) enhances the expansion of the bubbles.
  - The microbubbles collapse during the compression phase, and this generates localized shock waves and very high temperatures.
  - Transient cavitation is considered a threshold effect.
  - The lowest pressure for transient cavitation in tissue is not known.

TYPES OF BIOLOGIC DAMAGE

- Damage to the deoxyribonucleic acid (DNA) in the solution is attributed to cavitation.
- Neoplastic transformation of cultured cells has been reported.
- Lung hemorrhage in mammals has been observed at a pressure threshold of 1 to 2 megapascals (MPa) for the frequency range 0.5 to 5 MHz.
- Little evidence of biologic damage in mammals exists for I(SPTA)—spatial-peak temporal-average intensity—less than 100 milliwatts per centimeters squared (mW/cm^2).
- The mutagenic potential of ultrasound is relatively weak.
- Fetal abnormalities in mammals are associated with tissue heating.
  - Thermal damage is a threshold effect.
  - No damage is observed unless the temperature elevation exceeds a particular value for a minimum duration.
  - A temperature rise of 3°C to 4°C present for 1 hour can cause fetal abnormalities in small animals.
  - At higher temperatures, the time necessary to induce damage is shortened dramatically.
- Results of some research that studied the reflex response in rodents suggests that ultrasound exposure in utero affects prenatal growth and development.

EPIDEMIOLOGIC STUDIES

- Epidemiologic studies have the ability to link biologic damage with a potentially causative agent.
- If the relative risk from a causative agent is small, then a large sample size is necessary to distinguish agent-induced effects from disorders that occur spontaneously in the population.
- Confounding factors from different population groups and epidemiologic studies may be the reasons for the conflicting results.
- Results from multiple epidemiologic studies must, essentially, be in agreement to form recommendations or influence the formation of guidelines.
- The most important consideration is whether ultrasound exposure in utero at diagnostic intensity levels is harmful to the unborn child.
  - The RADIUS (Routine Antenatal Diagnostic Imaging with Ultrasound) trial found that routine ultrasound screening did not reduce perinatal morbidity and mortality.
  - No association between in utero ultrasound exposure and fetal chromosome abnormalities, cancer, and hearing disorders has been demonstrated.
  - Positive and negative findings regarding low birth weight and impaired neurologic development have been reported.
  - Results from epidemiologic studies have been generally negative, implying that biologic damage, if any, is subtle, delayed, or infrequent.

OUTPUT DISPLAY STANDARD (ODS)

- Two acoustic output parameters, thermal index and mechanical index, have been adopted as indicators for potential adverse biologic effects.
- The thermal index (TI) calculates the maximum temperature rise (°C) in tissue caused by energy absorption.
- The mechanical index describes the possibility of cavitation, which is more likely to occur at high acoustic pressure and low frequency.
  - Cavitation has been demonstrated at peak pressures and frequencies within the operational range of diagnostic medical ultrasound.

THERMAL MECHANISM

- Acoustic energy is converted to heat as the beam propagates through tissue.
- The rate of heat production depends on the absorption coefficient and the local time-averaged intensity.
- High-frequency ultrasound with a high absorption coefficient is readily converted to heat.
- Bone is a very effective absorber of ultrasound and ultimately becomes a heat source.
- Heat removal by conduction and perfusion mediates the rate of temperature rise.

- The rate of energy transmission by the transducer (power in milliwatts [mW]) is critically important in predicting the temperature rise in tissue.
- Temperature profiles can be generated for a given set of conditions (medium, frequency, aperture, focusing, power, time-averaged intensity, absorption coefficient, and rate of perfusion).
  - At each point in the ultrasonic field, the maximum temperature rise is calculated.
  - The acoustic power (designated as the reference value) that causes a maximum temperature rise of 1°C at any point in the ultrasonic field is determined.
  - The actual acoustic power setting is compared with the acoustic power reference value to predict the temperature rise in tissue during ultrasound examination.
- An increase in transducer aperture raises the acoustic power reference value (energy is distributed over a wider area).
- An increase in transducer frequency lowers the acoustic power reference value (ultrasound energy is more readily absorbed).

THERMAL INDEX

- The ODS enables the same point of reference to be applied to all sonographic equipment regardless of manufacturer.
- Thermal index is the ratio of the in situ acoustic power to the acoustic power required to raise tissue temperature by 1°C.
- The numerical value of the TI is, in essence, the maximum temperature rise in degrees Celsius within the ultrasonic field.
- The in situ acoustic power depends on instrument settings (frequency, aperture, focus zone[s], power, and pulse repetition frequency).
- The in situ acoustic power is calculated from the measured power in water corrected for attenuation by tissue.
- A derating factor assumes a conservative attenuation rate of 0.3 decibel per centimeter–megahertz (dB/cm-MHz) (overestimates the in situ acoustic power).
- Three thermal indices (TIs) based on models of soft tissue and bone composition within the scanned region have been developed to emulate clinical situations.
  - TIS is applied if the ultrasound beam passes through soft tissue only and bone is not present (abdomen and fetus during first trimester).
  - TIB is applied if the ultrasound beam, after passing through soft tissue, impinges on bone, which is located within the focal zone (fetus during second and third trimesters).
  - TIC is used if bone is encountered near the transducer (pediatric and adult head).

- An underestimation of the TI may occur if fluid or nonlinear propagation is present.
- An overestimation of the TI may occur if the scan path is long.

MECHANICAL INDEX

- Mechanical index (MI) is a dimensionless quantity and is directly proportional to the derated peak negative pressure (p_r) in megapascals and inversely proportional to the square root of the frequency (f) in MHz:

$$MI = \frac{p_r}{\sqrt{f}}$$

  - The derated peak rarefactional pressure is determined by the measurement of the peak rarefactional pressure in water, corrected for attenuation along the equivalent tissue path.
- Cavitation in water has not been observed for a mechanical index <0.7.
- The U.S. Food and Drug Administration (FDA) guidelines permit the introduction of new equipment if the mechanical index is <1.9.
- The operator does not know the location of highest peak rarefaction pressure within the scanned volume.
- An underestimation of the MI may occur if fluid or nonlinear propagation is present.
- An overestimation of the MI may occur if the scan path is long.

INDICATIONS OF RISK

- TI is a conservative estimate of temperature rise that is based on a worst-case scenario.
- Insonation of long duration is necessary to reach the steady state temperature rise predicted by the TI.
- The presence of pre-existing gas bodies enhances cavitation.
- Aerated lung, undissolved gas in the gastrointestinal tract, and gaseous contrast agents are potential sources of cavitation.
- According to the National Council on Radiation Protection and Measurements, an index value <0.5 is considered below the threshold level for adverse biologic effects.
- If the index value is >0.5, then risks associated with the examination must be considered relative to the diagnostic information to be gained.
- TIBs for commercial units range from 0.1 to 10 for fetal scanning.
- At high TIBs, insonation of short duration may cause harm.
- Exposure time should be limited when the TI exceeds 1.
  - No fetal abnormalities have been associated with a temperature rise of 3°C for 10 minutes.

RISKS VERSUS BENEFITS

- Diagnostic ultrasonography should be conducted only when medically indicated.
  - The phrase *medically indicated* means that the patient would receive some benefit from the information obtained (patient management is improved).
  - Objective criteria should be applied in the selection of patients for ultrasound examination.
- The "as low as reasonably achievable" (ALARA) principle should be practiced in diagnostic medical sonography.
  - The lowest power consistent with the objectives of the examination should be used.
  - The duration of active ultrasound transmission should be short, but it should be sufficient to obtain the necessary information.
  - The examination should not be limited in time and power to compromise its validity.

AMERICAN INSTITUTE OF ULTRASOUND IN MEDICINE (AIUM)

- The statement on mammalian in vivo biologic effects concludes that no adverse thermal effects in mammalian tissues exposed in vivo have been independently confirmed for I(SPTA) below 100 mW/cm^2 (unfocused) and 1 watt per centimeter squared (W/cm^2) (focused).
- The statement on mammalian in vivo biologic effects also concludes that no adverse biologic effects in mammalian tissues that contain well-defined gas bodies are induced if the mechanical index is <0.3.

CLINICAL GUIDELINES

- Nonmedical use of ultrasound for psychosocial and entertainment purposes is discouraged.
- Use of ultrasonography for merely viewing the fetus or determining the sex of the fetus without medical indication is inappropriate.
- Improved management and outcome of a pregnancy by routine screening with ultrasound has not been demonstrated in randomized research studies.
- Routine screening of every pregnancy has not been recommended by the National Institutes of Health (NIH).
- Perinatal mortality and morbidity have been reduced by *selective* ultrasound imaging during pregnancy.
- The eye is susceptible to high levels of heating, as the lens readily absorbs ultrasound and heat removal by perfusion is slow.
- For each application, the default settings should be reviewed and documented by the user.

MULTIPLE CHOICE QUESTIONS

1. According to the statement on mammalian in vivo biologic effects from the American Institute for Ultrasound in Medicine (AIUM), what intensity of an unfocused beam is considered the threshold for thermal effects?
   A. 1 W/cm^2
   B. 1 mW/cm^2
   C. 100 W/cm^2
   D. 100 mW/cm^2

2. According to the AIUM statement on mammalian in vivo biologic effects, what intensity of a focused beam is considered the threshold for thermal effects?
   A. 1 W/cm^2
   B. 1 mW/cm^2
   C. 100 W/cm^2
   D. 100 mW/cm^2

3. According to the AIUM statement on mammalian in vivo biologic effects, what value of mechanical index is considered the threshold for cavitation if well-defined gas bodies are present?
   A. 0.01
   B. 0.3
   C. 1.0
   D. 2.0

4. What effect is associated with the complete collapse of microbubbles during the high-pressure phase of the ultrasound cycle?
   A. Stable cavitation
   B. Transient cavitation
   C. Absorption
   D. Bremsstrahlung

5. What is the major finding of the RADIUS (Routine Antenatal Diagnostic Imaging with Ultrasound) study regarding in vivo exposure to ultrasound?
   A. Low birth weight
   B. Impaired neurologic development
   C. No change in perinatal morbidity or mortality
   D. Cancer induction

6. Which ultrasound parameter change would likely produce the highest rate of heating in soft tissue?
   A. Increase in transmitted frequency
   B. Decrease in pulse repetition frequency
   C. Decrease in duty factor from 0.08 to 0.05
   D. Increase in the width of the field of view

7. Which is an example of ALARA ("as low as reasonably achievable")?
   A. Free ultrasound viewing of the fetus at the local mall
   B. Ultrasound scanning of a model during a convention
   C. Selection of patients based on their ability to pay
   D. Selection of patients based on their medical conditions

8. According to the National Council on Radiation Protection and Measurements, what is considered the threshold output display standard (ODS) index for potential adverse effects?
   A. 0.1
   B. 0.5
   C. 10
   D. 100

9. If the thermal index exceeds 1.0 during fetal scanning, what is the proper response from the sonographer?
   A. Immediately stop scanning and file an incident report
   B. Immediately stop scanning with no administrative action
   C. Continue scanning with appropriate power and scan time to obtain the desired diagnostic information
   D. Continue scanning after placing ice packs on the patient

10. What does a thermal index of 1.5 indicate?
    A. Scan time is limited to 1.5 minutes
    B. Decrease the power setting by 1.5 decibel
    C. A temperature rise of 1.5°C may occur within the scanned volume
    D. Decrease frame rate by a factor of 1.5

11. Which medium is most likely to become a heat source within the ultrasonic field?
    A. Soft tissue
    B. Bone
    C. Water
    D. Air

12. What is the purpose of the derating factor?
    A. Calculates correction for attenuation in tissue
    B. Gives the scan time for thermal index above 1.0
    C. Calculates the effect of aperture on reference power level
    D. Gives the reduction in transmit power to achieve a thermal index of 1.0

13. Which thermal index model is applicable to fetal scanning during the second trimester?
    A. TIB
    B. TIC
    C. TIS
    D. TIF

Performance Testing

PHANTOMS

- A test object is usually composed of material that has an acoustic velocity of 1540 meters per second (m/s) (same as soft tissue), but its scattering and attenuation properties differ from those of soft tissue.
- The American Institute for Ultrasound in Medicine (AIUM) test object, because of poor scattering by the medium, has been replaced by tissue-mimicking (TM) phantoms.
- TM material has similar properties as those of tissue with respect to velocity, scattering, and attenuation.
- Small, strong reflectors (nylon pins) are placed in well-defined geometric patterns within the TM phantom to assess the spatial mapping of echoes.
- General-purpose TM phantoms commonly test for dead zone, axial resolution, lateral resolution, penetration, image uniformity, distance accuracy, focal zone, and cyst characteristics (Figures 18-1 and 18-2).
- Special-purpose TM phantoms are designed to accommodate specialized transducers or to assess parameters not included within the realm of general-purpose TM phantoms (contrast resolution, slice thickness, and beam width).
- Quality control testing with a rubber-based urethane phantom monitors the consistency, but not necessarily the accuracy, of the measured parameter (examples include ATS Model 539 and CIRS Model 42 phantoms).
  - The acoustic velocity of 1460 m/s is less than the assumed 1540 m/s in soft tissue, which may result in distance inaccuracy in some measurements.
  - Rubber-based urethane exhibits a nonlinear attenuation response at high frequencies, which will cause an underestimation of the penetration in soft tissue.
  - The advantages of rubber-based urethane include stability, ruggedness, ease of transport, and long lifetime.

PERFORMANCE TESTING

- TM phantoms are recommended for acceptance or performance testing.
- Clinically appropriate settings (power, frequency, receiver gain, time gain compensation [TGC], dynamic range, scan range, transmit focal zone(s), and gray-scale map) should be used for each performance test.

DEAD ZONE

- The dead zone is the region near the transducer where echo-induced signals are not spatially registered (Figure 18-3).
- Spatial pulse length (SPL) and reverberations from the transducer–phantom interface affect the depth of the dead zone.
- The depth of the dead zone is expected to decrease when the transducer is operated at higher frequencies.
- The depth of the dead zone for a properly functioning transducer under well-defined conditions should remain unchanged.

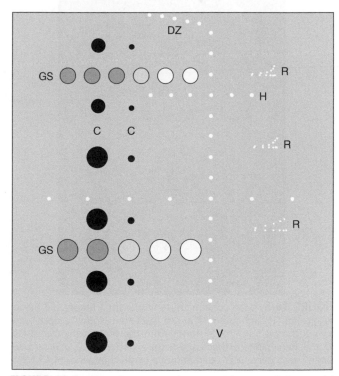

FIGURE 18-1 General purpose phantom. Diagram of the Model 40 GSE tissue-mimicking (TM) phantom. Vertical rod group (V), horizontal rod groups (H), dead zone rod group (DZ), axial/lateral resolution rod group (R), simulated cysts (C), and gray-scale targets (GS) are indicated.

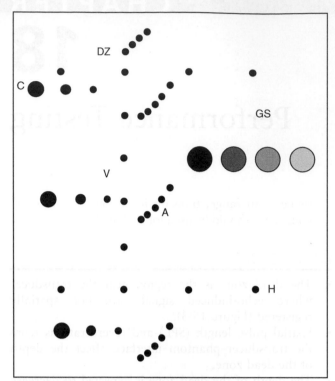

FIGURE 18-2 General purpose phantom. Diagram of the Model 403GS tissue-mimicking (TM) phantom. Vertical rod group (*V*), horizontal rod groups (*H*), dead zone rod group (*DZ*), axial resolution rod groups (*A*), simulated cysts (*C*), and gray-scale targets (*GS*) are indicated.

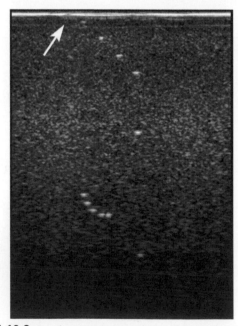

FIGURE 18-3 Dead zone measurement with a Model 403 tissue-mimicking (TM) phantom. The rod placement shows a dead zone of less than 4 mm. The distance from the face of the transducer to the beginning of the tissue-texture pattern is 2 mm (*arrow*). Linear array transducer operating at a center frequency of 11 MHz.

- The visualized rod, the shallowest in depth within the dead zone target group, demonstrates the axial extent of the dead zone.

- The depth at which "normal tissue texture" first appears when scanning the TM phantom also indicates the depth of the dead zone.

VERTICAL DISTANCE ACCURACY

- Vertical distance is measured along the axis of the beam and is based on the echo-ranging principle.
- The acoustic velocity used to convert elapsed time to distance is assumed to be constant (usually 1540 m/s).
- The known separation between the rods in the vertical target group of the phantom is compared with the measured distance in the image (Figure 18-4).
- Vertical distance indicators should be accurate within 2% of the actual distance or 2 mm, whichever is less restrictive.

HORIZONTAL DISTANCE ACCURACY

- Horizontal distance is measured perpendicular to the central beam axis within the scan plane.
- The placement of each scan line in the image is controlled by the autoscanning mechanism, which, in turn, governs the horizontal mapping of echo-induced signals.
- An accurate representation of spatial relationships in the horizontal direction primarily depends on scan line density and beam width.
- The known separation between the rods in the horizontal target group of the phantom is compared with the measured distance in the image (Figure 18-5).
- Horizontal distance indicators should be accurate within 3% of the actual distance or 3 mm, whichever is less restrictive.

LATERAL RESOLUTION

- Narrow beam width and high line density improve lateral resolution.

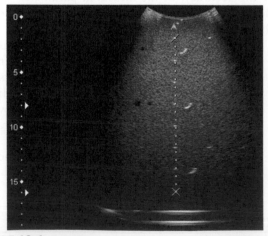

FIGURE 18-4 Assessment of vertical distance accuracy, in which the measured separation includes several rods in a Model 403 tissue-mimicking (TM) phantom over the scanning range. For a known distance of 140 mm, the internal calipers indicate 140 mm. The curvilinear array transducer is operating at a center frequency of 4 MHz.

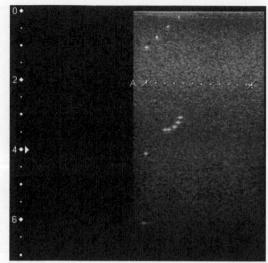

FIGURE 18-5 Assessment of horizontal distance accuracy, in which the measured separation includes horizontal rods in a Model 403 tissue-mimicking (TM) phantom at a scan depth of 2 cm. For a known distance of 30 mm, the measured separation is 30 mm. The linear array transducer is operating at a center frequency of 7 MHz.

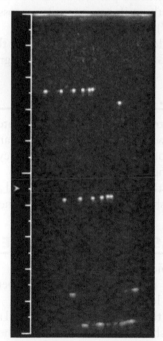

FIGURE 18-6 Effect of placement of a single transmit focal zone on lateral resolution within the field of view. The lateral resolution within the single focal zone at a depth of 5.5 cm is 2 mm as measured with the Model 40 tissue-mimicking (TM) phantom. The lateral resolution often deteriorates markedly when the focal zone is displaced distally from the region of interest. In this sonogram, the lateral resolution rod group at a depth of 10 cm is blurred. The linear array transducer is operating at a center frequency of 4 MHz.

- To quantify lateral resolution, the rods oriented horizontally with variable spacing (e.g., 5 mm, 4 mm, 3 mm, 2 mm, and 1 mm apart) are scanned (Figure 18-6).
- The smallest separation between any two resolvable rods measures the lateral resolution.

- The lateral resolution is expected to improve (gap between resolvable rods becomes smaller) when the transducer is operated at a higher frequency.
- Focusing alters the beam width, and, thus, lateral resolution is depth dependent.
- Lateral resolution rod groups located at multiple depths in the phantom enable the assessment of the lateral resolution with different transmit focal zones and operating frequencies.
- Lateral resolution, when measured under identical conditions, should not vary by more than the next largest increment in rod spacing above the normal value.

FOCAL ZONE

- A reflector, smaller than the beam width, is spatially represented in the image with a lateral extent equal to the beam width.
- Scanning equally spaced rods in the vertical target group depicts the beam width at various depths.
- The imaged rod with the minimum horizontal extent indicates the depth of the focal zone (Figure 18-7).
- The location of the measured focal zone should agree with the manufacturer's specifications and should not change with time.
- Dynamic receive focusing reduces the horizontal extent of all vertical rods, resulting in a less noticeable transmit focal zone.

AXIAL RESOLUTION

- To quantify axial resolution, the rods oriented vertically with horizontal offset and variable spacing (e.g., 2 mm, 1 mm, 0.5 mm, and 0.25 mm apart) are scanned.

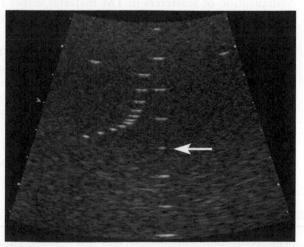

FIGURE 18-7 Write zoom of the vertical rod group within the Model 539 rubber-based phantom using a single focal zone placed at 7 cm. The vertical rod at a depth of 8 cm is the narrowest, indicating the location of the focal zone (*arrow*). Note that the rods above or below this focal region are depicted with a broader lateral extent. The curvilinear array operated at a center frequency of 6 MHz.

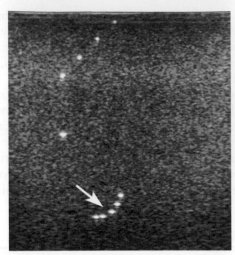

FIGURE 18-8 Assessment of axial resolution using the Model 403 TM phantom. At a depth of 3 cm, the axial resolution is 0.5 mm (*arrow*). The linear array transducer operated at a center frequency of 14 MHz.

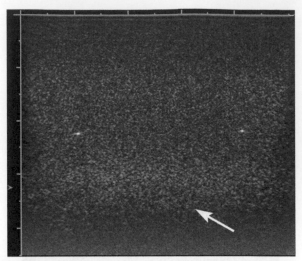

FIGURE 18-9 Sensitivity testing using the Model 403 TM phantom. The fading of parenchyma scatterers indicates the maximum depth of penetration of 3.7 cm (*arrow*). The linear array transducer operated at a center frequency of 14 MHz.

- The smallest separation between any two resolvable rods measures the axial resolution (Figure 18-8).
- The axial resolution is expected to improve (gap between resolvable rods becomes smaller) when the transducer is operated at a higher frequency.
- Axial resolution, when measured under identical conditions, should not vary by more than the next largest increment in rod spacing above the normal value.

SENSITIVITY

- The term *sensitivity* describes the ability of an instrument to detect weak echo signals, which approach noise levels.
- An indicator of sensitivity is the maximum depth of visualization of scatterers in TM material, either tissue texture pattern or weakly echoic spherical objects (Figure 18-9).
- The maximum depth of penetration is affected by frequency, power, focal zone, attenuation by medium, reject control, dynamic range, and electronic noise.
- Specified operating conditions (usually an application preset for the transducer) must be reproduced for all tests of sensitivity.
- A shift of more than 1 cm in the maximum depth of visualization for a particular transducer signifies a loss in sensitivity.

UNIFORMITY

- The term *uniformity* describes the ability of an instrument to display scatterers with equal reflectivity with the same brightness in the image.
- Artifacts attributed to defective scan lines, improper sampling, or signal loss are detected by scanning a TM phantom.

- The tissue texture pattern of the TM material should present with uniform intensity across the field of view (FOV) at a constant depth.
- Brightness levels must be compared at the same depth because TGC modifies the received signal level.

CYST SIZE, SHAPE, FILL-IN

- Anechoic structures within the TM material should be portrayed with the proper size, shape, and signal level.
- Fill-in is observed with simulated cysts displaced from the mechanical focal zone.
- The size of the structure in both vertical and horizontal directions should be within 1 mm of the stated value.

SOLID MASS SIZE AND SHAPE

- Hyperechoic structures within the TM material should be portrayed with the proper size, shape, and signal level.
- The size of the structure in both vertical and horizontal directions should be within 1 mm of the stated value.

SLICE THICKNESS

- Mechanical focusing in the elevation direction fixes the focal length to a specific depth.
- The measurement of slice thickness over a continuous range of scan depths is accomplished with an inclined plane phantom.
- The inclined plane phantom is composed of two uniformly attenuating materials with and without backscattering particles that form a flat interface oriented at 45 degrees.
- The axial length of the 45-degree interface in the image equals the slice thickness.

CONTRAST DETAIL

- Multiple conical targets with varying reflectivities (echo amplitudes) embedded in the TM material compose the contrast detail phantom.
- The visualization of an object depends on the echo intensity and object size.
- The visualization of small objects with similar reflectivity indicates excellent system sensitivity.
- Contrast detail phantoms can be used to compare the system sensitivity of different scanners.

HARD COPY IMAGE RECORDING

- The recorded image must be a faithful reproduction of the image viewed on the display monitor.
  - The display monitor and hard copy recording device must be matched in response so that image information is preserved (full range of gray levels, between black and white, with multiple intermediate shades).
  - Geometric relationships in the displayed image must be maintained on the recorded film.
- The SMPTE (Society of Motion Picture and Television Engineers) test pattern is the most appropriate means to evaluate the display monitor and the hard copy recording device (Figure 18-10).
  - The background is a uniform gray with a 50% signal level.
  - The range of signal levels is represented in 11 steps from 0% to 100% with 10% increments.
  - A patch with 5% contrast is inset within the 0% and 100% boxes.

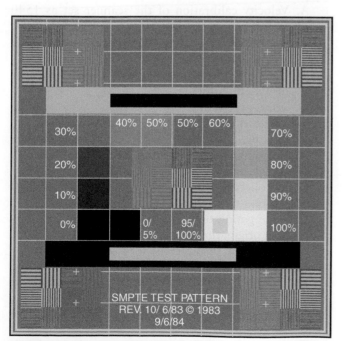

FIGURE 18-10 The SMPTE (Society of Motion Picture and Television Engineers) test pattern.

- Low-contrast and high-contrast bar patterns are at the center and each corner.
- White borders of evenly sized boxes form a grid to assess spatial distortion.

PURPOSE OF QUALITY CONTROL

- Quality control (QC) is the routine testing of medical devices to obtain objective assessment of performance and stability.
- The goal of the QC program is produce high-quality images consistently.
- An effective QC program must be simple to implement and easy to maintain.
- Basic QC tests are designed to identify common equipment problems.
- Periodic testing under well-defined conditions (i.e., specified instrument settings using appropriate phantoms) is essential to detect gradual degradation of system performance.
- Initial results of QC tests serve as baseline values for future comparisons.
- The documentation should include the result of each test and associated control limits (range of acceptable values for the measured parameter).

QUALITY CONTROL FOR B-MODE SCANNERS

- Tests for penetration, vertical and horizontal distance accuracy, image uniformity, fidelity of image display, and fidelity of image recording are considered the most sensitive indicators of the performance of B-mode scanners (Figure 18-11).
- A general-purpose phantom (either TM or rubber-based urethane) is recommended for routine QC testing (penetration, distance accuracy, and image uniformity).
- The SMPTE test pattern is the most appropriate means to evaluate the display monitor and the hard copy recording device.
- The transducer, the cable, and the connector should be inspected for damage on each day of use.
- Frequently used transducers should undergo QC testing at least every 6 months.

MULTIPLE CHOICE QUESTIONS

1. What parameter is not evaluated with a tissue-mimicking (TM) phantom?
   A. Axial resolution
   B. Dead zone
   C. Distance accuracy
   D. Output power

					Scanner
Manufacturer					
Model					
ID					

					Transducer
Model					
Frequency					
S/N					

Date	Image uniformity (OK)	Penetration (CM)	Distance accuracy		SMPTE (Gray levels)			Initials
			Vertical	Horizontal	Monitor	Hard copy	PACS	

FIGURE 18-11 Quality control form for recording the results of transducer testing.

2. How is the test for sensitivity performed using a general-purpose TM phantom?
   A. Signal strength (pixel value or brightness level) at 4 cm depth
   B. Maximum depth of visualization of TM material
   C. Smallest separation visualized in the axial rod group at a depth of 4 cm
   D. Depth of the rod closest to the surface visualized in the dead zone group

3. Why is the attenuation rate of TM phantoms often specified as 0.7 decibel per centimeter–megahertz (dB/cm-MHz)?
   A. Approximates the attenuation of soft tissue
   B. Innate characteristic of the TM material
   C. Optimal for measured distance accuracy
   D. Reduces the depth of the dead zone

4. What is the advantage of urethane general-purpose phantoms?
   A. Same acoustic velocity as soft tissue
   B. Expect lifetime of many years
   C. Accurate indication of sensitivity
   D. Accurate indication of distance

5. What test pattern or device best allows the assessment of the performance of the display monitor?
   A. Electronic calipers
   B. Hydrophone
   C. Society of Motion Picture and Television Engineers (SMPTE) test pattern
   D. TM phantom

6. Why is distance accuracy evaluated in both horizontal and vertical directions for a linear array transducer?
   A. Spatial mapping of echo-induced signals requires two independent processes

   B. Echo ranging must be calibrated correctly in both horizontal and vertical directions
   C. Beam width is not constant at all depths within the field of view
   D. Autoscanning must be calibrated correctly in both horizontal and vertical directions

7. The distance between the vertical rods in the TM phantom image measured using a Picture Archiving Communication System is not correct. What is a potential cause of this error?
   A. Velocity calibration of the scanner set as 1540 meters per second (m/s)
   B. Inaccurate workstation calibration of distance per pixel
   C. Geometric distortion introduced by the scanner display monitor
   D. Improper setting of dynamic range during acquisition

8. What is the dead zone?
   A. Region near the transducer where echo-induced signals are not spatially registered
   B. A collection of crystal elements that do not respond to pressure waves
   C. Time gating of receiver signals to eliminate signals originating at a specific depth
   D. The region distal to the focal zone

9. In the diagram of a TM phantom (Figure 18-12), which rod group is used to evaluate axial resolution?
   A. A
   B. B
   C. C
   D. D
   E. None of the above

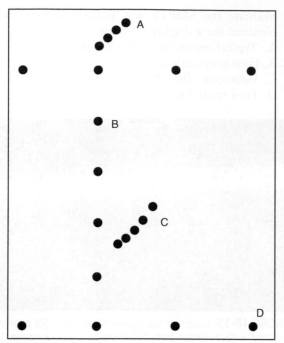

FIGURE 18-12 Diagram of a simplified tissue-mimicking (TM) phantom. The phantom is configured with multiple rod groups to test different parameters.

10. In the diagram of a TM phantom (see Figure 18-12), which rod group is used to evaluate the dead zone?
    A. A
    B. B
    C. C
    D. D
    E. None of the above

11. In the diagram of a TM phantom (see Figure 18-12), which rod group is used to evaluate lateral resolution?
    A. A
    B. B
    C. C
    D. D
    E. None of the above

12. In the diagram of a TM phantom (see Figure 18-12), which rod group is used to evaluate vertical distance accuracy?
    A. A
    B. B
    C. C
    D. D
    E. None of the above

13. In the diagram of a TM phantom (see Figure 18-12), which rod group is used to evaluate horizontal distance accuracy?
    A. A
    B. B
    C. C
    D. D
    E. None of the above

14. Why is the American Institute for Ultrasound in Medicine (AIUM) test object not appropriate to evaluate scanner performance?
    A. Does not mimic the acoustic properties of soft tissue
    B. Does not demonstrate long-term stability
    C. Visualization of rods in the presence of high background scattering is difficult
    D. Rods are not firmly held in place in a water-based medium

15. When scanning a TM phantom, the center frequency of the transducer is changed from 3.5 MHz to 6 MHz. What is most likely to deteriorate?
    A. Depth of the dead zone
    B. Axial resolution
    C. Vertical distance accuracy
    D. Sensitivity

16. Which design is most appropriate for a contrast detail phantom?
    A. Uniform TM material throughout the phantom
    B. High-density 0.1-mm rods distributed throughout the TM phantom
    C. Multiple hypoechoic objects embedded throughout the TM phantom
    D. TM material in which the rate of attenuation increases with depth

17. How often should a transducer be evaluated for distance accuracy using a TM phantom?
    A. Each day of use
    B. Every week
    C. Every 6 months
    D. Never

18. What routine quality control (QC) test is an excellent indicator of B-mode scanner performance?
    A. Maximum depth of penetration
    B. Intensity measurement
    C. Bandwidth of the transmitted pulse
    D. Slice thickness

19. How often should a mechanical inspection of the transducer be conducted?
    A. Each day of use
    B. Weekly
    C. Every 6 months
    D. Never

20. What routine QC test is performed using a TM or urethane general-purpose phantom?
    A. Uniformity
    B. Slice thickness
    C. Power output
    D. Signal-to-noise ratio

21. What is the primary goal of a QC program for B-mode imaging?
    A. Train student sonographers to scan
    B. Acquire consistent, high-quality images
    C. Compare scanners from different manufacturers
    D. Match the performance of multiple scanners at a facility

22. Why are instrument settings standardized for QC testing?
    A. Allows comparisons between scanners
    B. Permits long-term comparisons of QC results
    C. Permits comparison of results with published values
    D. Allows automatic processing of images

23. A radiology department is conducting weekly phantom imaging for every transducer. Why is this QC program likely to fail?
    A. Labor intensive
    B. Results not reproducible
    C. Extensive scanning shortens phantom lifetime
    D. Extensive scanning modifies phantom response

24. The display monitor shows a full range of signal levels (weak to strong), but the laser film image shows a loss of weak signals. What problem would you suspect?
    A. Brightness and contrast settings for the monitor are not correct
    B. Monitor and recording device are not matched in response
    C. The dynamic range on the scanner is set too high
    D. During normal operation, weak signals are typically not shown in the laser film image

25. The internal electronic calipers show the correct distance horizontal separation of 60 mm, but the laser film image measures 75 mm with hand-held calipers. What problem would you suspect?
    A. Incorrect brightness and contrast settings for the monitor
    B. Improper assumed acoustic velocity for echo ranging
    C. Too high gain for horizontal direction in laser film recorder
    D. During normal operation, the aspect ratio for the film is different from that for the monitor

26. Evaluate the image of the TM phantom (Figure 18-13) obtained during routine QC testing of a vector transducer used for abdominal scanning.
    A. Typical image; no problem detected
    B. Loss of axial resolution
    C. Poor uniformity
    D. Poor penetration

27. Evaluate the SMPTE test pattern (Figure 18-14) obtained for a display monitor.
    A. Typical result; no problem detected
    B. Poor gray-scale contrast
    C. Geometric distortion
    D. Poor spatial resolution

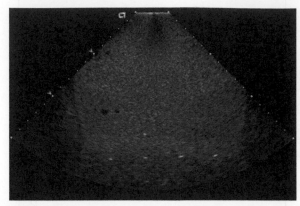

FIGURE 18-13 Image of the tissue-mimicking (TM) phantom obtained with a vector transducer operating at a center frequency of 4 MHz.

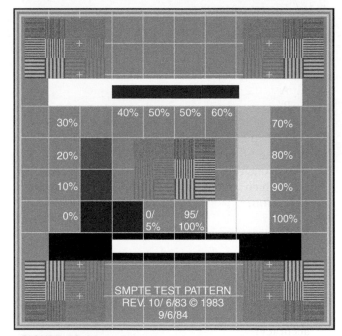

FIGURE 18-14 SMPTE (Society of Motion Picture and Television Engineers) test pattern obtained during quality control testing of the monitor.

CHAPTER 1

Review Questions
1. Hertz (Hz) or megahertz (MHz)
2. Density and bulk modulus
3. 10 MHz
4. 1540 m/s
5. 1540 m/s

Problems
1. 0.31 mm
2. 0.82 mm
3. 1600 m/s
4. 0.17 μs
5. 3.4 MHz

Multiple Choice Questions
1. A
2. D
3. A
4. C
5. C

CHAPTER 2

Review Questions
1. 5 MHz
2. None
3. Wavelength is increased
4. Bend toward normal
5. Continues on straight line path

Problems
1. 1.63 Mrayl
2. 0.69%
3. 99.31%
4. 8 cm
5. 65 μs
6. 27.4°
7. 9.5°

Multiple Choice Questions
1. D
2. C
3. C
4. B
5. A
6. C
7. A
8. C
9. A
10. B
11. B

CHAPTER 3

Review Questions
1. 0.5 to 0.8 dB/cm-MHz
2. Losses expressed in dB are additive
3. mW/cm^2 or W/cm^2
4. Megapascal or pascal
5. Absorption, scattering, reflection, divergence
6. Highest frequency (6 MHz)
7. 0.5 or reduced by a factor of 2

Problems
1. 3.6 dB/cm
2. 1.8 dB
3. 26 dB
4. 28 dB + 3.7 dB = 31.7 dB
5. 21 dB + 2.8 dB = 23.8 dB
6. 0.00001
7. 96 mW
8. $2 mW/cm^2$
9. 1024 or 1000
10. 7 dB
11. 7 dB/cm
12. 9 dB

Multiple Choice
1. C
2. A
3. D
4. B
5. D
6. C
7. B
8. C
9. A
10. D
11. B

CHAPTER 4

Review Questions
1. Convert electrical energy to sound energy (during transmission) and convert returning echo (sound energy) to electrical signal (during reception)
2. 2 MHz to 20 MHz
3. Spatial detail depends on wavelength of sound, which is dictated by the frequency.
4. Piezoelectric effect
5. PZT (lead zirconate titanate)
6. Crystal thickness
7. Shorten the transmitted pulse ultrasound wave and improve transmission of ultrasound energy from transducer into patient
8. Backing material and matching layer

9. Depth information is possible by measuring the time between transmission and reception via the echo ranging principle
10. The number of transmitted ultrasound pulses per second
11. The number of cycles in the pulse and the wavelength
12. Reduce the divergence of the ultrasound beam and thereby minimize the beam width
13. Bandwidth
14. Shorter pulse duration has increased bandwidth
15. The fraction of time that the transducer generates an ultrasound pulse
16. One microsecond
17. PRP equals the reciprocal of PRF
18. Restrict the region for which echoes can be generated which enables the reflector to be located
19. Restrict the region for which echoes can be generated which enables the reflector to be located more accurately
20. A-insulating case, B-crystal, C-backing layer, D-matching layer.

Problems

1. 9625 pulses per second
2. 104 µs
3. 1.1 mm
4. 0.7 µs
5. 0.001
6. 0.4
7. 0.5 µs
8. 6 MHz
9. 2 MHz

Multiple Choice Questions

1. D
2. B
3. A
4. B
5. A
6. A
7. A
8. B
9. C
10. D
11. A
12. C
13. A
14. C
15. A
16. D
17. B
18. B
19. B
20. B

CHAPTER 5

Review Questions

1. Beam width is most narrow within the near field
2. Near-field depth is increased
3. TGC
4. Time or depth
5. Acoustic lens and curved crystal
6. Reduce the beam width at a particular distance from the transducer
7. Variations in signals unrelated to reflectivity
8. Detection of weak echoes

Problems

1. 8.1 cm
2. 11.7 cm
3. 5.7 cm
4. 2.2 degrees
5. 1.8 degrees
6. 3.1 degrees
7. 100 or 20 dB

Multiple Choice Questions

1. D
2. A
3. B
4. C
5. A
6. D
7. A
8. A
9. A
10. C
11. D
12. C
13. C

CHAPTER 6

Review Questions

1. One
2. PRF
3. Two
4. One
5. At a depth of 3 cm, because attenuation along the path reduces intensity
6. At a depth of 5 cm, which is within the focal zone
7. One
8. Two
9. Digital scan converter, registration arm, and position generator
10. Hundreds of scan lines
11. None, because the spatial pulse length and beam width are much greater than pixel size

12. Focal length for a static B-mode transducer is fixed and cannot be changed except by changing the transducer
13. Interrogated by multiple scan lines, which allows for normal incidence at different points along the curved surface
14. Scan data acquisition time is long (a few seconds)

Problems
1. 91 μs
2. 0.14 mm × 0.15 mm
3. 0.7 dB/cm-MHz × 10 cm × 5 MHz = 35 dB or 3250 times

Multiple Choice Questions
1. A
2. B
3. C
4. A
5. B
6. D

CHAPTER 7

Review Questions
1. Echo ranging
2. Must be able to measure the time between transmission of the ultrasound beam and detection of the returning echo
3. Limit the region of echo formation, so that spatial mapping is improved
4. Each B-mode frame is composed of multiple scan lines and each scan line requires a transmitted pulse
5. Brightness level or gray level
6. Propagation path for one transmitted pulse with narrow beam width
7. Transmitted wave travels in a straight-line path, echo travels in a straight-line path back to the transducer, acoustic velocity is constant along the propagation path, narrow beam dimensions
8. Three
9. One
10. If good spatial detail for stationary structures is desired

Problems
1. 64 fps
2. 0.0156 second
3. 2400 pulses per second
4. 2400 pulses per second
5. 200 scan lines
6. 130 μs
7. 140 scan lines

8. 19.25 cm
9. 12.8 cm
10. 14 fps

Multiple Choice
1. B
2. B
3. B
4. A
5. B
6. C
7. D
8. D
9. C
10. A

CHAPTER 8

Review Questions
1. Electronic focusing in the elevation direction
2. Annular phased arrays require mechanical steering
3. Single crystal element with mechanical focusing
4. Curvilinear arrays typically have increased width of the field of view at depth
5. Narrows the beam width in the elevation direction

Problems
1. 2
2. 0.019 second
3. 0.019 second

Multiple Choice
1. D
2. A
3. A
4. C
5. C
6. A
7. C
8. B
9. A
10. C
11. D
12. A
13. A
14. A
15. B
16. B
17. C
18. D
19. D
20. C

CHAPTER 9

Multiple Choice
1. A
2. B
3. C
4. C
5. B
6. B
7. B
8. A
9. B
10. D
11. B
12. C
13. B
14. C
15. D
16. B
17. A
18. D
19. B
20. C

CHAPTER 10

Multiple Choice
1. C
2. A
3. D
4. C
5. C
6. A
7. A
8. C
9. A
10. B
11. A
12. B

CHAPTER 11

Multiple Choice
1. C
2. A
3. D
4. A
5. C
6. B
7. B
8. B
9. C
10. A
11. D

CHAPTER 12

Review Questions
1. Fill-in or partial volume
2. Straight line path from transducer to reflector
3. PRF
4. Strong reflector
5. High or low acoustic impedance compared with surrounding tissue
6. Reverberation

Multiple Choice
1. B
2. B
3. B
4. C
5. C
6. D
7. B
8. A
9. C
10. A

CHAPTER 13

Problems
1. 337 Hz
2. 275 Hz
3. 1012 Hz
4. 675 Hz
5. 24 cm/s
6. 36 cm/s
7. 47 cm/s
8. 29 cm/s
9. 1687 pulses/s
10. 3374 pulses/s
11. 1377 pulses/s
12. 843 pulses/s

Multiple Choice
1. B
2. D
3. B
4. A
5. B
6. C
7. C

CHAPTER 14

Review Questions
1. Fast Fourier transform (FFT)
2. Time
3. Velocity

4. FFT repeated in short time segments
5. Black region from 30 to 50 cm/s
6. One
7. Inaccurate representation of flow velocities exceeding the velocity limit
8. A time-dependent trace of the maximum velocity obtained by each FFT spectral analysis
9. Measures all Doppler shifts present in the sampling volume
10. Sampling volume is limited in size so that global flow is not depicted
11. 62 cm/s

Multiple Choice
1. A
2. C
3. D
4. B
5. C
6. A

CHAPTER 15

Multiple Choice
1. A
2. B
3. D
4. C
5. A
6. A
7. B
8. B
9. B
10. C

CHAPTER 16

Multiple Choice
1. A
2. B
3. C
4. A
5. B
6. B
7. B
8. C
9. D
10. D
11. A
12. D

CHAPTER 17

Multiple Choice
1. D
2. A
3. B
4. B

5. C
6. A
7. D
8. B
9. C
10. C
11. B
12. A
13. A

CHAPTER 18

Multiple Choice
1. D
2. B
3. A
4. B
5. C
6. A
7. B
8. A
9. C
10. A
11. E
12. B
13. D
14. A
15. D
16. C
17. C
18. A
19. A
20. A
21. B
22. B
23. A
24. B
25. C
26. C
27. B

APPENDIX A

Review Questions
1. 8 bits in one byte
2. RAM has faster access time than magnetic disk drive
3. Analog to digital converter
4. 2 gigabytes
5. Easier to write source code and debug, same program can run on computers from different manufacturers, user developed programs

Problems
1. 1100
2. 13
3. 10010
4. 29

5. 245,000
6. 7
7. 32
8. 011 and 011

Multiple Choice
1. B
2. B
3. B
4. A
5. C
6. B
7. B
8. C
9. C
10. A
11. D
12. A
13. C
14. C
15. A
16. A
17. B
18. D

APPENDIX B

1. Laminar flow is the most energy efficient way for blood to flow.
2. The difference between pressure at the proximal end of the vessel and the distal end of the vessel.
3. Rayleigh scatterer.
4. Parabolic velocity profile.
5. Short vessel length, pulsatile flow, elastic walls, and down-stream branching of the vessel.
6. Blood velocity increases in response to ventricular systole and decreases with ventricular relaxation (diastole). Blood flow may cease in diastole if the pressure gradient goes to zero or reverse in direction due to peripheral resistance.
7. Q is the flow in volume per unit time, L is the length of the tube, η is viscosity of the fluid (blood) in poise, p_1-p_2 is the pressure differential, r is the radius of the vessel, and π is a constant.

8. The vessel radius because it is raised to the 4th power.
9. The 3 mm radius represents about 5 times the flow capacity of the 2 mm radius; therefore approximately an 80% reduction in flow volume.
10. Pressure from contraction of the heart, static filling pressure, and hydrostatic pressure.
11. An equivalent increase in pressure occurs within the veins as well.
12. Potential energy (pressure).
13. The length of the tube (minimal effect), viscosity of the blood, the pressure differential, and the radius of the vessel.
14. Turbulence.
15. Blood viscosity, flow velocity, vessel diameter, and blood density.
16. Proximal to stenosis: laminar flow
At point of stenosis: jet, high velocity, uniform velocity
Immediately distal to stenosis: broadened velocity components, decreased velocity from jet.
Distal to stenosis: turbulence
Further downstream: laminar flow with permanent pressure loss
17. Pumping action of the heart (minimal), hydrostatic pressure (gravity), and static filling pressure (only if vein is near fully distended).
18. Tumor or mass, soft tissue, and muscle contraction.
19. Return of oxygenated blood to the heart, regulation of temperature, regulation of body fluid volume, storage reservoir for blood.
20. Transmural pressure.

APPENDIX C

1. Increased backscatter from microbubbles
2. Fundamental, harmonics, and subharmonics
3. Application of high power
4. Zero
5. Frequency selection based on harmonics (2 times the fundamental frequency)

Computer Fundamentals

Binary Representation

- The binary format has two possible states represented by 0 and 1.
- A *bit* is a single binary digit.
- Bits are combined in a group to increase number of possible configurations.
- The term *word* refers to the number of bits that are manipulated as a group by the computer.
  - Instructions are encoded by the sequence of 0s and 1s in the word.
  - Longer word length makes more digits available for computation.
  - Word length (number of bits in a word) is fixed for specific computer.
- A *byte* is a group of eight binary digits.
  - One byte encodes a single character.
  - Number of bytes indicates storage capacity.
- The placeholder value for a multi-digit binary number (e.g., one byte) is shown below:

Power of 2	2^7	2^6	2^5	2^4	2^3	2^2	2^1	2^0
Decimal value	128	64	32	16	8	4	2	1

- The *base* is two with an integer exponent.
- The integer exponent increases by 1 for each column right to left.
- The binary number 00110001 codes for 49 (32 + 16 + 1) as indicated below.

Power of 2	2^7	2^6	2^5	2^4	2^3	2^2	2^1	2^0
Binary Number	0	0	1	1	0	0	0	1

- The maximum value of eight bits is 11111111 or the decimal number 255.
- The number of different combinations of 0 and 1 that can be assembled using *n* bits is 2^n.
- For one byte, the number of combinations is 2^8 or 256.
- For 10 bits, the number of combinations is 2^{10} or 1024.
- Wider dynamic range, greater precision, or both are possible when the number of bits is increased.

Computer Hardware

- The central processing unit (CPU) executes program instructions, performs calculations and logic comparisons, and controls data transfers to other hardware devices.
- The read-only memory (ROM) cannot be changed.
- The random access memory (RAM) provides temporary, erasable storage of instructions and data with fast access.
- A wide variety of input/output (I/O) devices are interfaced to and controlled by the computer (e.g., keyboard, mouse, disk drive, and printer).
  - I/O devices provide a means of communication between the operator and the computer.
  - The results of computations can be kept in a more permanent form by output devices.
- Standardized formats are necessary for data transfer from and to the computer (9-pin serial, 25-pin serial, universal serial bus [USB], firewire, modem, and Ethernet).
- Digital cameras, printers, scanners, and flash drives typically use USB.
  - USB is a high-speed communication port, with a data transfer rate of 480 megabits per second (Mbps) for version 2.0, and 12 Mbps for version 1.1.
  - Devices can be connected to or removed from the port without power shut-down (hot swappable).
  - Multiple devices can be interfaced to a single computer port.
- The modem allows data transmission via telephone lines.
  - *Baud rate* is the number of bits transmitted per second.
  - The maximum transmission rate is 56 kilobits (kb) per second.
- The term *buffer* refers to the internal memory in a device for temporarily holding information until it is processed.
- The buffer compensates for differences in speed between hardware devices (CPU can send pages faster than the printer can print).
- Data capacity, transfer rate, cost, portability, ease of use, and long-term stability characterize the performance of storage devices (magnetic disk, optical disk, compact disk [CD], digital video disk [DVD], and USB flash drive).
- Inkjet and laser printers produce hard-copy printouts of text, graphics, and photographs in black and white or in color.

Software

- The *operating system* is a set of programs such as Windows for PC, OS X for Apple, or Linux, which controls the activities of the computer as directed by the user.
- An application program is designed specifically for a particular imaging modality or task.
- Programming languages offer a means for the user or software developer to solve specific problems and expand applications.
  - An *algorithm* is a step-by-step solution to a problem.
  - Machine language and assembly language have the fastest execution time but are computer specific.
  - High-level programming languages provide the greatest flexibility across different computer platforms.
  - Each programming language has a well-defined set of symbols, words, letters, and syntax that direct computer operation.
  - Interpreters, translators, or compilers convert high-level language source code to machine code (binary).

Computer Operation

- The execution of instructions follows a step-by-step planned sequence.
  - The program to be executed is loaded into the memory.
  - Each location in the memory holds one instruction or datum.
  - The first instruction is transferred from the memory to the CPU, where it is decoded and then executed.
  - This process is repeated for the next instruction held in the memory.
  - If additional data are required to complete the execution of an instruction, then those data are retrieved from the memory.
- *Memory capacity* is the total number of storage locations.
  - Each location has a specific address.
  - The term *random access* refers to the 0s and 1s at a specific storage location that can be read without examining other storage locations.
  - Capacity is usually designated in megabyte (MB), which equals 2^{20} locations, or gigabyte (GB), which equals 2^{30} locations.
  - Increased capacity results in faster execution times.
- The clock synchronizes the movement of data and operations applied to those data.
  - The term *computer speed* refers to the number of clock ticks per second, expressed in gigahertz.
  - Increased clock speed results in faster execution times.

Overview of the Picture Archiving and Communication System

- Images are stored electronically for retrieval, display, processing, interpretation, and distribution to other locations.

- Patient demographic data and reports must be associated with stored images.
- The computer network is interfaced to multiple imaging modalities.
- The network configuration provides redundancy of hardware devices (e.g., printers, workstations, storage devices, and document scanners), but with improved efficiency a single device can serve multiple imaging modalities.
- DICOM (Digital Imaging and Communication in Medicine) establishes the standards for file formats (patient data and images) as well as the criteria for the transfer, storage, and display of information.

Objectives of the Picture Archiving and Communication System

- Data transfer through the network must be controlled.
- Patient demographics and reports from multiple locations are available to the authorized user.
- Modality worklists of patients scheduled for examination are generated in real time.
- The network is continuously updated with new imaging data from patient examinations.

Topology

- Each device on the network has an Internet protocol (IP) address (unique identifier).
- All the devices or computers are interconnected by cables for data transmission.
- Data are transferred in packets with the destination and source specified.
- The server is a computer that performs a specific task for the other devices on the network.

Data Transmission

- The data transfer rate depends on the bandwidth, which is determined by the speed of the devices and the type of cabling.
- The bandwidths for Ethernet, fast Ethernet, and gigabit Ethernet are 10 Mbps, 100 Mbps, and 1000 Mbps, respectively.
- The most common cabling is optical fiber (100 to 1000 Mbps) and CAT 5 cable (1000 Mbps).

Interface

- Data from the imaging device must be communicated to the network.
- DICOM output from the imaging device provides proper format to be recognized by the PACS.

Data Archive

- Images and patient records (linked database) can be stored for the long term.
- The PACS requires rapid access to stored information (previous studies).
- The workload for hospital radiology departments is 10 to 80 GB per day.
- Advantages of electronic storage compared with hardcopy recording include less labor intensive, fewer lost films, lower cost, and easier access.
- Types of archival storage devices include magnetic disk, magnetic tape, and optical disk jukebox.

- Redundant array of independent disks (RAID) has redundancy, high capacity (100 terabytes [TB]), and short access time.
- By coding an image in a new format, data compression reduces the number of bytes required to represent image data.
  - Compression reduces archival storage requirements and increases the speed of image transfer.
  - The compressed image must be converted into the matrix format before viewing.
  - Lossless compression allows for a completely faithful regeneration of the image with no change in information content.
  - Lossy compression regenerates an image, which has changed information content but, ideally, has no impact on diagnostic interpretation if the compression factor is relatively low.

Workstations

- The *workstation* is an interactive computer for the review, manipulation, and interpretation of images.
- Images from any modality are displayed in the proper viewing format.
  - Hanging protocols designate the selection, positioning, and sequencing of images from standardized examinations.
- A high-resolution monitor (2–5 megapixels) is necessary for accurate interpretation.
- Access to all studies stored in the PACS allows comparisons with previous studies, with short retrieval times of 1 to 2 seconds.
- Image processing includes window/level, gray-scale mapping, zoom, panning, smoothing, and edge enhancement.

Security

- Images and reports must be readily available to designated health care professionals.
- Unauthorized access to patient information must be prohibited.
- The database must be protected from modification or loss.
  - A *firewall* is designed to limit flow of information to and from sources outside the network.
  - Encryption encodes transmitted information at the source, which must be converted by the recipient.
  - Authentication verifies that the identification of the sender or the recipient is correct.

Quality Control (QC)

- Routine evaluation of monitor performance is essential.
- QC tests include maximum luminance, minimum luminance, uniformity of luminance across viewing area, and video test patterns to access image quality.

Summary of the Advantages of the Picture Archiving and Communications System

- Decreased film costs
- Few lost films
- Current list of patients for imaging procedures
- Current list of studies for interpretation
- Prompt access to images from multiple modalities
- Access to images from previous studies
- Ability of multiple clinicians to view the same images simultaneously
- Compact storage of patient data
- Image processing
- Computer-aided detection
- Electronic transfer of information to remote locations
- Reduction in the number of file room personnel

Summary of the Disadvantages of the Picture Archiving and Communication System

- Capital costs of equipment
- Recurring equipment costs
- Labor cost for technical personnel
- Conversion to digital format
- Monitor viewing of images (light levels, dynamic range)
- Need to interface equipment from different manufacturers
- Constantly changing technology
- Security of patient information

REVIEW QUESTIONS

1. How many bits compose one byte?
2. Compare the access time for main memory (RAM) with that of storage devices such as magnetic disk drives.
3. What device digitizes analog signals?
4. Computer memory has a capacity of 2000 megabytes. What is the capacity in gigabytes?
5. What are the advantages of high-level programming languages?

PROBLEMS

1. Express the decimal number 12 in the binary number system.
2. Express the binary number 01101 as a decimal number.
3. Express the decimal number 18 in the binary number system.
4. Express the binary number 11101 as a decimal number.
5. How many pixels compose an image in which the matrix is described as 350×700?
6. How many bits are necessary to represent 128 different combinations of 0s and 1s?
7. How many numeric combinations are possible with 5 bits?
8. Suppose that the analog-to-digital converter (ADC) is set to digitize voltage signals from 1 to 2.59 volts according to the following table. What is the digital representation of a signal that is 1.66 volts? What is the digital representation of a signal that is 1.68 volts?

Digital Signal Strength	Voltage Range
000	1.0 to 1.19
001	1.2 to 1.39
010	1.4 to 1.59
011	1.6 to 1.79
100	1.8 to 1.99
101	2.0 to 2.19
110	2.2 to 2.39
111	2.4 to 2.59

MULTIPLE CHOICE QUESTIONS

1. What device is used to transmit data over telephone lines from one computer to another computer?
   A. CD-R (write once compact disk)
   B. Modem
   C. RAM (random access memory)
   D. Scanner
2. What is the capacity of computer memory?
   A. Speed of information retrieval
   B. Number of storage locations
   C. Address of storage location
   D. Number of bits at each storage location
3. What is a characteristic of RAM?
   A. Must be assessed in sequence
   B. Can be changed (written to)
   C. Contains the control unit
   D. Has slower access time than magnetic disk
4. How can the accuracy of the digitization of the analog signal from a detector be improved?
   A. Increasing the bit depth
   B. Using a higher capacity memory
   C. Changing the clock frequency
   D. Increasing the voltage of the analog signal
5. How many different numerical combinations of 0s and 1s can be represented by a byte?
   A. 8
   B. 16
   C. 256
   D. 1024
6. Which of the following is a characteristic of ROM?
   A. Functions as a buffer for the printer
   B. Read but cannot be changed
   C. Stores alphanumeric characters only
   D. Stores image in a matrix format
7. What is the disadvantage of a 256 × 256 image format compared with a 64 × 64 image format?
   A. Requires longer acquisition time to fill matrix
   B. Requires more storage locations in memory
   C. Number of shades of gray is decreased
   D. Contrast sensitivity is decreased

8. What is *baud rate*?
   A. RAM access time
   B. Central processing unit (CPU) clock speed
   C. Bits per second that are transmitted
   D. Program execution time
9. Which of the following describes a pixel?
   A. Allows multiple gray levels (shading) across the pixel
   B. Image display using a gray-scale map alters the pixel value
   C. Smallest spatial component of a digital image
   D. Is circular in shape
10. Which of the following describes word length?
    A. Number of bits treated as a group by CPU
    B. All computers have same word length of 64 bits
    C. Word length is variable for a specific computer depending on application
    D. Word length for PCs is, by definition, 8 bits
11. What software classification is appropriate for Microsoft Word?
    A. Operating system
    B. High-level programming language
    C. Low-level programming language
    D. Application program
12. What component of the computer performs numerical calculations?
    A. CPU
    B. RAM
    C. ADC
    D. ROM
13. What configuration name is given to a computer with high-resolution monitors used for image interpretation?
    A. Bus
    B. RAID (redundant array of independent disks)
    C. Workstation
    D. Server
14. What specifies the standard pertaining to file formats in the Picture Archiving and Communication System (PACS)?
    A. SMPTE (Society of Motion Picture and Television Engineers)
    B. USB (universal serial bus)
    C. DICOM (Digital Imaging and Communication in Medicine)
    D. ASCII (American Standard Code for Information Interchange)
15. What is lossless compression?
    A. Image data represented with fewer bytes
    B. Image acquired with pressure applied by the transducer
    C. Spatial smoothing of image data at the workstation
    D. Reduced field of view to improve spatial resolution

16. In the PACS, how many laser film printers are required to print images from four ultrasound scanners interfaced to the network?
    A. One
    B. Two
    C. Three
    D. Four

17. What security measure controls access to the PACS from outside sources?
    A. Encryption
    B. Firewall
    C. Internet protocol (IP) address
    D. DICOM

18. The PACS is accepted because of all of the following EXCEPT:
    A. High film costs
    B. Ready access to previous studies
    C. Accountability of films
    D. Superior image spatial resolution

Hemodynamics

Hemodynamic Characteristics of Blood

- Blood is a viscous fluid consisting of cells and plasma.
- Viscosity is the physical parameter that characterizes a fluid's ability to resist any change in its shape.
- Blood is propelled along a vessel by a pressure drop or pressure differential along its path.
- The major component of blood is the red blood cell, or erythrocyte, which is approximately 7 μm in its largest dimension.
- Viscosity of blood at normal hematocrit is 0.03 poise (dyne-seconds per cm^2), or approximately about four times that of water.
- Because of their small size, red blood cells interact with ultrasound waves as Rayleigh scatterers.

Arterial Blood Flow: Velocity Profiles

- During laminar flow, blood moves in layers, or laminae, in order to minimize energy losses.
- In a straight tube of uniform diameter, the layers closest to the vessel wall travel at the slowest velocities, and the layers near the center of the vessel travel at the highest velocities.
- In a relatively long tube with constant pressure differential, the flow velocity in each respective layer is constant over time.
  - The velocity distribution across the vessel lumen is known as *parabolic velocity profile* (Figure B-1).
  - Velocity profile is three-dimensional within a three-dimensional vessel, forming "layers" that are actually cylindrical in shape (cylindrical laminae), as depicted in Figure B-2.
  - Arterial blood flow is not uniform in velocity over time but increases and decreases during the heart cycle.

- As blood flow accelerates, the velocities of blood layers become closer to one another in value resulting in a "flattening" of the velocity profile.
- This flattened, or blunted, velocity profile is often referred to as "plug flow," as shown in Figure B-3.
- A three-dimensional depiction of the layers of a flattened velocity profile is shown in Figure B-4.
- Plug flow contains a large central core of blood within the vessel where the flow velocities are very similar.
- The flow layers near the walls still maintain a range of velocities, with the slowest blood flow being closest to the walls.
- The degree of flattening changes throughout the heart cycle, depending on the length of the vessel and the presence of branching.

Laminar flow
Parabolic velocity profile 3D view

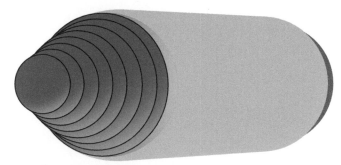

FIGURE B-2 Three-dimensional view of laminar flow. Blood flows in layers and does not mix.

Laminar flow parabolic velocity profile

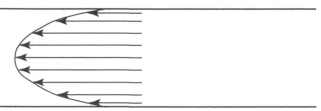

FIGURE B-1 Laminar flow in a vessel giving rise to a parabolic velocity profile.

Laminar flow flattened or "plug" velocity profile

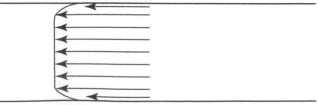

FIGURE B-3 Flattened or "plug" velocity profile.

Laminar flow
Flattened or "plug" velocity profile 3D view

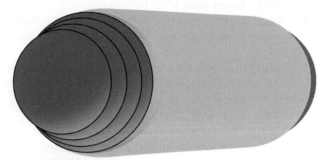

FIGURE B-4 Three-dimensional view of plug flow.

TABLE B-1	Effect of Radius on Volume Blood Flow Rate
Radius (r)	Factor (r⁴)*
0.5	0.062
1	1
2	16
3	81
4	256

*Note the dramatic change in the multiplication factor in Poiseuille's equation with small changes in the vessel radius.

Pressure–Flow Relationship
- Poiseuille's law describes the flow of a fluid.
  - Poiseuille's law specifically applies to continuous flow through a rigid-walled, straight tube of moderate-to-long length (does not directly pertain to flow within a large artery).
  - Flow in both settings is similar, and examining them individually provides insight into their effect on arterial blood flow.
- Factors that determine arterial blood flow are expressed in Poiseuille's equation:

$$Q = \frac{\pi(p_1 - p_2)r^4}{8L\eta}$$

where Q is the flow in volume per unit time, L is the length of the tube (most tubes in the body are considered to be "short" from a hemodynamic point of view), η is viscosity of the fluid (blood) in poise, $p_{1/2}$ is the pressure at a designated location, r is the radius of the vessel, and π is a constant.
  - The expression $(p_1 - p_2)$ represents the pressure difference between the pressure at the proximal end of the tube, p_1, and pressure at the distal end of the tube, p_2.
  - Where $p_1 = p_2$, there is no pressure differential and, thus, no flow.
- Because the radius is to the fourth power, the volume flow (Q) changes exponentially as the radius changes (Table B-1). Note the dramatic change in the multiplication factor in Poiseuille's equation with small changes in vessel radius.
- The calculation of volume flow rate is complex because of the pulsatile nature of arterial blood flow, the elasticity of the vessel walls, and the varied velocities of the blood laminae across the lumen.
- For most diagnostic applications, blood flow velocity, rather than volume flow rate, is measured.

Intravascular Pressure
- Contraction of the heart, static filling pressure, and hydrostatic pressure contribute to the overall intravascular pressure.

- The contraction of the heart produces pressure in a cyclical fashion.
  - Pressure varies from a systolic peak to a diastolic low (usually called *end diastolic*).
- Static filling pressure: After the arterial walls stretch to accommodate more blood volume, a force is generated by the elastic vessel walls to "push back" in an effort to return to their position of equilibrium (similar to a coiled spring).
- Hydrostatic pressure is pressure contributed by the relative position in a gravitational field.
  - For the general circulation, the right atrium is considered the reference point.
  - Blood at the level of the right atrium has zero hydrostatic pressure.
  - Below the right atrium, the hydrostatic pressure is positive (increases the intravascular pressure).
  - Above the right atrium, the hydrostatic pressure is a negative (decreases the intravascular pressure).
  - A six-foot man standing upright will have approximately +110 mm Hg in hydrostatic pressure contributing to the overall intravascular pressure at his ankles.

Fluid Energy and Bernoulli's Principle
- Kinetic energy and potential energy contribute to the total energy of blood.
- Kinetic energy is present in the form of flowing blood; as velocity increases, kinetic energy increases.
- Potential energy exists in the form of intravascular pressure.
- Factors, which contribute to intravascular pressure, also affect potential energy.
- Bernoulli's principle describes the inverse relationship between potential energy (pressure) and kinetic energy (blood velocity), as shown in Figure B-5.

Conduit Vessels and Resistance Vessels
- Blood vessels are hemodynamically classified into two general types: conduit vessels and resistance vessels.
- *Conduit vessels* are large vessels, which carry blood cells to their destinations.
  - Small changes in the vessel radius do not appreciably affect volume flow rate, as velocity will usually increase or decrease to compensate for a change in the radius.

Energy and Pressure

As the velocity of the blood decreases,

Kinetic energy
is converted back to
Potential energy

↓Velocity = ↓Kinetic energy, and
↑Potential energy

Energy and Pressure

As the velocity of the blood increases,

Potential energy
is converted to
Kinetic energy

↑Velocity = ↑Kinetic energy, and
↓Potential energy

FIGURE B-5 Relationship between energy and pressure.

- The flow through a conduit vessel is not determined by the vessel but by changes in the pressure differential.
- A change in either the proximal pressure (p_1) or the distal pressure (p_2) affects flow.
- *Resistance vessels* are very small, less than 1 mm in size, and include the vessels of the microcirculation (arterioles, capillaries, and venules).
  - A small change in the radius of a resistance vessel results in a large change in resistance to flow and, hence, in p_2 pressure.
  - Changes in p_2 pressure in the form of altered resistance within these vessels determine the character and volume of flow through the more proximal conduit arteries.

Modifications of Velocity Profile
- The flattened velocity profile characteristic of laminar flow within normal, straight arteries of uniform diameter is altered by structural changes in the vessel.
- Mild flow disturbance may occur in the presence of mild disease or when there is a change in the diameter or the direction of the vessel.

- *Flow disturbance* is generally accepted to mean a shift away from purely laminar flow but without the energy losses seen with turbulence.
  - Disturbed flow usually reverts readily to purely laminar flow as the area causing the disturbance is passed.
  - Disturbed flow often contains areas of eddy currents and helical flow.
- Severe turbulence occurs in the presence of hemodynamically significant stenosis.
- *Turbulence* is complete loss of laminar flow and represents a state in which the movement of blood cells is often at right angles or even 180 degrees to the axis of the vessel (reversed).
  - Turbulent flow is often described as chaotic flow.
  - Large energy losses in the form of a pressure drop occur in the vessel beyond the region of turbulent flow.
- *Reynolds' number* is a dimensionless metric, which represents the likelihood of turbulence.
  - Factors affecting the potential for turbulence include blood viscosity, flow velocity, vessel diameter, and blood density.
  - A Reynolds' number of around 2000 is generally thought to represent the threshold for the onset of turbulence; however, this is not universal.
  - Under certain conditions, turbulence may occur at a Reynolds' number less than 2000, and conversely, laminar flow may be maintained at higher values.

Obstruction
- Arterial obstruction is usually caused by a locally formed atherosclerotic plaque.
- A plaque presents a mechanical obstruction within the vessel, causing an effective narrowing of the vessel lumen.
- Stenosis occurs when the vessel lumen is narrowed to the point where blood flow is affected (described as "hemodynamically significant stenosis").
- Mild plaque initially results in disturbed flow, with some characteristics of laminar flow still maintained.
- As the plaque continues to develop, with more pronounced narrowing of the lumen, blood flow velocity through the area of obstruction becomes steadily higher until turbulence occurs.

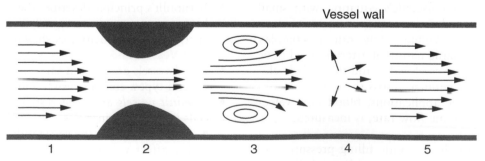

FIGURE B-6 Disruption of flow caused by stenosis (*shaded regions*). Velocity profiles include (1) laminar flow, (2) jet, (3) flow reversal, (4) turbulence, and (5) laminar flow.

- A hemodynamically significant stenosis alters the flow characteristics within the vessel (1) proximal to or upstream from the stenosis, (2) at the point of maximum stenosis, (3) immediately distal to or at the exit of the stenosis, (4) distal to the stenosis, and (5) further downstream from the stenosis (Figure B-6).

Velocity Profiles in the Vicinity of a Stenosis (see Figure B-6)

- Proximal to or upstream from the stenosis (region 1): laminar flow and evidence of increased downstream resistance (decreased or absent diastolic flow).
- At the point of maximum stenosis (region 2): abrupt increase in maximum velocity and jet flow through stenosis itself.
- At the exit of the stenosis (region 3): abrupt decrease in velocity (except in the path of the jet) and loss of laminar flow with eddy currents.
- Distal to the stenosis (region 4): abrupt decrease in velocity and turbulence with a total loss of laminar flow, which may extend far downstream.
- Downstream from the stenosis (region 5): eventual return to laminar flow with a permanent energy loss (pressure drop).

Venous Function

- The primary function of veins is the return of deoxygenated blood to the heart (or oxygenated blood in the case of pulmonary veins).
- As well as acting as a storage reservoir for blood, the venous system also plays an important role in the regulation of body temperature and fluid volume.
- Veins are elastic-walled, collapsible tubes that frequently exist in the body in a partially collapsed state.
- Because of low intravascular pressure in the venous system, blood flow tends to be more a function of factors external to the veins themselves.

Venous Pressure

- Venous pressure is composed of the residual intravascular pressure created by the pumping of the left ventricle, hydrostatic pressure produced by the weight of the column of blood, and static filling pressure.
- *Intravascular venous pressure* attributable to the pumping action of the heart is very low, approximately 15 mm Hg, without any evidence of the pulsatile flow that is seen within the arterial system.
- Because of the low pressure within the vessels, veins are not fully distended into a circular shape but frequently exist in a partially collapsed state.
- Little change in intravascular venous pressure can cause an enormous variation in the venous volume.
- As in arteries, hydrostatic pressure is increased in veins below the heart and is decreased in veins above the position of the heart.
- An upright, six-foot man will have an approximate +110 mm Hg hydrostatic pressure added to *both* arterial and venous pressures at the level of the ankles.

- The balance between arterial and venous pressures remains constant with different patient positions.
- *Static filling pressure* is a significant contributor to venous pressure only when increased volume distends the lumen to its full circular shape.
- When the vein walls are fully distended, any further increase in blood volume results in a rapid increase in venous pressure within the already distended vein.
- An example of increased venous pressure caused by static filling pressure would be venous valvular incompetence in a person standing in an erect position.
  - The veins in the legs are already distended because of the hydrostatic pressure occurring in the standing position; incompetent (leaking) proximal valves will cause a backflow of venous blood into the leg veins, greatly increasing the pressure.
- *Transmural pressure* is the difference between intralumenal pressure and tissue pressure external to the vein.
- Intralumenal pressure acts to expand the vein, whereas tissue pressure acts to collapse the vein.
- External tissue pressure may be in the form of soft tissue, muscular contraction, a mass exerting extrinsic pressure on the vein (in fact, a distended urinary bladder can exert enough pressure to reduce flow in the iliac veins), or a manual limb compression done by an examiner by hand or with a transducer.
- Intralumenal pressure may increase or decrease with respiration, abdominal contraction (Valsalva maneuver), patient general or limb position, venous valvular insufficiency, or intrinsic obstruction such as thrombus.

REVIEW QUESTIONS

1. Why does arterial blood flow in layers or laminae?
2. What causes blood to move through an artery?
3. What type of reflector of sound is the red blood cell?
4. What velocity profile is exhibited by blood flowing at a constant rate through a long, straight tube with rigid walls?
5. List three reasons why arterial blood flow in the large arteries of the body has a flattened velocity profile.
6. Describe the changes to peak blood velocity throughout the heart cycle.
7. List the factors in Poiseuille's equation and what they represent.
8. According to Poiseuille's equation, a small change in which factor has the greatest influence on volume flow rate?
9. Compare the flow rate for a vessel with a radius of 3 mm to one with a radius of 2 mm. What is the

percentage reduction in blood flow through the smaller lumen? Assume that the pressure differential, length, and viscosity are the same for each vessel.

10. List the three types of pressure that contribute to intravascular pressure.

11. What is the reason that an increase in intravascular arterial pressure at the ankles does not change the arterial–venous pressure relationship when a patient stands up?

12. According to Bernoulli's principle, what energy decreases when blood velocity is increased?

13. Describe the factors that influence volume flow rate through an unobstructed conduit vessel.

14. What term describes the complete loss of laminar flow distal to stenosis?

15. List three factors that comprise Reynolds' number.

16. List and describe the flow characteristics present at each of the five referenced points on Figure B-6.

17. List the three types of pressure that contribute to intravascular venous pressure.

18. List three conditions that could result in extrinsic pressure on a vein.

19. What are the four main functions of the venous system?

20. What term describes the pressure difference between internal pressure within a vein and external pressure?

Contrast Agents

Techniques

- Image contrast is enhanced by the increased reflectivity of tissues in which the contrast agent resides.
- Displacement of air by the contrast agent allows the transmission of ultrasound to underlying tissues.
- Monitoring signals from contrast agents as a function of time provides information regarding physiological function.

Types of Contrast Agents

- Contrast agents must demonstrate the properties of preferential tissue uptake, stability during measurement, low toxicity, and safe elimination.
- Free gas bubbles, encapsulated gas bubbles, particulates, emulsions, and aqueous solutions have application as contrast agents.
  - Free gas bubbles may pre-exist in a liquid or may be formed by rapid injection of a liquid through a narrow passage.
  - Encapsulated gas bubbles, the most common contrast agent, are gas-filled microspheres with a thin outer chemical coating.
  - Small particles, 1 μm (micrometer) in diameter, are phagocytized by the reticuloendothelial system.
  - Emulsions such as brominated fluorocarbon in lecithin are stable in blood for several hours and may have preferential uptake by hepatic metastases.
  - Aqueous solutions raise the acoustic impedance of blood.

Microbubbles

- Microbubbles must be stable to reach the desired site following intravenous administration.
- The size of the microbubble must be less than 6 μm to cross the pulmonary capillary bed.
- Free gas bubbles are relatively large compared with capillary vessels and have a fast dissolution rate in water.
- Methods to stabilize the gas bubble include:
  - Microspheres of albumin, lipids, or polymers form a capsule of entrapped gas.
  - A sugar matrix has gas-trapping sites on the particle surface.
  - Replacement of air with a perfluorocarbon gas lowers the diffusion rate.

- Large differences in density, acoustic velocity, and compressibility between the gas and the liquid contribute to the dynamics of the bubble.
- Peak scattering cross-section (probability) occurs at a resonant frequency set by bubble size (resonant frequency decreases as bubble size increases: 4 MHz for radius of 1 μm and 1 MHz for radius of 3 μm).
- Scattering decreases rapidly for frequencies above and below the resonant frequency.
- The presence of the capsule or matrix shifts the resonant frequency to a value higher than that of free air.
- Harmonic scattering is maximized at the resonant frequency and only occurs at frequencies near the resonant frequency.
- The second harmonic scatter component from microbubbles, in which the frequency is two times the fundamental frequency, generally has a higher intensity than the harmonics formed by nonlinear propagation through tissue.
- High-intensity ultrasound causes microbubbles to break apart after a few oscillations.

Imaging Techniques

- B-mode imaging detects the presence of a contrast agent by the concentration of strong scattering centers.
- Reperfusion imaging destroys the contrast agent within the field of view (FOV) by an application of high power and then monitors the return of the contrast agent by subsequent sampling at low power levels over time.
- Intermittent imaging shows the contrast agent present within the FOV by sampling at high power levels that simultaneously destroys the contrast agent.
  - Between images, perfusion replenishes tissues with the contrast agent.
  - The sampling rate is slowed to allow perfusion to occur (1–4 frames per second [fps]).
  - This technique emphasizes the rate of change of perfusion for the monitored regions.
- Contrast harmonic imaging differentiates tissues on the basis of the presence or absence of microbubbles.
  - Tissue devoid of contrast agent scatters sound only at the fundamental frequency.
  - Scattering from encapsulated bubbles contains fundamental as well as harmonic components.

- Signal processing isolates the echo-induced signals based on frequency.
- The signals from tissue *at* the transmitted frequency are suppressed, and signals at *twice* the transmitted frequency (second harmonic) are selected.
- Color flow imaging of contrast agent destroyed by high-power insonation shows a color mosaic.
- Autocorrelation processing of the harmonic component yields a power Doppler image showing the concentration of the contrast agent.
- Pulse inversion harmonic imaging provides gray-scale imaging of the microbubble concentration in real-time and at low-power settings.
  - Along each scan line, consecutive transmit pulses are reversed in phase.
  - Echo-induced signals from two transmit pulses are added together.
  - In the absence of microbubbles and motion, the sum signal is zero.
  - If harmonic scattering is present, then the sum signal has a net value.
- Power pulse inversion harmonic imaging combines a background gray-scale B-mode image obtained at the fundamental frequency, with pulse inversion sum signals encoded in color.

Clinical Applications

- Encapsulated microbubbles injected intravenously act as vascular contrast agents.
- Differential uptake of the contrast agent by tissues may identify neoplasms and other lesions.
- Microspheres at the desired site are destroyed by high-power ultrasound causing a release of

TABLE C-1	Clinical Applications of Contrast Agents
Technique	**Application**
Improved Doppler sensitivity	Small vessels, low-volume flow, deep-lying vessels, poor insonation angle
Perfusion imaging	Liver and renal lesions, myocardial perfusion
Contrast enhanced signal	Traumatic parenchyma damage of the kidneys, spleen, liver
Directly to body cavity (bladder)	Renal reflux
Blood pool tracers	Functional indices
Therapeutic applications	Site-specific administration of drugs

fibrinolytic or chemotherapeutic drugs contained within the microspheres.

- Clinical applications are summarized in Table C-1.

REVIEW QUESTIONS

1. Why are stabilized microbubbles used as contrast agents?
2. What frequency components are present in the backscatter from microbubbles?
3. How can one instigate the controlled destruction of microbubbles?
4. What is the sum of the in-phase and out-of-phase signals from pulse inversion in the absence of harmonics?
5. How is signal from tissue suppressed in contrast harmonic imaging?

Laboratory Exercises

Introduction to Laboratory Exercises, 104

Display Depth, Frame Rate, Freeze Frame, Cine Loop, 105

Overall Gain and Output Power, 108

Time Gain Compensation, 110

Transmit Frequency: Resolution and Penetration, 113

Transmit Focus, 116

Magnification (Write Zoom), 119

Dynamic Range, 122

Persistence (Frame Averaging), 124

Gray-Scale Mapping, 126

Distance and Area Measurements, 128

Doppler Controls 1, 131

Doppler Controls 2, 135

Doppler Angle to Flow, 139

Nyquist Limit and Aliasing, 143

Color Doppler Controls: Part 1, 147

Color Doppler Controls: Part 2, 152

Application Presets, 155

Tissue-Mimicking Phantom, 159

Introduction to Laboratory Exercises

With the continual advancement of ultrasound technology, including the more sophisticated implementation of application presets, why do sonographers need to know the function of each individual control? Why not allow the system to set all the parameters automatically, as many of them are programmed to do? Don't all manufacturers now have a "magic button" that optimizes every control for a perfect image?

The argument is similar to that with regard to modern digital cameras. The camera has an automatic setting so that most of the pictures "come out perfectly." If that were truly the case, why does every high-end camera advertise "full manual control" as an advanced user option? Absolute control over every detail in the imaging process is essential for the serious operator who wants a perfect image every time, even in the most complex and difficult situations.

The same is true in diagnostic imaging. Sonographers possess a very sophisticated "camera" costing many thousands of dollars. These technologically advanced machines are programmed to provide a satisfactory *starting point* for each examination type. Similar to automatic digital cameras, they do reasonably well (sometimes very well) under average conditions on average patients.

However, as with digital cameras, ultrasound devices require human input for unique or changing circumstances. How many "average" patients does the sonographer really scan? Within each examination type, control settings vary from patient to patient on the basis of age, size, weight, body habitus, and disease process. Within a single sonographic examination of the abdomen, the sonographer may scan the liver, the kidneys, the gallbladder, and the great vessels. Focus, display depth, gain, and transmit frequency must all be adjusted repeatedly to obtain the best possible images. Indeed, the time gain compensation (TGC) control must be verified or adjusted each time the transducer is oriented to a new imaging plane.

Knowledge, competency in scanning technique, attention to detail, and caring are the characteristics of a good sonographer. Sonographers should aspire to provide the best possible images for the benefit of every patient.

The lab exercises in this book are intended to guide the reader through the process of understanding the functions of the major controls available to the operator of the ultrasound machine. The section labeled DISCUSS describes the physical principles and concepts related to each control. The EXPLORE section provides an opportunity to experiment with the specific group of controls under consideration. Rather than producing a specific result, these exercises are intended to allow the sonographer to explore the range of adjustments for each control, to observe the effect when a control is turned on and off or turned from the maximum to the minimum value. Finally, the DOCUMENT section is designed as an assignment, where a very specific result is expected with each exercise. Hard-copy documentation is required, which may be evaluated and graded when this text is used as a classroom resource.

We have taken great care to include exercises for students in every sonographic discipline. Therefore, OPTION #1 was formulated to emphasize general sonography and basic vascular applications. OPTION #2 concentrates on cardiac applications. Cardiac sonographers should not feel limited to OPTION #2 only, as many of the exercises in OPTION #1 are also of benefit to those working in a cardiac lab.

Display Depth, Frame Rate, Freeze Frame, and Cine Loop

OBJECTIVES

1. To understand the function of depth control and the inverse relationship between scan range and real-time frame rate.

2. To be familiar with the location and function of the freeze frame and cine controls.

DISPLAY DEPTH

The *display depth* control allows the sonographer to adjust the scan range to best represent the anatomy of interest (Figure L1-1). Generally, display depth should be set one to a few centimeters beyond the deepest part of the organ of interest.

The display depth control may alter the real-time frame rate. As the scan range is extended, more time is required for the ultrasound pulse to travel to and the echo to return from the maximum depth (time of flight). As a consequence, the transducer transmits fewer pulses in a given period, and the time to complete one image frame (one complete set of scan lines across the field of view [FOV]) is longer. Increased time to compose a frame lowers the maximum frame rate. Manufacturers often automatically adjust pulse repetition frequency (PRF) or scan line density to maintain a constant frame rate. These automatic adjustments may not be obvious to the sonographer.

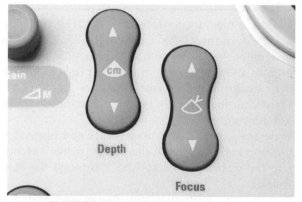

FIGURE L1-1 Depth control adjustment.

OPTION #1

EXPLORE

- Choose a medium-frequency (3–5 megahertz [MHz]) curvilinear array or sector transducer suitable for abdominal imaging. Select an abdominal application preset.
- Set the display depth for 20 cm.
- Obtain a sagittal image of the right hepatic lobe at this depth setting.
- Note the 2D frame rate (may be listed as "PRF").
- Change the display depth to 10 cm.
- Note the change in the 2D frame rate displayed on the screen.

DOCUMENT

- Choose a medium-frequency (3–5 MHz) curvilinear array or sector transducer suitable for abdominal imaging. Select an abdominal application preset.
- Obtain a sagittal image of the proximal abdominal aorta, with correct adjustment for the appropriate display depth. Acquire a hard-copy image of the proximal aorta.
- Obtain a sagittal image of the mid-abdominal aorta, with correct adjustment for the appropriate display depth. Acquire a hard-copy image of the mid-aorta.
- Obtain a sagittal image of the distal abdominal aorta, with correct adjustment for the appropriate display depth. Acquire a hard-copy image of the distal aorta.

OPTION #2

EXPLORE

- Choose a medium-frequency (2.5–3.5 MHz) sector transducer suitable for cardiac imaging. Select an adult cardiac application preset.
- Set the display depth for 20 cm.
- Obtain a parasternal long axis view of the heart at this depth setting.
- Note the 2D frame rate (may be listed as "PRF").
- Change the display depth to 10 cm.
- Note the change in the 2D frame rate displayed on the screen.

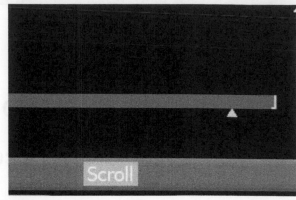

FIGURE L1-3 Playback display, with cursor showing the frame location in the stored sequence.

DOCUMENT

- Choose a medium-frequency (2.5–3.5 MHz) sector transducer suitable for cardiac imaging. Select an adult cardiac application preset.
- Obtain a parasternal long axis view of the heart.
- Set the display depth at the level of the pericardium. Obtain a hard-copy image or video clip at this depth setting.
- Set the display depth 3 cm deeper than the pericardium. Obtain a hard-copy image or video clip at this depth setting.
- Note that the shallower image would not allow visualization of the pathology outside the heart, such as pleural effusion.

FREEZE FRAME AND CINE LOOP

With *freeze* control, current scanners make it possible to store and review still images and real-time video clips (Figure L1-2). After freezing the image, the sonographer can recall the most recently acquired frames from the system memory (typically 100–200 frames). Activation

of this function is usually done by simply scrolling the trackball backward to view stored images frame-by-frame (Figure L1-3). Stored images can also be viewed in temporal sequence by activating the *cine loop* function.

Correct operation of the "freeze" button requires discipline and timing. During live scanning, the sonographer's hand that is not on the transducer should be on or near the freeze button. Effective use of this control requires proper timing and coordination with patient respiration and organ movement. The sonographer has the ability to scroll backward through stored frames, which can help obtain a usable image, particularly in the case of a difficult patient; however, this should not be used to compensate for a sloppy freeze technique. Activating the review function routinely on every stored image extends the examination time and may not result in optimal quality image.

OPTIONS #1 AND 2

EXPLORE

- Choose a medium-frequency (3–5 MHz) curvilinear array or sector transducer suitable for abdominal imaging. Select an abdominal application preset.
- Obtain a sagittal image of the right upper abdomen, demonstrating the inferior vena cava.
- Place your hand lightly on the freeze button (but do not activate yet).
- Have the patient take a deep breath and suspend respiration and then freeze the image within 3 seconds.
- Use the trackball to scroll back through the stored frames.
- Activate the loop playback mode, and watch the image loop in real-time.

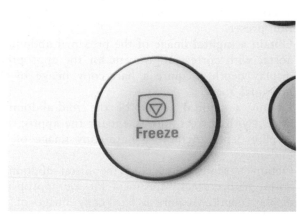

FIGURE L1-2 Freeze control.

DOCUMENT

- Choose a medium-frequency (3–5 MHz) curvilinear array or sector transducer suitable for abdominal imaging. Select an abdominal application preset.
- Obtain a sagittal view of the distal abdominal aorta. Have the patient breathe normally (normal shallow respiration).

- Freeze the image.
- Using the trackball, scroll through the stored images until the optimal frame is located. Acquire a hard-copy image.
- Repeat the exercise, freezing and unfreezing until you obtain a sharp frozen image without using the scroll-back function. Acquire a hard-copy image.

Overall Gain and Output Power

OBJECTIVES

1. To observe the visual effect of overall gain and output power adjustments on the B-mode image.

2. To understand the functional difference between gain control and output power control.

GAIN (OVERALL GAIN)

The *overall gain* control (Figure L2-1) amplifies the received signals equally throughout the display depth. The amount of amplification is quantified as the ratio of the output signal to the input signal. The gain control is adjusted when an increase or decrease in image brightness is desired. Within certain limitations (weak signals), the visual effect of increasing the gain is the same as increasing the output power.

Teaching point: Changing the gain has no direct effect on the rate of ultrasound energy delivered into the patient.

POWER (OUTPUT POWER)

The *output power* control (Figure L2-2) varies the excitation voltage applied to the transducer element(s). An increase in excitation voltage results in a higher-intensity sound pulse transmitted into the patient, which subsequently produces stronger echoes. A high power setting improves the sensitivity of the system to detect weak reflectors but also causes increased image brightness. The visual effect on a B-mode image is similar to an adjustment of the overall gain. Some systems automatically adjust the overall gain in conjunction with a changed power setting to maintain the overall image brightness at a constant level.

Teaching point: Raising the output power also increases the rate of ultrasound energy delivered into the patient. Conversely, reducing the output power decreases the rate of ultrasound energy delivered into the patient.

Obtaining the correct image brightness is a balance between output power and overall gain. The ability to correctly adjust image brightness to the optimal level with gain control depends on an adequate power setting (Figure L2-3). Ideally, the system should be set at the minimum output power necessary to image the structure at the depth of interest. Any additional increase in image brightness is achieved by increasing the overall gain.

The following guidelines should always be used when adjusting the overall gain and output power:

If an increase in image brightness is required, increase the overall gain first. If that does not result in adequate image brightness, then increase the output power.

If a decrease in image brightness is required, decrease the output power first. If that is not sufficient, then decrease the overall gain.

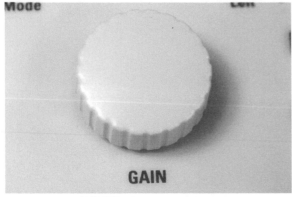

FIGURE L2-1 Gain control

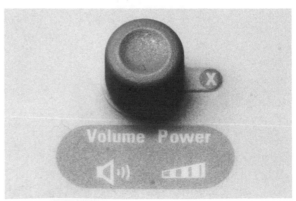

FIGURE L2-2 Transmit power control.

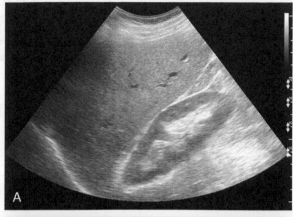

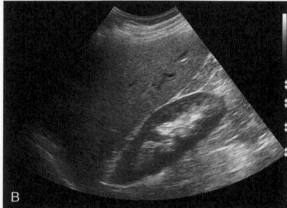

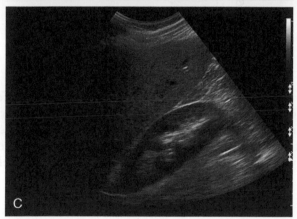

FIGURE L2-3 Effect of overall gain. **A,** Gain too high. **B,** Correct gain. **C,** Gain too low.

Each of the above procedures results in the lowest possible patient exposure to ultrasound energy.

OPTION #1

EXPLORE

- Determine whether the scanner has a user-accessible output power control. If this control is present, complete this exercise.

- Choose a transducer suitable for abdominal imaging, such as a 3–5 MHz curvilinear array. Select an abdominal application preset.
- Obtain a sagittal image of the right hepatic lobe with a 75% or –3 dB power setting.
- With the overall gain set correctly, *decrease the output power* until the image brightness is too low.
- Then, *increase the overall gain* until the image brightness is again correct.

DOCUMENT

- Choose a transducer suitable for abdominal imaging, such as a 3–5 MHz curvilinear array. Select an abdominal application preset.
- Set the output power control for a medium value. By varying only the overall gain control, obtain three hard-copy sagittal images of the right hepatic lobe, to demonstrate the following:
  - Gain too low
  - Gain correctly adjusted
  - Gain too high

OPTION #2

EXPLORE

- Determine whether the scanner has a user-accessible output power control. If this control is present, complete this exercise.
- Choose a transducer suitable for cardiac imaging such as a 2.5–3.5 MHz sector. Select an adult cardiac preset.
- Obtain a parasternal long axis view of the heart with a 75% or –3 dB power setting.
- With the overall gain set correctly, *decrease the output power* until the image brightness is too low.
- Then, *increase the overall gain* until the image brightness is again correct.

DOCUMENT

- Choose a transducer suitable for cardiac imaging, such as a 2.5–3.5 MHz sector. Select an adult cardiac application preset.
- Set the output power control for a medium value. Obtain a parasternal long axis view. By varying only the overall gain control, capture three video clips or obtain hard-copy images to demonstrate the following:
  - Gain too low
  - Gain correctly adjusted
  - Gain too high

Time Gain Compensation

OBJECTIVES

1. To understand the function and correct use of the time gain compensation (TGC) control.

2. To investigate the relationship between the TGC control and the overall gain control.

TIME GAIN COMPENSATION

Attenuation causes the sound wave to lose energy as it travels through tissue. Without compensation for attenuation, an echo originating from a deep-lying reflector would appear less bright (darker shade of gray) than an echo created from that same reflector at a shallower depth. Ideally, structures with identical reflectivity appear as the same shade of gray on the display unrelated to depth.

The *time gain compensation (TGC)* control enables the sonographer to selectively amplify echoes returning from different depths. Each slider control on the TGC panel corresponds to a specific depth and simultaneously to a specific region on the screen associated with that depth. Each slider may be individually adjusted, as necessary, to apply the appropriate amplification so that a uniformly bright image is produced. The depth of the echo-producing structures is determined by the time delay between the transmitted pulse and the echo return time, hence the name *time gain compensation*. TGC controls are adjusted on the basis of the visual appearance of an image, rather than by specific numeric values.

Adjusting each TGC slider control to a set value results in a *gain curve*, which is a graph of the applied gain or amplification plotted versus the time (depth) of the returning echo (Figure L3-1). This gain curve is often represented on the display alongside the two-dimensional image so that points along the depth axis correspond visually to the image. The gain curve may also be pictured by observing the relative position of the slider controls, as demonstrated in Figure L3-2.

Figures L3-1 and L3-2 illustrate the gain curve in a homogeneous medium, which is not representative of the human body. A sound wave transmitted from the transducer into the body must first pass through the abdominal wall or the chest wall, which is composed of muscle, fat, and connective tissue. Sound must then travel through the organ(s) being examined, such as the liver or the heart. These organs may have heterogeneous as well as homogeneous regions, including fluid-filled structures such as blood vessels or heart chambers.

Time Gain Compensation

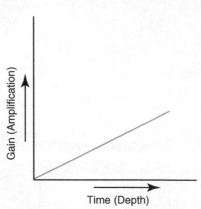

FIGURE L3-1 The gain curve.

Organs and other structures attenuate sound at different rates, and therefore a uniquely adjusted TGC curve is required. In addition, other signal-generating sources often occur in certain regions, such as immediately beyond the transducer face and in the extreme far-field.

Time Gain Compensation

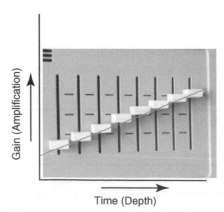

FIGURE L3-2 Gain curve with superimposed slider controls. The time gain compensation (TGC) control is rotated 90 degrees for comparison.

The TGC control can be used to minimize the effects of these distracting signals in the display.

In practice, a "standard" TGC curve based on the type of examination is often used to address all of the above issues. This results in a curve that is nonlinear and emphasizes or de-emphasizes certain sections of the two-dimensional image (Figures L3-3 and L3-4).

- *Near Gain.* Applied during the first few centimeters of the sound path. Examples are the body wall and the "dead zone" near the transducer face.
- *Slope.* The midportion of the gain curve, which theoretically corresponds to the organ(s) of interest. Examples are the liver and the heart. (Technically, each point of the curve has a value for slope, but the term is usually applied only to the middle section.)
- *Break Point.* The point at which the rate of amplification-per-depth is decreased and theoretically is set to correspond to the deepest border of the organ(s) of interest. Examples are the diaphragm in the abdomen and the posterior pericardium of the heart.
- *Far Gain.* Applied just beyond the organ(s) of interest. The proper choice of scan range should limit this region to a few centimeters in length.

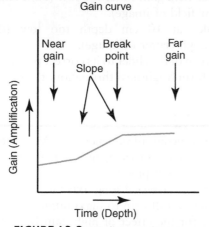

FIGURE L3-3 Nonlinear gain curve.

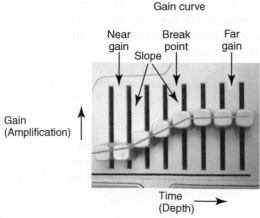

FIGURE L3-4 Correct adjustment of time gain compensation (TGC).

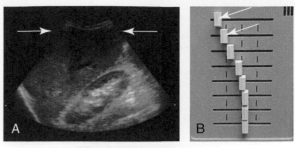

TGC incorrectly adjusted:
Near gain too low

FIGURE L3-5 Nonlinear gain curve superimposed on slider controls. The time gain compensation (TGC) control should be rotated 90 degrees counter clockwise for comparison with the graph in Figure L3-3..

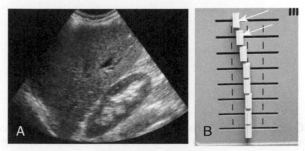

TGC correctly adjusted

FIGURE L3-6 Improper time gain compensation (TGC) adjustment.

TGC is adjusted by visual comparison with the two-dimensional image. In Figure L3-5, TGC is adjusted incorrectly (*arrows on frame A*). Note the low position of the first two sliders (*arrows on frame B*).

TGC is corrected by increasing the gain by moving the first two sliders to the right (*arrows on frame B* in Figure L3-6). Note the uniform image brightness in the near-field (*frame A*).

Although the TGC control affects sectional bands of the image according to depth, moving all of the TGC sliders by the same amount results in a change similar to adjusting the overall gain control. Thus, the overall gain and TGC controls are interdependent. If the overall gain is set too high or too low, the TGC sliders must then be positioned to the upper or lower limits of their ranges to compensate for the improper setting of the overall gain (Figure L3-7). The capability to set TGC to the correct configuration is limited.

OPTION #1

EXPLORE

- Choose a medium-frequency (3–5 MHz) curvilinear array or sector transducer suitable for abdominal imaging. Select an abdominal application preset.

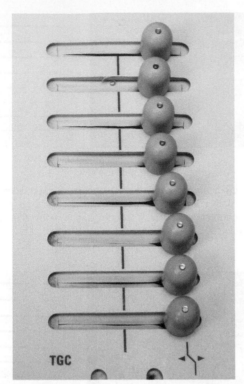

FIGURE L3-7 The time gain compensation (TGC) sliders positioned at near-maximum settings because of improper low overall gain.

- Set the scan range to show the most posterior aspect of the liver.
- Locate the TGC control. If possible, select the option that allows the gain curve to be visible on the screen.
- Obtain three sagittal images of the right hepatic lobe, to demonstrate the following:
  - Near-field gain slider too low (dark band through near field of image).
  - Slider control at 10 cm set too high (bright band through center of image).
  - Proper TGC setting showing uniform brightness throughout the image.

DOCUMENT

- Choose a medium-frequency (3–5 MHz) curvilinear array or sector transducer suitable for abdominal imaging. Select an abdominal application preset.
- Scan the right hepatic lobe in the sagittal plane. Turn the overall gain to the maximum. Attempt to compensate by decreasing all the TGC sliders. Create a hard-copy still image with these settings.
- Scan the right hepatic lobe in the sagittal plane. Turn the overall gain to the minimum. Attempt to compensate by increasing all the TGC sliders. Create a hard-copy still image with these settings.
- Scan the right hepatic lobe in the sagittal plane. Set the TGC sliders at the midpoint of their ranges (straight line). Adjust the overall gain to achieve approximately correct image brightness.
- Adjust the TGC sliders into the appropriate TGC curve format.
- Fine-tune the TGC and overall gain controls to produce an image with nearly uniform brightness.
- Create a hard-copy still image at this setting.

OPTION #2

EXPLORE

- Choose a medium-frequency (3–5 MHz) sector transducer suitable for cardiac imaging. Select an adult cardiac application preset.
- Set the scan range to approximately 1 cm beyond the posterior pericardium.
- Locate the TGC control. If possible, select the option that allows the gain curve to be visible on the screen.
- Obtain a parasternal long axis view of the heart. Set the TGC controls to demonstrate uniform brightness throughout the image.
- While scanning in real-time, obtain the following images:
  - Near-field gain slider too low (dark band through near field of image).
  - Slider at 10 cm depth too low (dark band through center of image).
  - Return of the slider to its correct position, showing uniform brightness throughout the image.

DOCUMENT

- Choose a medium-frequency (3–5 MHz) sector transducer suitable for cardiac imaging. Select an adult cardiac application preset.
- Obtain a parasternal long axis view of the heart.
- Turn the overall gain to maximum. Attempt to compensate for the effect of high gain by decreasing all the TGC sliders. Create a hard-copy still image or video clip with these settings.
- Turn the overall gain to the minimum. Attempt to compensate for low gain by increasing all the TGC sliders. Create a hard-copy still image or video clip with these settings.
- Set the TGC sliders at the midpoint of their ranges (straight line). Adjust the overall gain to achieve approximately correct image brightness.
- Adjust the TGC sliders for the appropriate gain curve format.
- Fine-tune the TGC and overall gain controls to produce an image with uniform brightness.
- Create a hard-copy still image or video clip with these settings.

Transmit Frequency: Resolution and Penetration

OBJECTIVES

1. To observe the effect of transmitted frequency on spatial resolution.
2. To observe the effect of transmitted frequency on penetration.

3. To understand that the attenuation coefficient of tissue is strongly dependent on transmit frequency, which consequently impacts proper time gain compensation (TGC), gain, and output power control settings.

TRANSMIT FREQUENCY

Other terms for transmit frequency include *operating frequency, center frequency,* and *nominal frequency.* Current broadband transducers are capable of operating throughout a range of frequencies during both transmit and receive modes. Transducers are typically given a name or label that describes the frequency range within which the given transducer operates. For example, "L 6–10" would refer to a Linear array transducer with a frequency range of 6–10 MHz. Some manufacturers use a single frequency to denote the midpoint of the frequency range in which the transducer may operate. Other manufacturers specify the maximum operating frequency in the frequency range.

The first and most obvious way to select a transmit frequency is by choosing the most appropriate transducer for the examination. Transducer selection should be based on the type of examination to be performed and includes choosing the correct transducer design (sector, linear, curvilinear, endocavitary, etc.) and the correct frequency range. For example, an adult echocardiogram would dictate the choice of a sector transducer. However, the sonographer may have the choice between two different sectors, one with a range of 2.25–3.5 MHz and another with a range of 3.5–5.0 MHz.

Most scanners have the capability of operating at different frequencies within the specified frequency range for each transducer. Manufacturers have provided controls that enable the sonographer to adjust the transmit frequency up or down, but the terminology is often vendor specific. Labels for the frequency selection control include "Frequency Fusion," "Multihertz," and "Transmit Frequency." Incremental increases and decreases in the frequency control may be shown on the display as

a specific value such as "5 MHz" or may simply be indicated as "R" for resolution and "P" for penetration.

To obtain the best resolution, the sonographer should always scan at the highest practical frequency, while still obtaining adequate penetration to image the organ of interest (Figures L4-1 and L4-2).

An additional consideration is the effect that a change in transmit frequency has on the TGC control settings. A higher transmit frequency will cause an increase in the attenuation coefficient, requiring a greater slope of the gain curve. A lower transmit frequency will cause a decrease in the attenuation coefficient, requiring a less steep slope of the gain curve. Changes in the overall gain and output power may also be required to maintain proper image brightness.

Note: The frequency range selected applies only to imaging. If the transducer is also capable of operating in the Doppler mode, the Doppler frequency is usually somewhat lower than the selected imaging frequency.

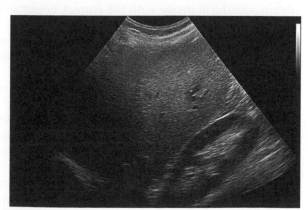

FIGURE L4-1 Transmit frequency of 5 megahertz (MHz). This frequency does not penetrate the liver adequately.

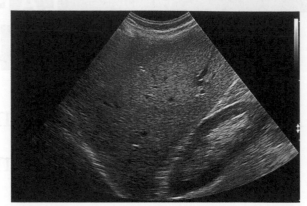

FIGURE L4-2 Transmit frequency decreased to 3 megahertz (MHz). Note the improved penetration of the liver.

The Doppler transmit frequency is indicated on the screen by some, but not all, manufacturers.

Note: The frequency selection control on some scanners also activates the harmonic imaging mode. As the control continues to be increased beyond the highest transmit frequency for the fundamental imaging mode, the system automatically switches to harmonic imaging. In the harmonic mode, the transmit frequency may be indicated as H1, H2, and so on or by some other labeling scheme.

OPTION #1

EXPLORE

- Select a transducer that is appropriate for abdominal imaging. A curvilinear array in the 3–5 MHz range is suggested. (A sector transducer in the same frequency range may also be used.) Choose an abdominal application preset.
- Set the transmit frequency control to the lowest frequency setting.
- Obtain a transverse image of the right hepatic lobe at the level of the main portal vein.
- Adjust the output power, overall gain, and TGC to obtain a uniform image with the correct brightness.
- Note the resolution throughout the image.
- Change the transmit frequency to the highest frequency setting. (Do not choose the harmonic mode, if that is an option with this control.)
- Re-adjust the TGC controls at the new transmit frequency setting.
- Re-adjust the overall gain control to optimize image brightness. For penetration, increase, as needed, the output power after the overall gain has been increased.
- Again, note the resolution throughout the image, and compare it with that obtained with the lowest transmit frequency.

- Repeat the above steps in the opposite order; begin with the image optimized for the highest frequency, switch to the lowest transmit frequency, and then re-adjust the TGC, output power, and overall gain controls to again optimize the image at the low transmit frequency.

DOCUMENT

- Select a transducer that is appropriate for abdominal imaging. A curvilinear array in the 3–5 MHz range is suggested. (A sector transducer in the same frequency range may also be used.) Choose an abdominal application preset.
- Obtain a transverse image of the liver at the level of the portal vein, using the lowest transmit frequency for that transducer. Adjust the TGC, output power, and overall gain controls to optimize the image at the low transmit frequency.
- When the optimum image has been acquired, freeze the image, and generate a hard copy to record the transmit frequency, output power, and overall gain settings.
- Increase the transmit frequency to its maximum setting, and optimize the image as above.
- Freeze the image, and generate a hard copy to record the transmit frequency, output power, and overall gain settings at the high transmit frequency.
- Record the values for the above settings on the laboratory worksheet.
- Make a visual comparison of the resolution in the two hard-copy recorded images.

OPTION #2

EXPLORE

- Select a transducer that is appropriate for adult cardiac imaging. A sector transducer in the 2.2–55 MHz range is suggested. Choose an adult cardiac preset.
- Set the transmit frequency control to the lowest frequency setting.
- Obtain an apical four-chamber view of the heart.
- Adjust the output power, overall gain, and TGC to obtain a uniform image with the correct brightness.
- Note the resolution throughout the image.
- Change the transmit frequency to the highest frequency setting. (Do not choose the harmonic mode, if that is an option with this control.)
- Re-adjust the TGC controls at the new transmit frequency setting.
- Re-adjust the overall gain control to optimize image brightness. For penetration, increase, as needed, the

output power after the overall gain has been increased.

- If the heart still cannot be adequately penetrated at this frequency, decrease the transmit frequency slightly until adequate penetration is obtained.
- Again, note the resolution throughout the image, and compare it with that of the lowest transmit frequency.
- Repeat the above steps in the opposite order; begin with the image optimized for the highest frequency, switch to the lowest frequency, and re-adjust the TGC, output power, and overall gain controls to again optimize the image at the low transmit frequency.

DOCUMENT

- Select a transducer that is appropriate for adult cardiac imaging. A sector transducer in the 2.25–3.5 MHz range is suggested. Choose an adult cardiac preset.

- Obtain an apical four-chamber view at the lowest frequency for that transducer. Adjust the TGC, output power, and overall gain controls to optimize the image at the low transmit frequency.
- When the optimum image has been acquired, freeze the image, and generate a hard copy to record the transmit frequency, output power, and overall gain settings.
- Increase the transmit frequency to its maximum setting, and optimize the image as above.
- Freeze the image, and generate a hard copy to record the transmit frequency, output power, and overall gain settings at the higher transmit frequency.
- Record the values for the above settings on the laboratory worksheet.
- Make a visual comparison of the resolution in the two hard-copy recorded images.

Transmit Focus

OBJECTIVES

1. To observe that lateral resolution is markedly affected by focal point location.
2. To appreciate that beam divergence beyond the focal point degrades lateral resolution and this effect is more pronounced as the focal point is moved closer to the transducer.
3. To understand the relationship between the number of focal zones, the number of pulses per scan line, and frame rate (or pulse repetition frequency).

LOCATION OF FOCAL POINT

Lateral resolution is closely related to the beam width at any given point along the scan line, while axial resolution is generally constant throughout the field of view (FOV). Lateral resolution is almost always greater in magnitude (poorer) than axial resolution, except at the focal point where lateral resolution may approach axial resolution.

Adjusting the depth of focus to improve the lateral resolution in one region of the image has the opposite effect of degrading the lateral resolution in other regions (Figure L5-1). Loss of detail beyond the focal point is caused by beam divergence, which results in a broader sound beam and, therefore, poorer lateral resolution.

Note: Although sonographers often use *focal point* and *focal zone* interchangeably, these terms have different meanings. The focal point is the *point* along the sound beam where the near-field (converging segment) ends and the far-field (diverging segment) begins. The focal point also corresponds to the location at which beam intensity is highest (in a nonattenuating medium) and beam width is narrowest. The focal zone extends some distance in either direction from the focal point until the intensity has decreased 3 decibels (dB) from the maximum.

MULTIPLE TRANSMIT FOCAL ZONES

Lateral resolution is best at the focal point and then deteriorates in either direction as the distance from the focal point increases. Each transmitted sound beam can have only one focal point. *Multiple transmit focus* divides the scan line in segments, whereby each segment includes the focal point of the transmitted beam. Sequential sound beams, each with a different focal point, are superimposed to create a single scan line of B-mode information. If three transmit focal zones are employed, three separate transmit pulses are required

to form a single scan line. Therefore, each scan line takes generally three times as long to form. This results in an approximate threefold reduction in the real-time frame rate. For example, a transducer operating at a maximum frame rate of 30 frames per second in the single-focal-zone mode would be reduced to 10 frames per second if three transmit focal zones were selected (assuming the display depth remains unchanged).

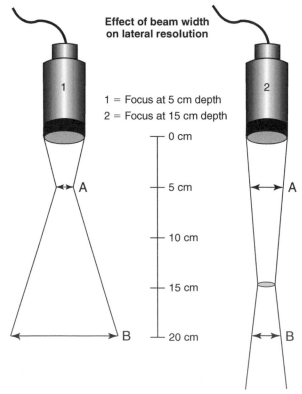

Effect of beam width on lateral resolution

1 = Focus at 5 cm depth
2 = Focus at 15 cm depth

FIGURE L5-1 The difference in beam width and, thus, the difference in lateral resolution at points A and B along each of the sound beams with different focal points. Beam 1 is focused at a depth of 5 cm, and beam 2 is focused at a depth of 15 cm.

OPTION #1

EXPLORE

- Choose a transducer suitable for abdominal imaging, such as a curvilinear array of 3–5 MHz. Select an abdominal application preset.
- Obtain a sagittal image of the right hepatic lobe, including the gallbladder, if possible.
- Set the number of focal zones on the display to one.
- Adjust the focal zone control so that the single indicator is positioned at a depth of 18 cm or just anterior to the diaphragm on the image (Figure L5-2).
- Observe the detail resolution in the region of the gallbladder (near-field), and in the deep right hepatic lobe (far-field) as shown in Figures L5-3 and L5-4.
- Now adjust the focal zone control gradually to a shallower depth so that the single indicator is positioned at 16 cm, 14 cm, 12 cm, 10 cm, 8 cm, 6 cm, and 4 cm.
- As the focal zone is moved from deep to shallow, observe the improving detail resolution in the region of the gallbladder (near-field), and the degrading resolution in the deep right hepatic lobe (far-field).
- Set the number of focal zones on the display to three or more.

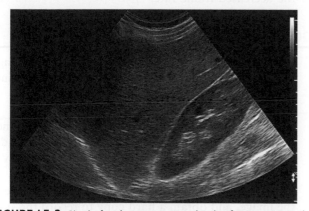

FIGURE L5-2 Single focal zone set at a depth of 14 cm. Note the improved spatial resolution at this depth.

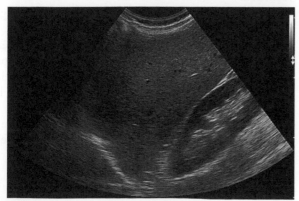

FIGURE L5-3 Single focal zone set at a depth of 4 cm. Note the improved spatial resolution near the transducer.

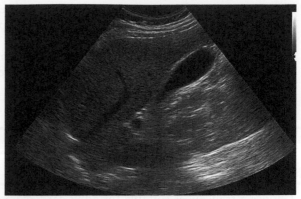

FIGURE L5-4 Single focal zone set at a depth of 4 cm, near the transducer. Note the improved spatial resolution of the anterior gallbladder wall showing a small polyp and the loss of spatial resolution in the far-field.

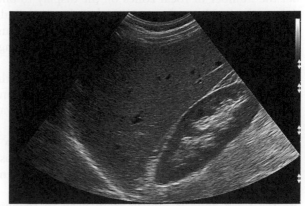

FIGURE L5-5 Four transmit focal zones distributed throughout the scan range denoted by arrows on right side. Note the improved spatial resolution throughout the image. The frame rate was slowed dramatically.

- Adjust the depth of each of the three focal zones so that they are fairly evenly spaced throughout the liver (Figure L5-5).
- Note the improved resolution throughout the image.
- Note the decrease in frame rate (temporal resolution).

DOCUMENT

- Choose a transducer suitable for abdominal imaging, such as a curvilinear array of 3–5 MHz. Select an abdominal application preset.
- Obtain a sagittal image of the right hepatic lobe, including the gallbladder, if possible.
- Set the number of focal zones on the display to one.
- Adjust the focal zone control so that the single indicator is positioned at a depth of 18 cm or just anterior to the diaphragm on the image.
- When the optimal image has been obtained, freeze the image, and obtain a hard copy to record the spatial resolution in the near-field and the far-field.
- Now adjust the focal zone control so that the single indicator is positioned at a depth of 4 cm or at the posterior gallbladder wall (see Figures L5-3 and L5-4).

- When the optimal image has been obtained, freeze the image, and obtain a hard copy to record the spatial resolution in the near-field and the far-field.
- Compare the two stored images, and note the change in spatial resolution in the near-field and the far-field with each focal zone setting.

OPTION #2

EXPLORE

- Choose a transducer suitable for adult cardiac imaging such as a 2.5–3.5 MHz sector. Select an adult cardiac application preset.
- Obtain a parasternal long-axis view of the heart.
- Set the number of focal zones on the display to one.
- Adjust the focal zone control so that the single indicator is positioned at a depth of 15 cm or just beyond the posterior pericardium on the image (Figure L5-6).
- Observe the detail resolution in the region of the anterior wall of the right ventricle (near-field) and in the region of the left ventricular posterior wall (far-field).
- Now adjust the focal zone control gradually to a shallower depth so that the single indicator is positioned at 16 cm, 14 cm, 12 cm, 10 cm, 8 cm, 6 cm, and 4 cm (Figure L5-7).
- As the focal zone is moved from deep to shallow, observe the improving detail resolution in the region of the right ventricle anterior wall (near-field) and the degrading resolution in the region of the left ventricle posterior wall (far-field).

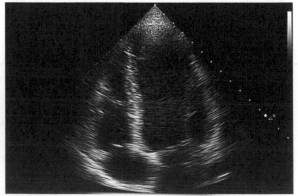

FIGURE L5-6 Apical four-chamber view, with the focal zone set at a depth of 15 cm. Note the lack of spatial resolution in the near-field within the cardiac apex.

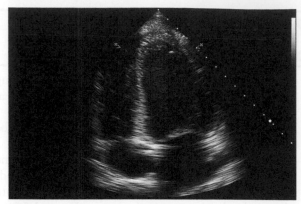

FIGURE L5-7 Apical four-chamber view, with focal zone set at a depth of 4 cm. Note the improved spatial resolution in the near-field within the cardiac apex.

- Set the number of focal zones on the display to three. (Depending on the model of the scanner, you may need to exit the cardiac preset and use an abdominal preset to be able to do this.)
- Adjust the depth of the three focal zones so that they are fairly evenly spaced throughout the heart.
- Note the improved detail resolution throughout the image.
- Note the degraded temporal resolution as a result of the decreased frame rate.

DOCUMENT

- Choose a transducer suitable for adult cardiac imaging such as a 2.5–3.5 MHz sector. Select an adult cardiac application preset.
- Obtain a parasternal long-axis view of the heart
- Set the number of focal zones on the display to one.
- Adjust the focal zone control so that the single indicator is positioned at a depth of 15 cm or at the level of the mitral valve.
- When the optimal image has been obtained, freeze the image, and obtain a hard copy to record the spatial resolution in the near-field and the far-field. Alternatively, a video clip of the heart may be recorded.
- Now adjust the focal zone control so that the single indicator is positioned at a depth of 4 cm.
- When the optimal image has been obtained, freeze the image, and obtain a hard copy to record the spatial resolution in the near-field and the far-field. Alternatively, a video clip of the heart may be recorded.
- Compare the two stored images or video clips, and note the change in detail resolution in the near-field and the far-field with each focal zone setting.

Magnification (Write Zoom)

OBJECTIVES

1. To recognize the advantages of image magnification.
2. To understand the difference between write zoom and read zoom.

3. To choose the most appropriate zoom method based on clinical application.

READ ZOOM VERSUS WRITE ZOOM

Image magnification has traditionally been thought of as a trade-off between using a "read" or postprocessing zoom and a "write" or preprocessing zoom. *Read zoom* magnifies the stored image with no change in pixel number or subsequent improvement in spatial resolution, whereas *write zoom* reassigns an increased number of pixels to the scanned region during data acquisition. Since the physical dimensions associated with each pixel are reduced, write zoom offers improved resolution compared with read zoom.

Classical wisdom has dictated that read zoom should be used only as a last resort, whereas write zoom should always be the method of choice, where practical. One of the few situations in which the use of read zoom would be justified is to magnify a difficult-to-obtain image for measurement purposes. For example, if the sonographer had just spent 10 minutes trying to obtain a suitable image of a common bile duct or a left ventricular wall and then wanted to enlarge the image for measurements, he or she would be reluctant to unfreeze the image to rescan at a higher magnification (write zoom). Therefore, clinical judgment would dictate that read zoom be employed in this situation, even though no improvement in spatial resolution is realized.

With today's technology, the practical distinction between read zoom and write zoom has become blurred, if not irrelevant, in actual practice. Indeed, this is true for all preprocessing and postprocessing functions in general. In the past, read zoom functioned only on a frozen (static) image, while write zoom had to be performed during live scanning. With modern equipment, individual frames are stored almost instantaneously, and all types of processing functions can be performed while the system is in the live scanning mode. Furthermore, the newest machines now continually store raw data and allow the sonographer to retroactively alter many of the original machine settings that have traditionally been thought of as preprocessing functions, such as gain, time gain compensation (TGC), dynamic range, and magnification, even after an image has been stored.

WRITE ZOOM AND DISPLAY DEPTH

The most basic control to alter image size is the display depth. Depth control is used frequently and, when properly set, is an important component of image optimization. Decreasing the display depth for the purpose of image magnification is appropriate in circumstances where (1) the area of interest is fairly close to the transducer, or (2) the anatomy between the specific area of interest and the transducer must be included in the image.

If the area of interest is deep in the body and the display depth is decreased for the purpose of magnification, the area of interest can be cut off at the bottom of the display. In this situation, write zoom is the control of choice. The name of this control is somewhat vendor specific, although most refer to it as "zoom." One manufacturer has labeled this function as "res." Some manufacturers use two separate controls: one for activating the "ROI cursor box" and one to apply the actual magnification. Other manufacturers assign a single control that toggles among "cursor on," "cursor size," and "cursor position." The trackball is then used to resize and reposition the cursor box. On some systems, the trackball may also scroll or pan the magnified image.

OPTION #1

EXPLORE

- Choose a transducer suitable for abdominal imaging such as a 3–5 MHz curvilinear array. Select an abdominal application preset.
- Obtain a transverse image of the right hepatic lobe, including the right kidney.
- Enable the zoom cursor box on the screen.

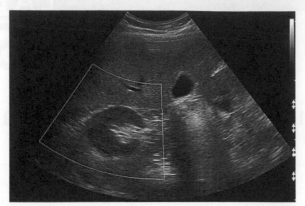

FIGURE L6-1 "Region of Interest" cursor box centered over the right kidney.

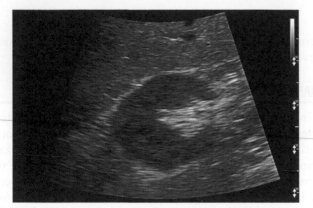

FIGURE L6-2 Magnified region of interest showing the right kidney.

- Adjust the size and position of the cursor box to include just the right kidney (transverse view) as shown in Figure L6-1.
- Zoom the image so that the right kidney nearly fills the screen (Figure L6-2).
- Exit the zoom mode.
- Decrease the display depth to attempt to show the transverse right kidney at the same magnification. (Note that the image is cut off before the same degree of magnification is achieved.)

DOCUMENT

- Choose a transducer appropriate for transabdominal gynecologic imaging. Select a GYN application preset.
- Using the full-bladder technique, obtain a sagittal image of the right ovary.
- Enable the zoom cursor box on the screen.
- Adjust the size and position of the cursor box to include just the right ovary.
- Obtain a hard-copy image, showing the full two-dimensional image, with the cursor box visible on the screen.
- Zoom the image so that the right ovary nearly fills the screen.
- Obtain a hard-copy image of the magnified right ovary.

OPTION #2

EXPLORE

- Choose a transducer suitable for cardiac imaging. Select an adult cardiac application preset.
- Obtain a parasternal long-axis view of the heart.
- In live scanning mode, enable the zoom cursor box on the screen.
- Adjust the size and position of the cursor box to cover the mitral valve.
- Zoom the image so that the moving image of the mitral valve nearly fills the screen.
- Exit the zoom mode.
- Decrease the display depth to attempt to show the mitral valve at the same magnification. (Note that the image is cut off before the same degree of magnification is achieved.)

DOCUMENT

- Choose a transducer suitable for cardiac imaging. Select an adult cardiac application preset.
- Obtain a parasternal short-axis view of the heart that includes the aortic valve (Figure L6-3).

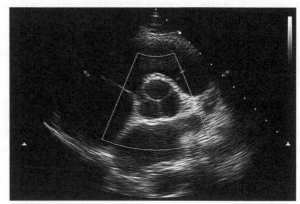

FIGURE L6-3 "Region of Interest" cursor box centered over the aortic valve.

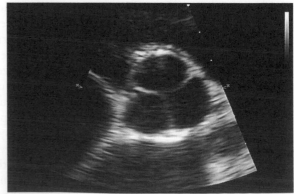

FIGURE L6-4 Magnified region of interest showing the enlarged view of the tri-leaflet aortic valve.

- In live scanning mode, enable the zoom cursor box on the screen.
- Adjust the size and position of the cursor box to include just the aortic valve.
- Obtain a video clip or a hard-copy image showing the full two-dimensional image, with the cursor box visible on the screen.

- Zoom the image so that the aortic valve nearly fills the screen.
- Obtain a video clip or hard-copy image of the magnified aortic valve (Figure L6-4).

Dynamic Range

OBJECTIVES

1. To observe the effect of dynamic range on displayed image contrast.

2. To understand the relationship between dynamic range and compression.

DISCUSS

Dynamic range expressed in decibels (dB) represents the ratio of the largest signal to the smallest signal that a system or component can process. Each returning echo is converted to an electrical signal that must be categorized according to its amplitude (strength) and stored as a digital value in the scan converter. The stored pixel value must then be translated to a shade of gray for display.

Because the range of analog signal levels (approximately 100,000:1 or more) exceeds the number of discrete digital values available in the scan converter matrix (usually 0–255), signals must be partitioned according to a logarithmic scale. This process is called *log compression*. The logarithmic translation is necessary, since linear translation limits the signal variation by a factor of 255. Consequently, with linear processing, the full range of signals from high to low cannot be retained. Log compression effectively increases the amplitudes of low signals and decreases the amplitudes of high signals so that all echo-induced signals are represented in the scan converter (0–255).

The dynamic range of the displayed image may equal the full dynamic range of echo-induced signals, *or* it may be more restricted by excluding some high or low signals. In either case, the dynamic range is reduced. A low dynamic range raises image contrast but usually with a loss of weaker echoes.

The operator control that varies the displayed dynamic range is called *dynamic range*, *compression*, or *log compression*. Although this control has been traditionally considered a preprocessing function, the most current scanners now allow the recapture and processing of raw data retroactively. If the control is labeled "compression," an *increase* in this control results in a *decrease* in dynamic range (dB is lowered). If the control is labeled "dynamic range," then an *increase* in the control results in *increased* dynamic range and *decreased* compression (dB is raised).

The displayed dynamic range may be described as wide or narrow. A wide dynamic range is considered to be 55–60 dB, while a narrow range is considered to be 40–45 dB. A wide dynamic range causes the image to appear low in contrast or "flat" because each gray level corresponds to large signal increments. A narrow dynamic range improves image contrast. Although theoretical differences with regard to the contrast resolution of wide and narrow dynamic range images do exist, in practice, the determining factor is personal preference. The ability to perceive informational content on the screen is also affected by the limited dynamic range of the monitor and the sensitivity of the human eye to distinguish slight differences in gray levels.

OPTION #1

EXPLORE

- Choose a transducer suitable for abdominal imaging, such as a 3–5 MHz curvilinear array. Select an abdominal application preset.
- Obtain a sagittal image of the right hepatic lobe, including the right kidney.
- Set the dynamic range control initially to 40 dB.
- Gradually increase the dynamic range by 5-dB increments to 60 dB (or the highest available setting on the machine).
- Perform the above in reverse order: Start at the highest setting for dynamic range, and decrease by 5 dB at a time until 40 dB is reached.
- Note the difference in contrast in the images obtained with the highest and the lowest dynamic range settings (Figures L7-1 and L7-2).

DOCUMENT

- Choose a transducer suitable for abdominal imaging, such as a 3–5 MHz curvilinear array. Select an abdominal application preset.

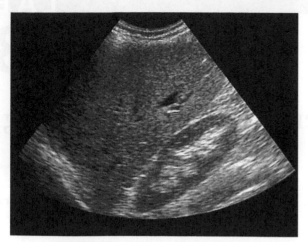

FIGURE L7-1 Dynamic range of 45 dB.

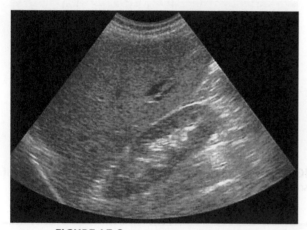

FIGURE L7-2 Dynamic range of 60 dB.

- Obtain a transverse image of the right hepatic lobe, including the right kidney.
- Set the dynamic range control initially to 45 dB.
- Acquire a hard-copy image at the 45-dB setting.

- Increase the dynamic range to 60 dB (or the highest available setting on the machine).
- Acquire a hard-copy image at the 60-dB setting.

OPTION #2

EXPLORE

- Choose a transducer suitable for cardiac imaging, such as a 2.5–3.5 MHz sector. Select an adult cardiac application preset.
- Obtain a parasternal long-axis view of the heart.
- Set the dynamic range control initially to 40 dB.
- Gradually increase the dynamic range by 5-dB increments to 60 dB (or the highest available setting on the machine).
- Perform the above in reverse order: Start at the highest setting for dynamic range, and decrease by 5 dB at a time until 40 dB is reached.
- Note the difference in contrast in the images obtained with the highest and the lowest dynamic range settings.

DOCUMENT

- Choose a transducer suitable for cardiac imaging such as a 2.5–3.5 MHz sector. Select an adult cardiac application preset.
- Obtain a parasternal short-axis view of the heart at the level of the aortic valve.
- Set the dynamic range control initially to 45 dB.
- Capture a video clip, or acquire a hard-copy image at the 45-dB setting.
- Increase the dynamic range to 60 dB (or the highest available setting on the machine).
- Capture a video clip, or acquire a hard-copy image at the 60-dB setting.

Persistence (Frame Averaging)

OBJECTIVES

1. To understand the concept of frame averaging.
2. To be able to determine the appropriate situations in which frame averaging is beneficial.

3. To recognize the effect of frame averaging on temporal resolution.

DISCUSS

Frame averaging, or *persistence*, is a noise reduction technique in which successive frames are temporarily stored in a buffer and then combined with a newly acquired frame for real-time display. Commonly, two to four (or more) frames are combined, with no change in the overall displayed frame rate. Because noise is random, whereas echoes from anatomic structures are consistent and repeatable, the merging of echo data from multiple scans of the field of view (FOV) helps reduce noise.

Since frame averaging uses several frames acquired at different times, the technique is most effective for structures that are not in rapid motion, such as the liver or the kidneys. Fast moving structures, such as the heart, are poor candidates for frame averaging because of the large variation in spatial position over short time intervals. Anatomic landmarks in successive frames are not superimposed at the same location in the averaged image, which results in the blurring of these structures.

Temporal resolution is the ability to differentiate or resolve the dynamic motion of structures. Obviously, good temporal resolution is most important for structures with rapid movement. As frame averaging is increased, temporal resolution is degraded. In the case of some applications such as imaging of the liver, temporal resolution is not particularly important, and the noise reduction achieved by frame averaging results in improved image quality. For other applications, such as imaging of the heart and blood vessels, the loss of temporal resolution is a significant consideration and far outweighs any advantage of frame averaging for noise reduction.

Frame averaging is also referred to as *persistence* by some manufacturers. This operator control is typically available for both B-mode and color flow imaging and ranges from zero to a maximum of usually four or five frames averaged together (Figure L8-1). High persistence settings enhance averaging but are more likely to cause "smeary-looking" structures in the image.

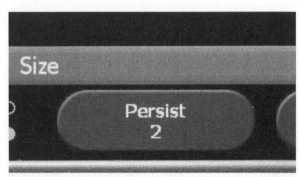

FIGURE L8-1 Selection of persistence control is by means of a "soft key" on the console.

OPTION #1

EXPLORE

- Choose a transducer suitable for abdominal imaging such as a 3–5 MHz curvilinear array. Select an abdominal vascular application preset.
- Obtain a sagittal image of the liver, including the inferior vena cava.
- While live scanning mode is activated, gradually increase persistence or frame averaging from the lowest value to the highest value.
- Note the blurred or "smeary" appearance of the image as persistence is increased, particularly in the case of the borders of the inferior vena cava.

DOCUMENT

- Choose a transducer suitable for abdominal imaging such as a 3–5 MHz curvilinear array. Select an abdominal vascular application preset.
- Obtain a sagittal image of the abdominal aorta.
- While live scanning mode is activated, gradually increase persistence or frame averaging from the lowest value to the highest value.

- Capture a video clip or a hard-copy image to demonstrate the blurred or "smeary" appearance of the aorta.
- Move the transducer to the patient's right to obtain an image of the right hepatic lobe.
- Increase persistence to the maximum, and have the patient suspend respiration to completely stop any movement within the scanned region.
- Capture a video clip or a hard-copy image to demonstrate the improved image quality for the right hepatic lobe.

OPTION #2

EXPLORE

- Choose a transducer suitable for cardiac imaging, such as a 2.5–5 MHz sector. Select an adult cardiac application preset.
- Obtain an apical four-chamber view of the heart.
- While live scanning mode is activated, gradually increase persistence or frame averaging from the lowest value to the highest value.
- Note the blurred or "smeary" appearance of the image as persistence is increased.

DOCUMENT

- Choose a transducer suitable for cardiac imaging, such as a 2.5–5 MHz sector. Select an adult cardiac application preset.
- Obtain an apical four-chamber view of the heart.

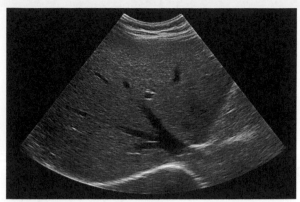

FIGURE L8-2 Transverse image of the liver with hepatic veins captured with persistence set at a high level (setting "5").

- While live scanning mode is activated, gradually increase persistence or frame averaging from the lowest value to the highest value.
- Now, adjust persistence to the lowest value.
- Capture a video clip to demonstrate the excellent temporal resolution, with persistence set to the lowest value.
- Using a subcostal approach during suspended deep inspiration by the patient, obtain a transverse image of the liver and hepatic veins.
- Increase persistence to the maximum, and have the patient suspend respiration to completely stop most movement within the scanned region.
- Capture a video clip or a hard-copy image to demonstrate improved image quality for the liver and hepatic veins (Figure L8-2).

Gray-Scale Mapping

OBJECTIVES

1. To understand the principle of gray-scale mapping.

2. To observe the effect of gray-scale mapping on image contrast.

DISCUSS

Digital scanners allow the manipulation of stored data after acquisition but before display. One such signal processing technique is the adjustment of image contrast by *gray-scale mapping*. Each pixel is displayed uniformly as a particular shade of gray, depending on the pixel value. The translation of signal amplitudes to gray levels (gray-scale mapping) may be altered to emphasize or de-emphasize a certain range of echo amplitudes. For example, if mid-range amplitudes are deemed to contain the most important echo data, the available shades of gray may be weighted so that more shades are assigned to mid-range echoes than to high-amplitude or low-amplitude echoes. Contrast is improved for mid-range echoes because the shades of gray are distributed over a narrower extent of signal levels (the range of pixel values associated with a particular shade of gray is reduced).

Most manufacturers include a wide selection of gray-scale maps or curves, each designed to emphasize a specific segment of echo amplitudes (Figure L9-1). These gray-scale maps are programmed into the system and can be selected by the sonographer. Typical gray-scale map controls offer individual maps labeled A through

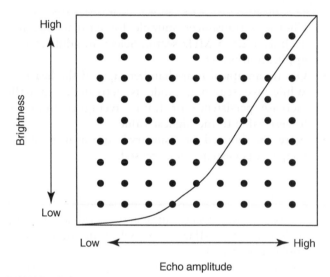

FIGURE L9-2 A user-programmable gray-scale map that enhances strong echoes.

Z, and often AA, BB, and so on. Most ultrasound systems also provide user-programmable gray-scale maps, although these are seldom used in clinical practice (Figure L9-2).

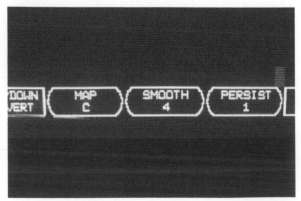

FIGURE L9-1 Gray-scale map "C" is selected.

OPTION #1

EXPLORE

- Choose a transducer suitable for abdominal imaging such as a 3–5 MHz curvilinear array. Select an abdominal application preset.
- Obtain a sagittal image of the right hepatic lobe, including the right kidney.
- Set the gray-scale map initially to the default setting.
- Using the gray-scale map control, select various gray-scale maps.
- Identify maps that are most appealing or that appear to best demonstrate the anatomy.

DOCUMENT

- Choose a transducer suitable for abdominal imaging such as a 3–5 MHz curvilinear array. Select an abdominal application preset.
- Obtain a transverse image of the right hepatic lobe, including the right kidney.
- Set the gray-scale map initially to the default setting.
- Acquire five hard-copy images demonstrating five different gray-scale maps.

OPTION #2

EXPLORE

- Choose a transducer suitable for cardiac imaging such as a 2.5–3.5 MHz sector. Select an adult cardiac application preset.

- Obtain a parasternal long axis view of the heart.
- Set the gray-scale map initially to the default setting.
- Using the gray-scale map control, select various gray-scale maps.
- Identify maps that are most appealing or that appear to best demonstrate the anatomy.

DOCUMENT

- Choose a transducer suitable for cardiac imaging such as a 2.5–3.5 MHz sector. Select an adult cardiac application preset.
- Obtain a parasternal short axis view of the heart at the level of the aortic valve.
- Set the gray-scale map initially to the default setting.
- Capture five video clips to demonstrate five different gray-scale maps.

Distance and Area Measurements

OBJECTIVES

1. To understand the importance of proper measurement techniques.

2. To perform linear distance, area, and circumference measurements on the acquired image.

DISCUSS

Measurement of linear distance, circumference, and area is an important part of sonography. The reader should consult the many comprehensive articles that describe the proper techniques for organ-specific measurements in various areas of sonography. This lab is not a substitute for the operator's manual, as each ultrasound machine has a somewhat different knobology to execute measurements. The goal of this lab is to help the student understand the basic principles of measurement and to apply appropriate measurement techniques in practice.

Most ultrasound systems have two options for making measurements. The first uses a software calculation package, which is application specific. Along with control default settings, the application preset determines the appropriate calculation package. For an obstetrics (OB) preset, selecting "Calc" from the menu initiates the OB calculation software. The measurement package guides the sonographer through the data acquisition process and, ultimately, creates a report of the results. In a similar fashion, the cardiac preset activates a cardiac calculation package.

The second option is stand-alone measurements of linear distance, area, or circumference. These measurements are made by pressing the "Caliper" button and positioning the onscreen cursor with the trackball (Figure L10-1). A "Select" key activates each caliper alternately so that the position of each caliper may be adjusted until the sonographer is satisfied with the position. Often, multiple sets of calipers can be displayed on the screen simultaneously.

A manual, single measurement, which is not part of the calculation package, is frequently performed for the gallbladder wall or the common bile duct. Manual measurements are also necessary for some subjects that have no pre-programmed calculation software, for example, the dimensions of the pancreas or the thickness of the abdominal wall. Often, single, on-the-fly

measurements are obtained in cardiac imaging for a quick estimation of the size of the left atrium or the thickness of the left ventricular wall.

For accurate linear measurements, the position of the caliper must be carefully chosen. Focus and display depth should be optimized for the organ of interest. Gain or time gain compensation (TGC) is reduced to minimize any ring-down artifact that might create an artifactually "thicker" interface such as the gallbladder wall (Figure L10-2).

Traditionally, most linear measurements were made "leading edge to leading edge." The belief was that the leading edge of a reflecting interface would be more faithfully reproduced than the trailing edge, regardless of equipment settings such as gain or TGC. Therefore, measurements such as the fetal biparietal diameter were made from the outer edge of the skull bone to the inner edge of the bone on the opposite side of the head. Other measurements, such as that of the common bile duct, were performed in the same way.

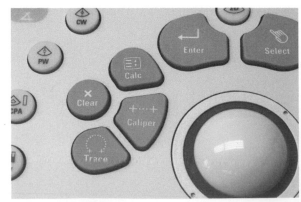

FIGURE L10-1 Measurement controls. On this particular instrument, the "Caliper" button and the "Select" button control the caliper position; the "Calc" button initiates the preset-specific calculation package software. The ellipse tool and the trackball are also shown.

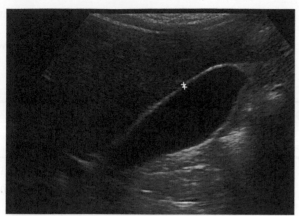

FIGURE L10-2 Linear measurement of the thickness of the gallbladder wall. Note that gain has been decreased slightly to minimize artifactual thickening of the wall and that the image has been enlarged to position the calipers accurately.

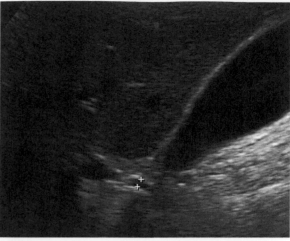

FIGURE L10-4 Common bile duct measured as 0.27 cm with the trailing edge–to–leading edge technique (measurement of the lumen). Note that this measurement differs by 30% from that in Figures L10-3.

Today, with continual improvements in image quality, the leading edge technique has been disregarded, and the calipers are generally placed on the outer or inner boundary of the organ. Measurement of the fetal biparietal diameter still requires the leading edge–to–leading edge method. This is not necessarily because of its better accuracy but, rather, because the existing biparietal diameter growth charts are based on this technique. If the "outer-to-outer" technique were now used, the growth charts would need to be revised.

Nevertheless, sonographic measurements must conform to the guidelines of the institution (e.g., leading edge–to–leading edge technique or others). The difference in measurement technique can result in small, but sometimes significant, errors (Figures L10-3 and L10-4).

Circumference and area measurements, whether performed within a calculation package or as stand-alone measurements, can be executed with free-hand tracing or with the ellipse tool.

With the free-hand tracing method, the sonographer positions one caliper at a start point and then manually draws, freehand, the boundary around the organ or structure. This can be somewhat awkward, and success depends to a large extent on the artistic ability and motor control of the sonographer.

The second method, which is available on many systems, employs an ellipse tool. The ellipse is positioned on the screen by locating two reference points (with calipers) until the ellipse coincides with the borders of the structure to be measured. If the structure is near-circular in shape, the measurement is complete at this point. If the structure is ovoid in shape, a third control allows the shape of the ellipse to be stretched into an oval. The oval ellipse is then manipulated by the trackball until it is superimposed on the structure (Figures L10-5 and L10-6).

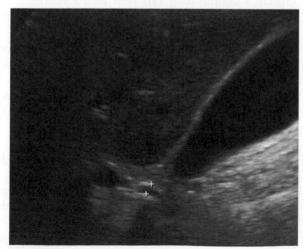

FIGURE L10-3 Common bile duct measured as 0.37 cm using the leading edge–to–leading edge technique.

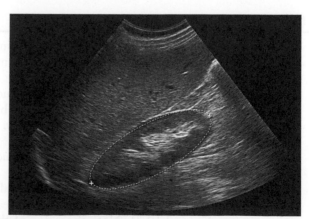

FIGURE L10-5 Measurement of the area and circumference of the right kidney using the ellipse tool. Note the two cursor anchor points.

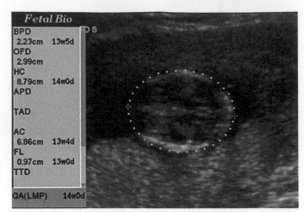

FIGURE L10-6 Measurement of the fetal head circumference with the ellipse tool.

- Reposition the calipers to measure only the duct lumen (see Figure L10-4).
- Obtain a hard-copy image. Compare the two measurements.

OPTION #2

EXPLORE

- Choose a transducer suitable for adult cardiac imaging such as a 2.5–3.5 MHz sector. Select an examination preset for adult cardiac imaging.
- Obtain a sagittal long axis view of the heart.
- Optimize gain, TGC, and display depth to display the left atrium and the aortic root. Freeze the image.
- Using the trackball, scroll until the left ventricle chamber appears to be at end-diastole (largest chamber size).
- Select the caliper control. Position the calipers to obtain a measurement of the left atrium.
- Return to live scanning mode.
- Optimize gain, TGC, and display depth to display the left ventricular posterior wall, the left ventricle chamber, and the interventricular septum. Freeze the image.
- Using the trackball, scroll until the left ventricle chamber (LV) appears to be at end-diastole (largest chamber size).
- Select the caliper control. Position the calipers to obtain measurements of the left ventricular posterior wall, the LV end-diastolic diameter, and the interventricular septal thickness.

DOCUMENT

- Choose a transducer suitable for adult cardiac imaging such as a 2.5–3.5 MHz sector. Select an examination preset for adult cardiac imaging.
- Obtain a sagittal long axis view of the heart.
- Optimize gain, TGC, and display depth. Freeze the image.
- Using the trackball, scroll until the LV chamber appears to be at end-diastole (the largest chamber size).
- Select the free-hand trace control. Position the start point at the apex, and trace all the way around the endocardium.
- Note the area value. Obtain a hard-copy image.
- Using the trackball, scroll until the LV appears to be at peak systole (the smallest chamber size).
- Select the free-hand trace control. Position the start point at the apex, and trace completely around the endocardium.
- Note the difference in area between the systolic and diastolic measurements.

OPTION #1

EXPLORE

- Choose a transducer suitable for abdominal imaging such as a 3–5 MHz curvilinear array. Select an examination preset for abdominal imaging.
- Obtain a sagittal image of the right kidney, including the right hepatic lobe.
- Optimize gain, TGC, focus, and display depth.
- Freeze the image. The renal borders should be distinct throughout the image.
- Select the freehand trace tool. Position the start point at the upper pole of the kidney, and manually trace the entire circumference. Note the values for area and circumference.
- Select the ellipse tool. Position the anchor points of the ellipse at opposite ends of the kidney.
- Select the oval adjustment control. Adjust the shape until the ellipse coincides with the borders of the kidney. Compare the area and circumference measurements with those obtained by the freehand method.

DOCUMENT

- Choose a transducer suitable for abdominal imaging such as a 3–5 MHz curvilinear array. Select an examination preset for abdominal imaging.
- Obtain an oblique image of the common bile duct just distal to the portal vein. The left lateral decubitus position of the patient may facilitate this view.
- Optimize gain, TGC, focus, and display depth.
- Freeze the image. The walls of the common bile duct should be distinct.
- Select the electronic caliper control. Position the calipers to make a leading edge–to–leading edge measurement (see Figure L10-3). Note the value of the measurement, and obtain a hard-copy image.

Doppler Controls 1

OBJECTIVES

1. To investigate the practical application of the Doppler effect in detecting blood flow.
2. To understand the function and appropriate use of Doppler controls (Doppler cursor, sample volume, sample volume depth, gain, power, velocity scale, baseline, audio volume, and spectral invert).

DOPPLER EQUATION

Doppler ultrasound enables the measurement of the velocity of flowing blood within the heart and blood vessels and, as such, is an important component of sonographic examination. The Doppler principle is based on the change in observed frequency, or *Doppler shift frequency*, when sound waves reflect from a moving object and then return to the transducer. The Doppler shift frequency (f_D) is calculated from the Doppler equation:

$$f_D = \frac{2vf}{c} \cos\theta$$

where θ is the Doppler angle to flow, f is the transducer frequency, v is the blood flow velocity, and c is the acoustic velocity.

The Doppler equation predicts the magnitude of the Doppler shift. Two parameters in this equation, *transmitted frequency* and the *angle to flow*, may be altered by the sonographer to facilitate blood flow measurement. (Doppler angle to flow is discussed in detail in Lab 13.)

The operator controls that allow the sonographer to specify these two factors are the *transmit frequency* and the *cursor angle*. In addition, the *angle correct* control allows the sonographer to input the flow direction so that the flow velocity can be more accurately determined. Other Doppler controls pertain to the display of the Doppler information, such as *velocity scale* and *baseline*, or to the process of sampling the blood flow, such as *gate size* and *gate position*. All standard Doppler controls are discussed in this Lab and in Labs 12 and 13.

All controls discussed below apply to both pulsed-wave (PW) Doppler and continuous-wave (CW) Doppler; the exception is the *sample volume*, which is specific only to pulsed-wave Doppler. (In these labs, nonimaging Doppler probes have been excluded, hence PW and CW Doppler refer to the duplex mode only.)

DOPPLER CURSOR

The *Doppler cursor* is a line superimposed on the B-mode image, and it indicates the path of the sound beam in the Doppler mode. The angle and the left-right position of the cursor may be controlled in a variety of ways, depending on the manufacturer and model of the machine. Most often, these controls include the trackball as well as a secondary knob or button. The Doppler cursor appears when the PW Doppler mode is selected. The CW Doppler mode also uses an onscreen cursor if the transducer has that capability.

SAMPLE VOLUME

Doppler sample volume defines the three-dimensional region from which the Doppler information is obtained and displayed. The sample volume is determined by beam width as well as by the size and position of the *range gate*. The range gate is displayed on screen as a small box or a double set of lines located along the Doppler cursor line. The terms *range gate*, *gate*, and *sample volume* are used interchangeably. Gate depth is usually controlled with the track ball and must be positioned such that the sample volume is located within the area of flow to be interrogated (Figure L11-1). Lab 12 examines sample volume and range gate in more detail.

DOPPLER GAIN

Doppler gain amplifies the received Doppler signal (Figure L11-2). Raising Doppler gain increases both the brightness of the Doppler spectral waveform and the volume of the audio signal. Doppler gain must be balanced with *Doppler output power*. Output power set too low results in the gain setting being near-maximum and high noise content in the display (Figures L11-3 and L11-4).

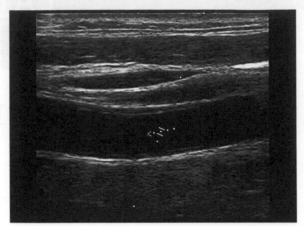

FIGURE L11-1 The Doppler cursor with 58-degree angle to flow and the sample volume in the center of the vessel. The "<" cursor indicates direction of flow.

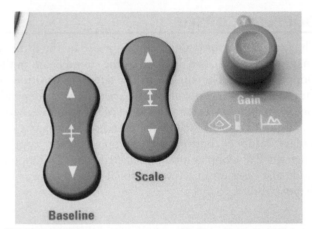

FIGURE L11-2 The Doppler gain, scale, and baseline controls.

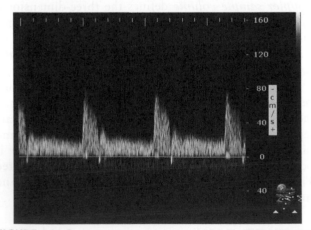

FIGURE L11-3 The Doppler spectral waveform with the Doppler gain set too high. Note the background noise and the fill-in of the spectral window.

DOPPLER OUTPUT POWER

The *Doppler output power* control (not available on some machines) also affects the brightness of the Doppler spectral waveform and the volume of the audio signal. However, this is accomplished by increasing excitation

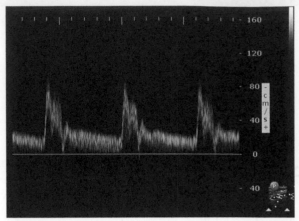

FIGURE L11-4 The Doppler spectral waveform with the proper Doppler gain setting. Note the absence of noise in the background and the clearly visible spectral window. The "+" and "−" axes on the display are inverted to display the waveform "right side up."

voltage to the transducer rather than by amplifying the received signal. Doppler output power should be kept to a moderate level, if possible, both from the standpoint of spectral quality (output power at maximum is usually unnecessary and may introduce noise) and from consideration of patient exposure.

VOLUME CONTROL

Nearly every Doppler instrument has a *volume control*. This control should be adjusted when the brightness of the spectral Doppler waveform is appropriate but the audio signal is either too loud or too soft. When gain or output power are set too high or too low, adjustments in gain or power should be made before changing the volume control. For example, if gain is too high and the audio signal is also too loud, reducing Doppler gain may resolve both problems. If gain is set correctly and the audio signal is too low, turning up gain boosts the audio level; however, this will cause the spectral display to be overgained.

VELOCITY SCALE

Most of the current spectral Doppler instruments depict flow in units of velocity (centimeters per second [cm/s]) rather than in units of the Doppler shift frequency (hertz [Hz]). The *velocity scale* control adjusts maximum displayed velocity in both positive and negative directions. On most of the current machines, the Doppler pulse repetition frequency (PRF) is coupled with the maximum displayed velocity. The upper limit of the velocity scale (in both positive and negative directions) is established by the Nyquist limit, which is equal to one-half of the Doppler PRF. The velocity scale may be increased to accommodate higher flow velocities until the maximum velocity limit is reached. The maximum velocity limit corresponds to the highest Doppler PRF available when sampling at the gate depth.

BASELINE (ZERO SHIFT)

The spectral Doppler display shows flow velocities toward and away from the transducer simultaneously. Often, the baseline is positioned in the center of the display to partition maximum velocity equally in both positive and negative flow directions. The *baseline* control may be adjusted up or down, positioning the baseline off-center, in order to expand the displayed maximum velocity in one direction, with subsequent reduction in the other direction.

SPECTRAL INVERT

Depending on the application and the anatomy being examined, the spectral Doppler waveform may be displayed primarily above the baseline (flow toward the transducer) or below (flow away from the transducer). In some circumstances, the spectral display is inverted to show an otherwise negative, or "upside-down" waveform as "right-side-up." Traditionally, cardiac Doppler signals have been displayed in the direction in which they occur, without inversion of the waveforms. In vascular applications, such as carotid artery scanning, the common practice is to display all normal waveforms above the baseline. If the waveform appears upside down because of the Doppler angle to flow, the *spectral invert* control "flips" the waveform for the right-side-up display. The notation for positive or negative axes on the spectral display is also simultaneously inverted, so the waveform is still depicted with the correct flow direction (see Figure L11-4).

OPTION #1

EXPLORE

- Choose a transducer suitable for abdominal imaging such as a 3–5 MHz curvilinear array with Doppler capability. Select an abdominal application preset.
- Obtain a sagittal image of the proximal abdominal aorta.
- Select the pulsed-wave Doppler mode.
- Angle the Doppler cursor toward the patient's head, thus creating an angle between the "Doppler beam" and the direction of flow in the artery. Use a heel-toe tilt of the transducer to add additional angle, if necessary, to achieve a Doppler angle to flow of approximately 60 degrees.
- Position the sample volume within the proximal abdominal aorta.
- Activate the spectral display to begin the Doppler interrogation of the proximal aorta.
- Adjust the Doppler output power, if available, to a medium value.
- Increase or decrease the Doppler gain until the waveform appears at the correct brightness level (see Figure L11-4).

- Adjust the audio volume to an appropriate level.
- Adjust the baseline control so the baseline is approximately one third of the way up from the bottom of the display. Approximately two thirds of the velocity scale should be reserved for the positive direction (the direction of flow in this case) and one third of the velocity scale for the negative direction.
- Invert the spectral display to observe the function of this control, and then invert again to return to the normal orientation.

DOCUMENT

- Choose a transducer suitable for abdominal imaging such as a 3–5 MHz curvilinear array with Doppler capability. Select an abdominal or abdominal vascular application preset.
- Obtain a sagittal image of the abdominal aorta.
- Select the pulsed-wave Doppler mode.
- Position the transducer to image the mid-distal portion of the abdominal aorta.
- Angle the Doppler cursor toward the patient's feet, and place the sample volume within the distal abdominal aorta.
- Use a heel-toe tilt of the transducer to add additional angle, if necessary, to achieve a Doppler angle to flow of approximately 60 degrees.
- Activate the spectral display to begin the Doppler interrogation of the aorta.
- Adjust the Doppler output power, if available, to a medium value.
- Increase or decrease the Doppler gain until the waveform appears at the correct brightness level (see Figure L11-4).
- Adjust the audio volume to an appropriate level.
- Adjust the baseline control so that the baseline is approximately one third of the way up from the bottom of the display.
- Invert the spectral display to flip the waveform above the baseline. Note the reversal of the "+" and "−" indicators on the spectral display.
- Adjust the velocity scale so that the waveform fills most of the above-baseline display area without cutting off the peaks of the waveforms.
- Increase the Doppler gain to a level that is too high, filling in any "window" in the spectral waveform and introducing noise into the display.
- Acquire a hard copy, and label it "Doppler gain too high."
- Decrease the Doppler gain to the correct setting. Any window in the waveform should be clearly visible, and there should be no extraneous noise in the spectral display.
- Acquire a hard copy labeled "Correct Doppler gain."

OPTION #2

EXPLORE

- Choose a transducer suitable for cardiac imaging such as a 2.5–3.5 MHz sector with Doppler capability. Select an adult cardiac application preset.
- Obtain an apical five-chamber view.
- Select the pulsed-wave Doppler mode.
- Position the Doppler cursor in the left ventricular outflow tract with the sample volume immediately proximal to the aortic valve leaflets.
- Activate the spectral display to begin the Doppler interrogation of the aortic valve.
- Adjust the Doppler output power, if available, to a medium value.
- Increase or decrease the Doppler gain until the waveform appears at the correct brightness level (see Figure L11-4).
- Adjust the audio volume to an appropriate level.
- Adjust the baseline control so that the baseline is approximately in the middle of the spectral display.
- Invert the spectral display to observe the function of this control, and then invert again to return to the normal orientation.

DOCUMENT

- Choose a transducer suitable for cardiac imaging such as a 2.5–3.5 MHz sector with Doppler capability. Select an adult cardiac application preset.
- Obtain an apical five-chamber view as above.
- Select the pulsed-wave Doppler mode.
- Position the Doppler cursor within the left ventricular outflow tract so that the sample volume is immediately proximal to the aortic valve leaflets.

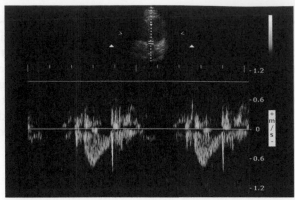

FIGURE L11-5 Spectral waveform of the aortic valve. Note that the flow is displayed below the baseline.

- Activate the spectral display to begin the Doppler interrogation of the aortic valve.
- Adjust the Doppler output power, if available, to a medium value.
- Adjust the audio volume to an appropriate level.
- Adjust the baseline control so that the baseline is approximately in the middle of the spectral display.
- Adjust the velocity scale so that the waveform fills most of the below-baseline (negative) display area, without cutting off the peaks of the waveforms. (Figure L11-5).
- Increase the Doppler gain to a level that is too high, filling in any window in the spectral waveform and introducing noise.
- Acquire a hard copy, and label it "Doppler gain too high."
- Decrease the Doppler gain to the correct setting. Any window in the waveform should be clearly visible, and there should be no extraneous noise in the spectral display.
- Acquire a hard copy labeled "Correct Doppler gain."

Doppler Controls 2

To understand the function and appropriate use of the following Doppler controls: sweep speed, wall filter, reject, Doppler transmit frequency, and update mode.

SWEEP SPEED

The *sweep speed* of the spectral display (Figure L12-1) may be adjusted to show more detail in each waveform (increased sweep speed) or multiple waveform cycles in each sweep (decreased sweep speed). For example, in a venous duplex examination of the lower extremity, a slow sweep speed is desirable because the venous response to several manual limb compressions can be

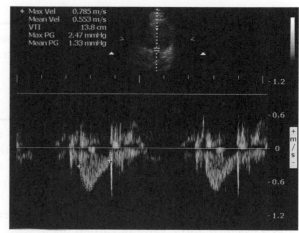

FIGURE L12-3 Rapid sweep speed showing more detailed tracing of the aortic valve waveform.

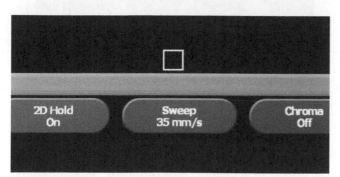

FIGURE L12-1 Adjustment of sweep speed control is by means of a "soft-key" on the console.

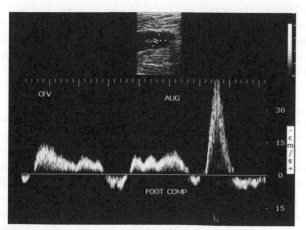

FIGURE L12-2 Slow sweep speed of the common femoral vein, which permits the documentation of manual limb compression and the resultant augmentation.

recorded in a single sweep (Figure L12-2). Conversely, in a carotid artery examination or an aortic valve evaluation with an echocardiogram, each waveform is expanded using high sweep speed for improved analysis of individual waveform characteristics and more accurate measurements (Figure L12-3).

WALL FILTER

Spectral data below a specific frequency set by the *wall filter* are removed from the waveform. Wall thump and other slow-motion Doppler artifacts are typically generated at frequencies below 100 hertz (Hz). Therefore, a wall filter setting of 100 Hz will eliminate these unwanted artifacts. However, at a too-high setting of the wall filter, slow-velocity flow information is also removed from the low-frequency portion of the waveform (Figure L12-4). This is usually an undesirable consequence and calls for the reduction of the wall filter to a lower frequency.

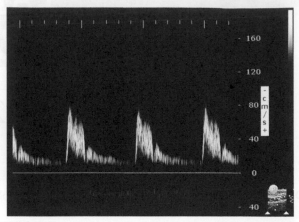

FIGURE L12-4 Example of wall filter set too high. Note the dark band just above the baseline where no information is displayed. The wall filter is set to 600 hertz (Hz).

REJECT

The *Doppler reject* control (rejection) eliminates low-amplitude signals to suppress noise in the spectral display.

DOPPLER TRANSMIT FREQUENCY

Some ultrasound systems allow the sonographer to change the *Doppler transmit frequency*. Lowering the Doppler transmit frequency is a useful technique to reduce aliasing by decreasing the Doppler shift frequency. A low Doppler transmit frequency can also be advantageous in evaluating difficult-to-penetrate areas such as a calcified aortic valve or carotid plaque.

UPDATE MODE

The Doppler pulse repetition frequency (PRF) dictates the highest velocity that can be displayed without aliasing (Nyquist limit). Operations that reduce the available Doppler PRF decrease the maximum velocity limit. Duplex scanning with "simultaneous" imaging plus Doppler requires that the imaging transmit pulses are interspersed with the Doppler pulses, effectively lowering the Doppler PRF. Acquisition is not really simultaneous but alternates back and forth between imaging and Doppler transmission. Switching to the *update mode* freezes the real-time B-mode image and allows the maximum Doppler PRF. The system then updates the B-mode image at regular intervals or whenever the update button is pushed.

PULSED-WAVE SAMPLE VOLUME SIZE (RANGE GATE)

As discussed in Lab 11, the *sample volume* is determined laterally by beam width and axially by the range gate aligned with the near and far sample boundaries. The size and position of the sample volume are denoted on

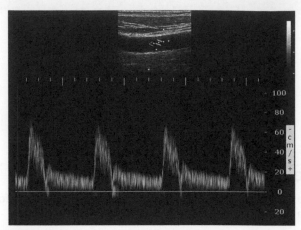

FIGURE L12-5 Small sample volume positioned in the center of the vessel.

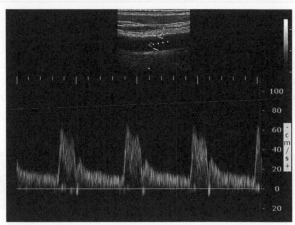

FIGURE L12-6 Large sample volume positioned to interrogate the entire cross-section of the vessel. Note the slightly broader spectral waveform than in Figure L12-5.

the display by a digitally superimposed "box" or double set of lines along the axis of the Doppler cursor. The size of the sample volume may be increased or decreased in the axial dimension, even though most duplex systems default to the smallest available sample size. The lateral dimension of the sample volume is fixed and cannot be changed. A large sample size can be used to improve sensitivity to flow or capture a wider flow profile (Figures L12-5 and L12-6).

HIGH-PRF MODE

The maximum Doppler PRF allowed at a given depth, and thus the Nyquist limit, is governed by the transit time required by each ultrasound pulse. As the depth of the sample volume is increased, the maximum Doppler PRF is reduced. Aliasing is far more likely when high-velocity flow at greater depths is encountered. An innovative method, called *high-PRF mode*, increases the Doppler PRF above the echo-ranging constraint to reduce the possibility of aliasing in this situation.

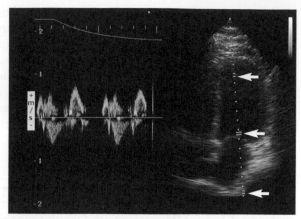

FIGURE L12-7 Apical four-chamber view in high-PRF mode. Note the primary sample volume (*middle arrow*) and two secondary sample volumes (*near and far arrows*). The Doppler waveform of the mitral valve (*left side of image*) was obtained from the primary sample. Note that the shallow secondary sample is positioned in the ventricular apex, where little flow is present and the deeper secondary sample is outside the heart altogether.

High PRF violates the basic tenet of range-resolution—that an ultrasound pulse is not transmitted until the echoes generated by the previous pulse have returned from the entire scan range. At a high Doppler PRF (e.g., twice the maximum Doppler PRF based on echo ranging), pulse transmission occurs before all the echoes have been received. Range ambiguity is introduced, and a second sampling area appears on screen. In most cases, by examining the positions of the two sample volumes compared with the anatomy on the screen, the origin of the high-velocity flow can be identified (Figure L12-7). At even higher Doppler PRFs, a third sample volume is displayed on the screen.

OPTION #1

EXPLORE

- Choose a transducer suitable for abdominal imaging such as a 3–5 MHz curvilinear array with Doppler capability. A sector in the same frequency range is also acceptable. Select an abdominal or abdominal vascular application preset.
- Obtain a sagittal image of the proximal abdominal aorta.
- Select the pulsed-wave Doppler mode.
- Angle the Doppler cursor toward the patient's head, thus creating an angle between the "Doppler beam" and the direction of flow in the artery. Use a heel-toe tilt of the transducer to add additional angle, if necessary, to achieve a Doppler angle to flow of approximately 60 degrees.
- Position the sample volume within the proximal abdominal aorta.
- Activate the spectral display to begin the Doppler interrogation of the proximal aorta.

- Optimize the gain, output power, velocity scale, and baseline of the spectral display.
- Decrease the sample volume size to the smallest dimension with the sample volume located in the center of the vessel lumen.
- Increase the sample volume size until it is equal to the diameter of the vessel. Note the increased fill-in of frequencies within the spectral window.
- Increase the Doppler reject control from the lowest to the maximum value. Note if true frequency information is eliminated from the waveform at the highest reject setting.
- Locate the update control. Switch back and forth between the live "simultaneous" imaging mode and the "frozen image" mode.
- While in the simultaneous mode, increase the velocity scale to the maximum value.
- Switch to the update mode, and again increase the velocity scale to the maximum value. The maximum velocity should be higher in the update mode than in the live simultaneous mode. Note that some instruments do not allow the system to increase the Doppler PRF above the maximum available in the simultaneous mode.

DOCUMENT

- Choose a transducer suitable for abdominal imaging such as a 3–5 MHz curvilinear array with Doppler capability. A sector in the same frequency range is also acceptable. Select an abdominal or abdominal vascular application preset.
- Obtain a sagittal image of the proximal abdominal aorta.
- Select the pulsed-wave Doppler mode.
- Angle the Doppler cursor toward the patient's head, thus creating an angle between the "Doppler beam" and the direction of flow in the artery. Use a heel-toe tilt of the transducer to add additional angle, if necessary, to achieve a Doppler angle to flow of approximately 60 degrees.
- Position the sample volume within the proximal abdominal aorta.
- Activate the spectral display to begin the Doppler interrogation of the proximal aorta.
- Optimize the gain, output power, velocity scale, and baseline of the spectral display.
- Locate the sweep speed control.
- Decrease the sweep speed to the lowest setting. Obtain a hard-copy image of the spectral display with the lowest sweep speed.
- Increase the sweep speed incrementally until the maximum setting is reached. Obtain a hard-copy image of the spectral display at the highest sweep speed.
- Note the default value for the wall filter (probably 50 or 100 Hz). Obtain a hard-copy image of the spectral display at the lowest wall filter setting.

- During live acquisition of the spectral Doppler, gradually increase the wall filter setting to the maximum setting. Obtain a hard-copy image of the spectral Doppler at the highest wall filter setting.
- Note the loss of low-frequency components, both in the audio signal and in the spectral display, at the highest wall filter setting.

OPTION #2

EXPLORE

- Choose a transducer suitable for cardiac imaging such as a 2.5–3.5 MHz sector with Doppler capability. Select an adult cardiac application preset.
- Obtain an apical four-chamber view.
- Select the pulsed-wave Doppler mode.
- Position the sample volume in the left ventricle, immediately beyond the mitral valve cusps.
- Activate the spectral display to begin the Doppler interrogation of the mitral valve inflow.
- Optimize the gain, output power, velocity scale, and baseline of the spectral display.
- Decrease the sample volume size to the smallest dimension. Note the narrow spectral waveform with the presence of a spectral window.
- Increase the sample volume size to 10 mm. Note the increased fill-in of frequencies within the spectral window.
- Increase the Doppler reject control from the lowest to the maximum value. Note whether true frequency information is eliminated from the waveform at the highest reject setting.
- While in the pulsed-wave Doppler mode, increase the velocity scale to the maximum value, and note the maximum velocity that can be displayed at that depth.
- With the Doppler cursor in the same position, switch to the continuous wave Doppler mode.

- As the Doppler samples along the full length of the line of sight, note the increase in flow information from the left ventricle and the left atrium. Also, note that the mitral valve flow pattern is still visible, even though some extraneous flow information is present.
- Increase the velocity scale to the maximum value in the continuous wave mode. Note the increased maximum velocity compared with that displayed in the pulsed-wave mode.

DOCUMENT

- Choose a transducer suitable for cardiac imaging such as a 2.5–3.5 MHz sector with Doppler capability. Select an adult cardiac application preset.
- Obtain an apical four-chamber view.
- Select the pulsed-wave Doppler mode.
- Position the sample volume in the right ventricle immediately beyond the tricuspid valve cusps.
- Activate the spectral display to begin the Doppler interrogation of the tricuspid valve inflow.
- Optimize the gain, output power, velocity scale, and baseline of the spectral display.
- Locate the sweep speed control.
- Decrease the sweep speed to the lowest setting. Obtain a hard-copy image of the spectral display at the lowest sweep speed.
- Increase the sweep speed incrementally until the maximum setting is reached. Obtain a hard-copy image of the spectral display at the highest sweep speed.
- Note the default value for the wall filter (probably 50 or 100 Hz). Acquire a video clip or a hard-copy image of the spectral display at the lowest wall filter setting.
- During live acquisition of the spectral Doppler, gradually increase the wall filter setting to the maximum value. Acquire a video clip or a hard-copy image of the spectral display at the highest wall filter setting.
- Note the loss of low-frequency components, both in the audio signal and in the spectral display, at the highest wall filter setting.

Doppler Angle to Flow

OBJECTIVES

1. To understand the relationship between the Doppler angle and the observed Doppler shift frequency.
2. To state the change in the Doppler signal for Doppler angles near 0 degrees, 60 degrees, and 90 degrees.
3. To be familiar with the methods to obtain a Doppler angle of 60 degrees or less, including machine controls and heel-toe probe maneuvers.
4. To understand the concept of "angle correction" and how to perform this function accurately.

DOPPLER ANGLE TO FLOW

The *Doppler angle to flow* (also commonly called *Doppler angle*) is a critical concept that must be understood to achieve a thorough working knowledge of Doppler ultrasound. The Doppler equation shows that the Doppler shift frequency is directly proportional to the cosine of the Doppler angle to flow (θ).

$$f_D = \frac{2vf}{c} \cos\theta$$

The Doppler angle is defined as the angle of the beam axis with respect to the direction of the moving reflector, in this case, red blood cells (Figure L13-1). The direction of the Doppler sound beam is indicated by the Doppler cursor. The Doppler angle to flow may be estimated by determining the angle between the Doppler cursor and a line parallel to the vessel walls or to the projected direction of flow within the heart. Alternatively, color flow imaging may identify the direction of flow more accurately. Defining the direction of flow in the vessels is much more important than defining the direction of flow in the heart due to differences in the angles of insonation.

The Doppler angle to flow must be determined correctly so that (1) an "adequate" Doppler angle (60 degrees or less) is attained and (2) flow velocity can be computed accurately by substituting a value for the angle θ into the Doppler equation. The sonographer must specify the angle by adjusting an *angle-correct* pointer on the screen to be parallel with the direction of flow. The concept of angle correction is used extensively in vascular applications but not in cardiac applications (discussed below).

The cosine of various angles shown in Table L13-1 demonstrates how the value for cos θ affects the Doppler shift frequency, f_D. The maximum Doppler shift occurs when the angle to flow is 0 degrees, where cos θ is equal to 1.0. The Doppler shift frequency decreases as the angle increases; at an angle of 60 degrees, the value for cos $\theta = 0.5$, and at an angle of 90 degrees the value for cos $\theta = 0$. With an angle to flow of 90 degrees, no Doppler shift occurs, and the transmitted frequency is equal to the received frequency (Figure L13-2).

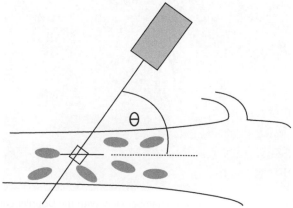

FIGURE L13-1 The Doppler angle to flow, shown here at approximately 60 degrees with the angle-correct indicator parallel to the vessel walls.

TABLE L13-1	Table of Values Representing Cos θ
Degrees	**Cos θ**
0	1.00
10	0.98
20	0.93
30	0.86
40	0.76
50	0.64
60	0.50
70	0.34
80	0.17
90	0.00

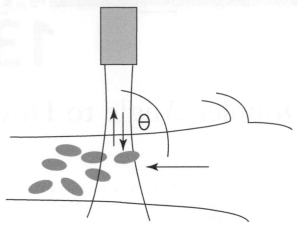

FIGURE L13-2 The Doppler angle to flow at 90 degrees. In this circumstance, cos θ is equal to zero, and no Doppler shift is observed.

Another important observation is the variation in cos θ with slight changes in Doppler angle to flow at orientations near 0 degrees compared with those near 60 degrees.

At 10 degrees, the Doppler angle to flow yields a value of 0.98 for cos θ compared with the value of 1.0 if the angle were reduced to 0 degrees. When the beam is near parallel to flow an error of 10 degrees in the estimation of the Doppler angle results in a 2% error in the calculation of flow velocity (angle is assumed to be 0 degrees but is really 10 degrees). Furthermore, an error of 20 degrees for Doppler angle to flow (angle is assumed to be 0 degrees but is really 20 degrees) produces a 7% error in the calculation of flow velocity (value for cos θ is 0.93).

The same comparisons for 10 degrees and 20 degrees offset to a true Doppler angle to flow of 60 degrees yield much higher errors in the velocity calculation. At 70 degrees, the cos θ value is equal to 0.34 compared with 0.50 for an angle of 60 degrees or a difference of 38%. At 80 degrees, the cos θ value is equal to 0.17 compared with 0.50 for an angle of 60 degrees or a difference of 66%.

Because of this angular dependence of the cosine function, the consideration of Doppler angle to flow in vascular and cardiac applications is fundamentally different. In vascular applications, Doppler angles near 60 degrees are most often used. The 60-degree angle has been found to be the most workable compromise between practical application and magnitude of Doppler shift. In most vascular applications, an angle of 60 degrees is readily obtained, whereas an angle of 0 degrees is not. However, when working with angles in the 60-degree range, the accurate estimation of the Doppler angle is critical, and the angle-correct pointer must be adjusted accordingly. Therefore, proper angle correction is mandatory in vascular applications (Figures L13-3 and L13-4).

Conversely, the majority of Doppler measurements in cardiac applications are performed with the sound beam parallel to the flow direction (Figure L13-5). The Doppler angle is assumed to be 0 degrees, even though in many instances it may be 10 degrees or even 20 degrees.

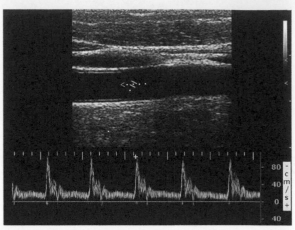

FIGURE L13-3 The Doppler angle at 60 degrees, with properly set angle correction. The peak systolic velocity is measured at 105 centimeters per second (cm/s).

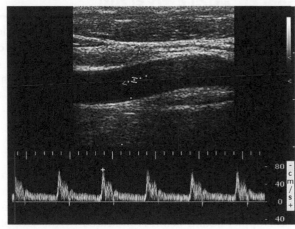

FIGURE L13-4 Doppler spectral analysis of the same vessel as Figure L13-3, with the angle correct improperly set to yield a Doppler angle to flow of 60 degrees, while actual Doppler angle to flow is closer to 70 degrees. Note the erroneously lower peak systolic velocity (74 centimeters per second [cm/s]).

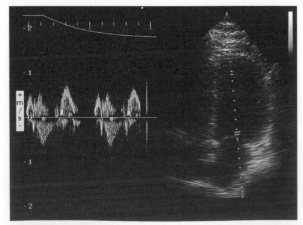

FIGURE L13-5 Apical four-chamber view with the Doppler cursor at 0 degrees, showing peak velocity measurement of the mitral valve inflow. Note the absence of the angle-correct device in the cardiac application.

As discussed above, the error in velocity measurement with an actual Doppler angle to flow of 20 degrees assumed to be 0 degrees is only about 7%. Therefore, cardiac sonographers rarely, if ever, use angle correction.

A Doppler angle to flow of 60 degrees or less may be obtained by (1) tilting the transducer using a heel-toe motion, (2) angling the Doppler cursor, or (3) using a combination of both these techniques. The Doppler cursor may be controlled with either the trackball or a separate knob or switch (Figure L13-6). The angle-correct control is usually a separate knob or switch. One manufacturer developed a unique system whereby the Doppler cursor automatically moves to maintain the 60-degree angle to flow as the angle-correct control is adjusted by the sonographer (Figures L13-7 and L13-8).

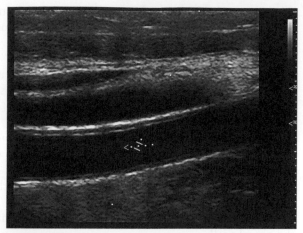

FIGURE L13-8 Heel-toe tilt of the transducer depicting the vessel at a slant across the display, facilitating the 60-degree Doppler angle to flow. Slight fine-tuning of the cursor angle results in a good Doppler angle.

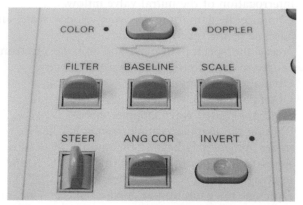

FIGURE L13-6 Doppler controls. Note the separate knobs for angle correct and cursor position or angle ("steer").

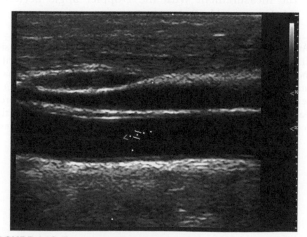

FIGURE L13-7 Without heel-toe tilt of the transducer, the initial transducer position is perpendicular to the vessel, making a 60-degree Doppler angle difficult to obtain.

OPTION #1

EXPLORE

- Choose a transducer suitable for vascular imaging such as a 7–10 MHz linear array. Select a carotid-vascular application preset.
- Obtain a sagittal image of the right common carotid artery with the vessel oriented horizontally across the screen (as in Figure L13-7).
- Select the pulsed-wave Doppler mode.
- Set the Doppler cursor so that the vessel is intersected at 90 degrees.
- Position the sample volume within the mid–common carotid artery (with the Doppler angle still at 90 degrees).
- Activate the spectral display. Note the poor quality of the Doppler signal at 90 degrees.
- With the spectral display active, gradually move the Doppler cursor from an angle of 90 degrees to 60 degrees.
- Note the improvement of the quality of the spectral display. Listen carefully to the audio to appreciate that the Doppler shift increases in frequency as the Doppler angle decreases.
- With the Doppler angle at 60 degrees, adjust the angle-correct indicator to be parallel to the vessel walls.
- Optimize the gain, output power, velocity scale, and baseline controls.
- Freeze the spectral display, and measure the peak systolic velocity with the electronic caliper.

DOCUMENT

- Choose a transducer suitable for vascular imaging such as a 7–10 MHz linear array. Select a carotid-vascular application preset.

- Obtain a sagittal image of the right common carotid artery, with the vessel oriented horizontally across the screen (as in Figure L13-7).
- Select the pulsed-wave Doppler mode.
- Using a heel-toe tilt of the transducer, obtain an image in which the more superior aspect of the vessel points to approximately 8 o'clock on the screen (as in Figure L13-8).
- Angle the Doppler cursor toward the patient's head, establishing a Doppler angle to the artery of 60 degrees.
- Position the sample volume within the center of the artery lumen.
- Adjust the angle-correct indicator to be parallel with the vessel walls.
- Activate the spectral display, and optimize the gain, output power, velocity scale, and baseline controls.
- Freeze the spectral display, and obtain a hard-copy image.
- Using a heel-toe tilt of the transducer, obtain an image in which the common carotid artery is angled away from the transducer in the opposite direction from the previous exercise.
- Angle the Doppler cursor toward the patient's feet, establishing a Doppler angle to the artery of 60 degrees.
- Position the sample volume within the center of the artery lumen.
- Adjust the angle-correct indicator to be parallel with the vessel walls.
- Activate the spectral display, and invert the spectrum so that the common carotid artery waveform appears above the baseline.
- Optimize the gain, output power, velocity scale, and baseline controls.
- Freeze the spectral display, and obtain a hard-copy image.

OPTION #2

EXPLORE

- Choose a transducer suitable for cardiac imaging such as a 2.5–3.5 MHz sector with Doppler capability. Select an adult cardiac application preset.
- Obtain an apical four-chamber view.
- Select the pulsed-wave Doppler mode.

- Position the Doppler sample volume in the left ventricle, immediately beyond the mitral valve cusps.
- Activate the spectral display to begin the Doppler interrogation of the mitral valve inflow.
- Optimize the gain, output power, velocity scale, and baseline of the spectral display.
- Freeze the spectral display, and use the electronic caliper to measure the peak systolic velocity.
- Obtain a parasternal long axis view (PLAX).

DOCUMENT

- Choose a transducer suitable for cardiac imaging such as a 2.5–3.5 MHz sector with Doppler capability. Select an adult cardiac application preset.
- Obtain an apical four-chamber view.
- Select the pulsed-wave Doppler mode.
- Position the Doppler sample volume in the left ventricle, immediately beyond the mitral valve cusps.
- Activate the spectral display to begin the Doppler interrogation of the mitral valve inflow.
- Optimize the gain, output power, velocity scale, and baseline of the spectral display.
- Freeze the spectral display, and use the electronic caliper to measure the peak systolic velocity.
- Obtain a hard-copy image.
- Obtain a (PLAX).
- Select the pulsed-wave Doppler mode.
- Position the Doppler sample volume in the left ventricle, immediately beyond the mitral valve cusps.
- Activate the spectral display to begin the Doppler interrogation of the mitral valve inflow.
- Optimize the gain, output power, velocity scale, and baseline of the spectral display.
- Freeze the spectral display, and use the electronic caliper to measure the peak systolic velocity.
- Obtain a hard-copy image.
- Note the difference in measured velocities between the measurement at an angle of 0 degrees, and the measurement with the Doppler angle between 45 degrees and 60 degrees.*

---

*Angle correction is not used in cardiac Doppler spectral analysis. The PLAX view is not suitable to quantify mitral flow velocity, since the relatively large Doppler angle to flow produces an inaccurate velocity measurement. In this lab, the purpose of the PLAX view is to demonstrate the effect of the Doppler angle on measured peak velocity, compared with the peak velocity measured when the Doppler angle is near 0 degrees as in the apical four-chamber view,

Nyquist Limit and Aliasing

OBJECTIVES

1. To understand the relationship between the Doppler pulse repetition frequency (PRF) and the maximum Doppler shift frequency that can be accurately displayed (Nyquist limit).

2. To investigate the effect of transmit frequency, Doppler angle to flow, blood flow velocity, sample depth, and simultaneous imaging mode on the presence or absence of aliasing.

DISCUSS

Aliasing is an artifact in pulsed-wave (PW) Doppler spectral analysis, in which ambiguous Doppler velocity information occurs when the Doppler shift frequency exceeds the Nyquist limit. Commonly, aliasing is expressed as a waveform whose uppermost portion is "cut off" and appears on the opposite side of the baseline (Figure L14-1). At a minimum, two Doppler transmit pulses are required for each cycle in order to accurately determine the Doppler shift frequency. Therefore, the Nyquist limit—denoting the maximum Doppler shift frequency that can be measured without aliasing—is equal to one-half of the Doppler pulse repetition frequency (PRF). For a Doppler shift frequency of 8 kilohertz (kHz), the PRF must be at least double that rate, or 16 kHz.

The factors that affect the instrument's ability to accurately analyze the Doppler signal generally fall into two categories: (1) those that affect the Doppler shift frequency and (2) those that affect the Doppler PRF.

FACTORS THAT AFFECT DOPPLER SHIFT FREQUENCY

Transmit Frequency

The Doppler transmit frequency is determined by the selected transducer and the transmit frequency range available in the Doppler mode. Note that the nominal frequency of a particular transducer refers only to the B-mode imaging frequency. For example, a transducer labeled as 6–10 MHz describes the range of imaging frequencies with no reference to the transmit frequency in the Doppler mode.

As mentioned in Lab 12, some ultrasound systems allow the sonographer to adjust the Doppler transmit frequency. Decreasing the Doppler transmit frequency correspondingly reduces the Doppler shift frequency, and this tactic becomes a potential method to eliminate aliasing (Figures L14-2 and L14-3). A low Doppler transmit frequency can also be useful for scanning difficult-to-penetrate areas, such as a calcified aortic valve or carotid plaque.

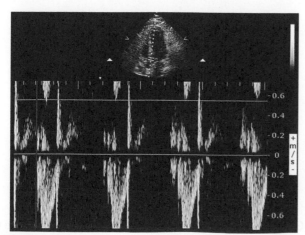

FIGURE L14-1 Spectral Doppler of aortic valve flow, which demonstrates aliasing.

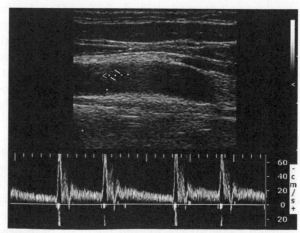

FIGURE L14-2 Aliasing with Doppler transmit frequency of 5.0 megahertz (MHz).

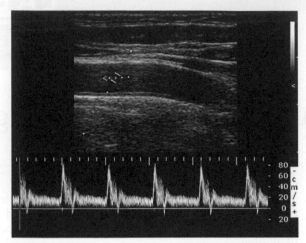

FIGURE L14-3 Doppler transmit frequency decreased to 3.8 megahertz (MHz), which eliminates the aliasing observed in Figure L14-2.

The control for Doppler transmit frequency may be labeled "transmit frequency" (when in the Doppler mode and located in the area reserved for Doppler controls or settings). The actual transmit frequency may be displayed, for example "3.5 MHz," or the transmit frequency settings may be indicated as "low–medium–high." Another possible scheme labels the Doppler transmit frequency as "penetration–resolution" or "penetration–normal–resolution" if two or three options are available.

Blood Flow Velocity

Blood flow velocity is obviously not under the control of the sonographer, but it is a very important consideration when working in the Doppler mode. At high velocity, the Doppler shift frequency is increased, and the operation choices (selection of transducers and equipment settings) become more limited.

Doppler Angle to Flow

The Doppler equation demonstrates that a steep Doppler angle (close to 0 degrees) yields the highest Doppler shift frequency from the sampled volume. In some circumstances, the sonographer has flexibility to adjust the Doppler angle. For example, an arterial stenosis can often be approached from various angles and insonation at a 60-degree angle has less likelihood for aliasing than does a 30-degree angle. In other situations, the sonographer has severe limitations in the manipulation of the Doppler angle.

In the heart, an aortic valve stenosis can generate velocities up to 6 meters per second (m/s) and must be insonated at an angle as close as possible to 0 degrees. In this case, the combination of very high velocity, the Doppler sound beam being parallel to flow (maximum value for cos θ), and relatively deep depth of the sample is an ideal recipe for aliasing. The only

solution that typically works is localizing the high-velocity valvular jet with color flow imaging and PW Doppler and then switching to continuous-wave (CW) Doppler in the duplex mode. Aliasing does not occur in CW Doppler, and thus, this Doppler mode has no limitation in representing high Doppler shift frequencies, which when encountered in PW Doppler produce ambiguous velocity information. Sonographers experienced in Doppler-only techniques with the CW Pitoff transducer may also choose to evaluate aortic stenosis by this method.

FACTORS THAT AFFECT DOPPLER PULSE REPETITION FREQUENCY

Velocity Scale and Baseline Controls

As the velocity scale is adjusted, the Doppler PRF and simultaneously the Nyquist limit are changed accordingly. The range of the velocity scale may be increased to reduce aliasing. However, if the velocity scale reaches the maximum and aliasing is still present, other options must be pursued. Aliasing may be eliminated by lowering (or raising, depending on the flow direction) the baseline, which partitions more (or all) of the available velocity scale to flow in that specific direction (Figure L14-4).

Depth

In order for PW Doppler to retain accurate range resolution, the transducer must delay the transmission of another Doppler pulse until echoes have returned from the sampling depth. This, of course, is true for imaging as well. The sampling depth is determined by the position (depth) of the sample volume. As the sampling depth is increased, the delay time between each pulse becomes longer, and, therefore, the maximum Doppler PRF is lower.

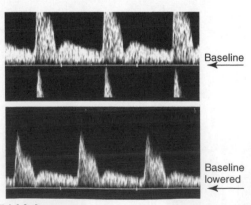

FIGURE L14-4 Spectral display showing adjustment of baseline to eliminate aliasing. With the low baseline, flow in the reverse direction is not displayed.

Sometimes, the patient or probe position can be manipulated to allow a shallower sampling depth. For example, optimizing the two-dimensional image of the carotid artery often requires increasing the distance between the transducer and the vessel. The image of a carotid artery may be best at a depth of 4 cm. However, when performing the Doppler portion of the examination, the transducer can often be positioned more anteriorly to decrease the depth of the vessel. This may result in a poorer B-mode image quality, but the shallower sample depth enables a higher Doppler PRF. In a high-velocity carotid stenosis, decreasing the depth in this way may be sufficient to eliminate aliasing.

Simultaneous Mode

As discussed in Lab 12, the simultaneous mode theoretically reduces the Doppler PRF by interspersing imaging, color flow imaging, or both with Doppler sampling. This can dramatically lower the Nyquist limit, depending on the instrument. The optimal duplex practice for most situations is to freeze the B-mode image during live Doppler acquisition, which preserves the quality of the B-mode image and, at the same time, ensures the maximum Doppler PRF.

OPTION #1

EXPLORE

- Choose a transducer suitable for vascular imaging such as a 7–10 MHz linear array. Select a carotid vascular application preset.
- Obtain a sagittal image of the right common carotid artery. Select the PW Doppler mode.
- Use a heel-toe tilt of the transducer, and angle the Doppler cursor toward the patient's head to obtain a Doppler angle to flow of 60 degrees within the distal common carotid artery.
- Position the sample volume within the center of the lumen.
- With the Doppler angle at 60 degrees, adjust the angle-correct indicator to be parallel to the vessel walls.
- Activate the spectral display to begin the Doppler interrogation of the distal common carotid artery. Select the invert function, if necessary, to position the waveform above the baseline.
- Optimize gain, output power, and audio volume.
- Position the baseline one third of the way up from the bottom of the spectral display.
- Set the velocity scale at 30 centimeters per second (cm/s). Observe the aliasing of the signal.
- Gradually increase the velocity scale until the systolic peak is clearly displayed within the upper boundary of the display and no evidence of aliasing is present.

DOCUMENT

- Choose a transducer suitable for vascular imaging such as a 7–10 MHz linear array. Select a carotid vascular application preset.
- Obtain a sagittal image of the right common carotid artery. Select the PW Doppler mode.
- Use a heel-toe tilt of the transducer, and angle the Doppler cursor toward the patient's feet to obtain a Doppler angle to flow of 60 degrees within the proximal common carotid artery.
- Position the sample volume within the center of the lumen.
- With the Doppler angle at 60 degrees, adjust the angle-correct indicator to be parallel to the vessel walls.
- Activate the spectral display to begin the Doppler interrogation of the proximal common carotid artery. Select the invert function, if necessary, to position the waveform above the baseline.
- Optimize gain, output power, and audio volume.
- Position the baseline one third of the way up from the bottom of the spectral display.
- Set the velocity scale so that the waveform is accurately displayed with the systolic peak just within the upper limit of the velocity scale. The waveform should fill approximately three fourths of the available area in the display.
- Locate the Doppler transmit frequency control. Adjust the Doppler frequency to the highest value.
- Obtain a spectral tracing of the common carotid artery, and freeze the spectral display.
- Using electronic calipers, measure the peak systolic velocity.
- Obtain a hard-copy image.
- Obtain a spectral waveform at the lowest Doppler transmit frequency setting.
- Using electronic calipers, measure the peak systolic velocity.
- Obtain a hard-copy image.
- Note the differences in the apparent heights of the spectral peaks and the frequencies (pitch) of the audio signals. The velocity measurements should be the same because the instrument compensates for the change in transmit frequency in the calculation of flow velocity.

OPTION #2

EXPLORE

- Choose a transducer suitable for cardiac imaging such as a 2.5–3.5 MHz sector with Doppler capability. Select an adult cardiac application preset.
- Obtain an apical four-chamber view.
- Select the PW Doppler mode.

- Position the Doppler cursor in the left ventricular outflow tract, with the sample volume just proximal to the aortic valve cusps (see Figure L14-1).
- Activate the spectral display to begin the Doppler interrogation of the aortic valve.
- Optimize gain, output power, and audio volume.
- Adjust the baseline so that it is in the center of the spectral display. The aortic valve waveform should be on the bottom half of the display (negative direction).
- Set the velocity scale to approximately 0.6 meters per second (m/s) in either direction or until aliasing occurs.
- Move the baseline in the positive direction (up) to allow more of the available velocity scale to be dedicated to flow away from the transducer (negative direction).
- Observe the decrease or elimination of aliasing on the display.

DOCUMENT

- Choose a transducer suitable for cardiac imaging such as a 2.5–3.5 MHz sector with Doppler capability. Select an adult cardiac application preset.
- Obtain an apical four-chamber view.
- Select the PW Doppler mode.

- Position the Doppler cursor in the left ventricle, with the sample volume in the left ventricle immediately beyond the mitral valve cusps.
- Activate the spectral display to begin the Doppler interrogation of the mitral valve inflow.
- Optimize the gain, output power, velocity scale, and baseline of the spectral display.
- Locate the Doppler transmit frequency control. Adjust the Doppler frequency to the highest value.
- Obtain a spectral tracing of the aortic valve flow, and freeze the spectral display.
- Using electronic calipers, measure the peak systolic velocity of the aortic waveform.
- Obtain a hard-copy image.
- Obtain a spectral waveform at the lowest Doppler transmit frequency setting. (If this control is not available in the cardiac PW preset, switch to the CW mode to perform this exercise.)
- Using electronic calipers, again measure the peak systolic velocity.
- Obtain a hard-copy image.
- Note the differences in the apparent heights of the spectral peaks and the frequencies (pitch) of the audio signals. The velocity measurements should be the same because the instrument compensates for the change in transmit frequency in the calculation of flow velocity.

Color Doppler Controls: Part 1

OBJECTIVES

1. To understand the similarities and differences between color flow imaging and pulsed-wave spectral Doppler.
2. To recognize the qualitative nature of color flow imaging and the inherent limitation in translating Doppler shift frequency to velocity.
3. To obtain an adequate color angle to flow.
4. To be familiar with the following color Doppler controls: color region of interest box, color gain, color velocity scale, color baseline, packet size, color map invert, and color frequency.

DISCUSS

Color flow imaging detects and displays blood flow velocity within a two-dimensional area defined by the *color box* or the *color ROI* (region of interest). The color flow information is superimposed on the two-dimensional B-mode image to depict blood flow within the borders of vessels or within the heart (Figure L15-1). The effective use of color flow imaging requires a thorough understanding of the relationship among B-mode imaging, color flow imaging, and pulsed-wave (PW) spectral Doppler. Although color flow imaging is fundamentally a method to show the Doppler frequency information, the process differs appreciably from that of spectral Doppler and is considered a third "modality." The modalities of B-mode imaging, color flow imaging, and PW spectral Doppler each have strengths and weaknesses.

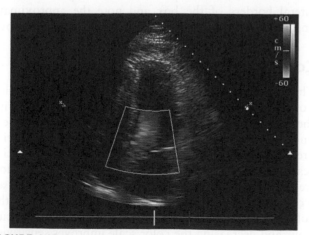

FIGURE L15-1 Apical five-chamber view of the heart obtained with a 3 MHz sector transducer. The color region-of-interest (ROI) box defines the portion of the 2D field of view for the color display (see Color Plate 1).

Multiple transmit pulses are required for each *color scan line* to measure the Doppler shift frequencies for reflectors at different depths along that scan line. The flow information is collected by a detection method called *phase shift autocorrelation*. Because autocorrelation slows the frame rate considerably, the ROI or the color box defines a subdivision of the 2D field of view (FOV) for color flow imaging. Color display does not encompass the entire screen but is restricted to a small region so that frame rate can be maintained. Blood flow within the ROI is depicted as shades of red or blue or multiple hues (violet, blue, green, yellow, orange, and red). In the red–blue scheme, the dark shades represent low Doppler shift frequencies, and the light shades (color saturation to white) represent high Doppler shift frequencies.

One of the pitfalls of color flow imaging is that the color for each pixel codes for a single metric, usually the mean Doppler shift frequency, which is converted to velocity without taking the Doppler angle into consideration. Recall that the Doppler angle and transmit frequency affect the Doppler shift frequency. A curved vessel within the color box presents different Doppler angles to the Doppler beam (sampling direction and flow do not maintain the same angular orientation along the vessel). Since angle correction is not applied, color flow imaging is qualitative and not quantitative in nature (Figure L15-2).

Color flow imaging depicts global flow over a relatively large two-dimensional area. Flow along the length of a vessel, as well as complex vasculature, can be demonstrated. One of the most important applications of color flow imaging is to identify regions of high-velocity flow, turbulence, or suspected absence of flow so that these may be further evaluated with spectral Doppler.

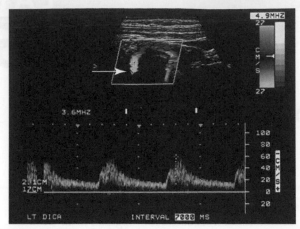

FIGURE L15-2 Linear array image with the color box showing increased brightness where the color angle to flow approaches 0 degrees (*arrow*). Spectral Doppler with angle correction shows correct flow velocity (see Color Plate 2).

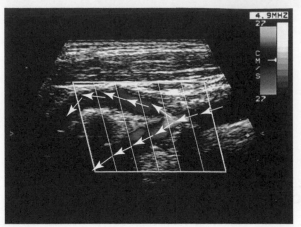

FIGURE L15-3 Linear array color flow image with color region-of-interest (ROI) box, which shows color angle to flow at the edges of the box and imaginary lines parallel to the color scan lines.

Color Field of View

The size of the color box or of the ROI, the *position (left-right)*, and *depth* are typically controlled by the trackball and a three-way selector switch that sequentially activates each function. To maximize the frame rate, the size of the color box should be kept reasonably small, setting the optimal width to include the organ of interest and no larger.

Color Box Angle or Steering

Color angle to flow is an important concept, which must be applied to properly interpret the color display. In cardiac applications, the color box is not "steered" (angled off-axis to the B-mode sound beam). This is typically true of any sector-type transducer. Color angle to flow is established by defining the probe position relative to the direction of flow as well as by positioning the cursor box to the left or right on the display. In other applications, the ROI box may be steered to the left or right by turning a knob to vary the steering angle in small increments or by selecting one of a fixed set of angles such as "Left," "Right," or "Center" (straight down).

One of the challenges of color flow imaging is to find out the approximate angle to flow so that color data may be obtained and interpreted. Color angle to flow close to 90 degrees produces no color, while a very steep angle (close to 0 degrees) results in very light shades of color that may be misinterpreted as high-velocity flow. A relatively simple method to determine the approximate color angle to flow is examining the apparent direction of flow with respect to the lateral borders of the ROI box (Figures L15-3 and L15-4). Although the angle to flow for a given vessel may change within the color box, the borders of the box create a starting point for angle estimation. For more precise assessment, the sonographer should mentally "draw" imaginary lines

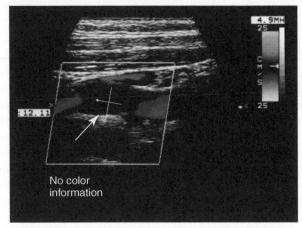

FIGURE L15-4 Linear array color flow image with color region-of-interest (ROI) box. A perpendicular color angle to flow in the center of the box shows an area of no color (*arrow*). Color flow is observed near the box edges where an adequate angle to flow exists (see Color Plate 3).

across the box, from top to bottom, and parallel to the lateral borders of the box and note the approximate angle at which each line intersects the direction of flow.

Color Velocity Scale

The *color velocity scale* is incorporated into the color flow display and is shown as the color scale bar with the maximum velocity indicated (in centimeters per second [cm/s]). Velocities less than the maximum velocity are shown without *color aliasing*. The color velocity scale is sometimes referred to as *color* pulse repetition frequency (PRF) because a change in this control causes a corresponding change in the color scale. Increasing the color scale enhances the ability to display high-velocity flow, and decreasing the color scale improves sensitivity to slow flow (Figures L15-5 to L15-7).

Color aliasing occurs when the flow velocity exceeds the Nyquist limit established by the color sampling rate.

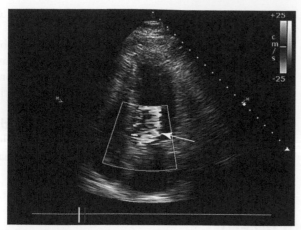

FIGURE L15-5 Color aliasing creates a "mosaic pattern" (*arrow*) that helps draw the viewer's eye to the high-velocity flow (see Color Plate 4).

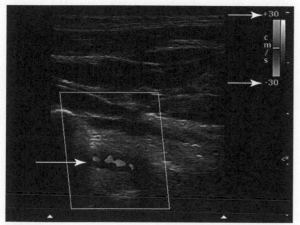

FIGURE L15-6 Color scale set to +/– 30 centimeters per second (cm/s) (*small arrows*). Note the poorly displayed color flow within the vertebral artery (*large arrow*) (see Color Plate 5).

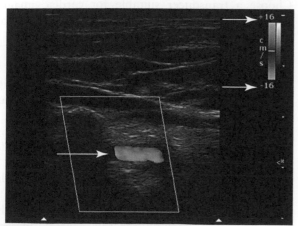

FIGURE L15-7 Color scale decreased to +/– 16 centimeters per second (cm/s) (*small arrows*). Note the color flow within the vertebral artery (*large arrow*) is more uniform than in Figure L15-6 (see Color Plate 6).

Because color flow imaging requires more pulses than does PW Doppler (resulting in a low color PRF per scan line), aliasing is unavoidable in many situations. This is especially true in the heart, where even normal velocities may cause color aliasing. However, aliasing is not considered a significant problem because color flow imaging does not provide a quantitative measurement of velocity. In fact, color aliasing creates a unique appearance, often referred to as a "mosaic pattern," which helps draw the viewer's attention to high-velocity flow patterns (see Figure L15-5).

Color Map Invert

The orientation of the color bar indicates the assignment of colors to positive and negative flow directions. The color at the top of the bar is assigned to depict flow toward the transducer. Flow in the opposite direction is represented by colors in the bottom half of the bar. A pair of acronyms can assist the sonographer to remember the red–blue color schemes: BART stands for "blue away, red toward," and RABT stands for "red away, blue toward." The *color map invert* control reverses the colors on the color scale bar as well as the colors where flow is present. This inversion may be applied to preferentially show the vessel or cardiac structure as red or blue.

Color Baseline

Color baseline, like the baseline in the spectral Doppler, defines the transition point between flow in the positive direction and flow in the negative direction. The red and blue colors on the color bar are separated by a thin, black line. The color baseline may be shifted toward the positive or negative flow direction, allocating more of the available color velocity scale to that flow direction.

Color Gain

The *color gain* control amplifies the color signals to increase the likelihood of a pixel being encoded in color. Color gain that is too low does not adequately "fill" the vessel. Color gain that is too high causes the occurrence of *color bleed artifact*, whereby the color extends outside the borders of the vessel or heart chamber (see Figure L15-8).

Packet Size or Ensemble Length

As discussed above, multiple transmit pulses are required for each color scan line. The group of pulses transmitted along a single color scan line is referred to as *packet* or *ensemble*. The number of pulses in the group is called *packet size* or *ensemble length*. A large packet size improves the accuracy of the Doppler shift

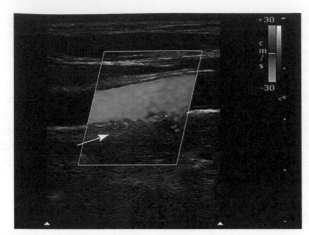

FIGURE L15-8 Color gain set too high, which causes color bleed outside the vessel walls (*arrow*) (see Color Plate 7).

frequency assessment, but with a resultant loss of temporal resolution (decreased frame rate). On some scanners, the sonographer can adjust the packet size. The optimal packet size for a given situation is a trade-off between accurate determination of Doppler shift frequency and temporal resolution.

Color Transmit Frequency

Some instruments allow the sonographer to vary the *color transmit frequency*. A lower color transmit frequency decreases the Doppler shift frequency, thereby reducing the potential for color aliasing. A low color transmit frequency can also be useful for evaluating difficult-to-penetrate areas such as a calcified aortic valve or carotid plaque.

OPTION #1

EXPLORE

*   Choose a transducer suitable for vascular imaging such as a 7–10 MHz linear array. Select a carotid artery preset.
*   Obtain a sagittal image of the right common carotid artery. Select the color flow imaging mode.
*   Angle the color ROI box cranially.
*   Use a heel-toe tilt of the transducer toward the patient's head to create an adequate color angle to flow within the distal common carotid artery.
*   Invert the color map, if necessary, so that flow within the common carotid artery is displayed as red.
*   Increase the color gain until color bleed occurs outside the vessel.
*   Decrease the color gain just until the color bleed disappears. This is the optimal color gain setting.
*   Set the color velocity scale to approximately 30 cm/s. Decrease the color velocity scale to 15 cm/s and then

to 10 cm/s. Note the difference in appearance of color within the vessel as color aliasing occurs.
*   Locate the control for packet size (or ensemble length) if your machine has this control. Increase packet size, and note the degradation in temporal resolution. Return the packet size control to the default value.
*   Activate the color box size controls, and use the trackball to adjust the height and width of the color box. Note the effect on frame rate by large and small sizes of the color box.

DOCUMENT

*   Choose a transducer suitable for abdominal imaging such as a 3–5 MHz curvilinear array. Select an abdominal vascular preset.
*   Obtain a sagittal image to the right of mid-line imaging the proximal inferior vena cava (IVC) and the liver. Select the color flow imaging mode.
*   Angle the color ROI box superiorly to create an adequate color angle to flow within the proximal IVC.
*   Invert the color map, if necessary, so that the flow within the IVC is displayed as blue.
*   Optimize the color gain.
*   Increase the color PRF to +/– 50 cm/s. Note the decrease or absence of color flow within the IVC.
*   Obtain a hard-copy image.
*   Decrease the color PRF to +/– 20 cm/s.
*   Optimize the color gain.
*   Obtain a hard-copy image.

OPTION #2

EXPLORE

*   Choose a transducer suitable for cardiac imaging such as a 2.5–3.5 MHz sector with Doppler capability. Select an adult cardiac preset.
*   Obtain an apical five-chamber view.
*   Optimize the gray-scale image.
*   Select the color flow imaging control, and position the color box in the region of the left ventricular outflow tract (LVOT) and the aortic valve.
*   Set the color scale to +/– 60 cm/s.
*   Increase the color gain control until obvious color bleed occurs in surrounding tissue.
*   Decrease the color gain just until the color bleed disappears. This is the optimal color gain setting.
*   Locate the control for packet size (or ensemble length) if your machine has this control. Increase packet size, and note the degradation in temporal resolution. Return the packet size control to the default value.

- Activate the color box size controls, and use the trackball to adjust the height and width of the color box. Note the effect on frame rate by large and small sizes of the color box.

DOCUMENT

- Choose a transducer suitable for cardiac imaging such as a 2.5–3.5 MHz sector with Doppler capability. Select an adult cardiac preset.
- Obtain an apical five-chamber view.
- Optimize the gray-scale image.

- Select the color flow imaging control and position the color box in the region of the LVOT and the aortic valve.
- Set the color scale to +/– 60 cm/s.
- Optimize the color gain.
- Acquire a video clip or a hard-copy image to show the color flow of the aortic valve and the LVOT.
- Decrease the color scale to +/– 25 cm/s, and observe the color aliasing.
- Acquire a video clip or a hard-copy image to demonstrate the color aliasing of the aortic valve flow.

LAB

16

Color Doppler Controls: Part 2

OBJECTIVE

To understand the function and application of the color Doppler controls: color priority, color map, color persistence, color line density, and color wall filter.

DISCUSS

In Lab 15, color flow imaging controls related to the acquisition of color data were studied. The controls that manipulate the display of color flow data, including color priority, color map, color persistence, color line density, and color wall filter, are examined in this Lab.

Color Priority

In color flow imaging, the ultrasound system must assess whether a given pixel will be displayed in gray-scale (no flow) or color (flow). The presence or absence of a Doppler shift frequency for that pixel is the primary determinant of color or gray assignment. The *color priority* control (Figure L16-1) increases the likelihood of a color being assigned to the pixel by shifting the emphasis toward blood flow. This primarily affects the returning echoes that contain minimal frequency shift information, which borders the system's cut-off point for flow or no flow.

Color Map

Similar to the gray-scale map in B-mode imaging, the *color map* assigns flow velocities to various shades of

red, blue, white, and black. Maps consisting of rainbow hues also encode flow information. Typically 10 to 15 different color maps are available. Some accentuate brighter colors; others emphasize slow or fast velocity flow. The *color variance map* displays the velocity distribution, rather than the mean velocity, within a given pixel.

Ultimately, color map selection is a matter of personal preference of the sonographer or physician viewing the studies. System presets specify default maps for specific applications based on the experience of multiple users.

Color Persistence

Color persistence averages color flow data in successive frames in a similar fashion to that of B-mode frame averaging. However, the result of color frame averaging is somewhat different. For 2D real-time frame averaging, the goal is to minimize noise by superimposing several frames of nearly identical composition. For best results, the organ(s) must remain relatively stationary. In color frame averaging, the blood flow changes from frame to frame, so this type of comparison between frames does not work very well. Instead, color persistence is employed to give a smoother appearance to blood flow. With frame averaging turned completely off, the color flow image often has a grainy and very transient appearance.

Slight frame averaging prolongs the color flow events on the screen and smoothes out the flow. This allows the sonographer to better appreciate the extent of a mitral valve regurgitant jet or a high-velocity carotid artery stenosis. Color persistence can obviously be excessive and lead to an inconsistency of color flow information. Also, as frame averaging is more pronounced, the temporal resolution is degraded. System presets include default values for color persistence based on specific examinations. These can also be adjusted according to sonographer preference.

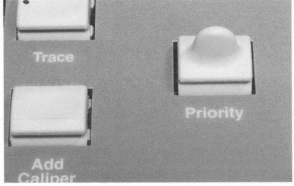

FIGURE L16-1 Console showing the color priority selection switch.

152

Copyright © 2013 by Mosby, an imprint of Elsevier Inc.

Color Line Density

Color flow imaging frame rate is affected by multiple factors such as *color line density*, which determines the length of time required for each frame. Increased color line density improves color lateral resolution; however, the acquisition time to complete each frame is more prolonged. Again, system presets include default values for color line density based on specific examinations. On some systems, color line density can be adjusted by the sonographer.

Color Wall Filter

Doppler frequencies below a specific frequency set by the *color wall filter* are eliminated from the color flow image. These low frequencies tend to represent slow-moving structures such as vessel walls and heart muscle. In most circumstances, colors generated from these structures would be considered artifactual. Wall-motion artifacts appear on the display if the color wall filter setting is too low (Figure L16-2). A too-high setting eliminates actual flow information.

OPTION #1

EXPLORE

- Choose a transducer suitable for vascular imaging such as a 7–10 MHz linear array. Select a carotid vascular preset.
- Obtain a sagittal image of the right common carotid artery.
- Enter color flow imaging mode, and center the color region-of-interest (ROI) box over the distal common carotid artery. Angle (steer) the box toward the patient's head.

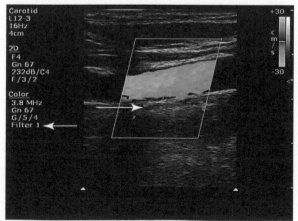

FIGURE L16-2 Color wall filter set on the lowest setting (*small arrow*) resulting in color wall motion artifact (*large arrow*) (see Color Plate 8).

- Use a heel-toe tilt of the transducer toward the patient's head to create an adequate color angle to flow within the distal common carotid artery.
- Invert the color map, if necessary, so that flow within the common carotid artery is displayed as red.
- Optimize the color gain and color scale.
- Locate the color persistence control. Turn the control to the maximum setting, and observe the "smeary" appearance of the color in the vessel. Now, turn the control to the minimum setting, and observe the grainy appearance of the color display. Finally, increase persistence to the optimal value.
- Locate the color line density control. Increase color line density until the maximum is reached. Observe changes in the color frame rate. Now, turn the control back to the minimum value. Again, observe the changes in frame rate and the quality of the color display.
- Locate the control for color map selection. Note the current map number (or letter). Select different color maps, and observe the differences in the color flow images. Return to the default color map.

DOCUMENT

- Choose a transducer suitable for vascular imaging such as a 7–10 MHz linear array. Select a carotid vascular preset.
- Obtain a sagittal image of the left common carotid artery.
- Enter color flow imaging mode, and center the color ROI box over the proximal common carotid artery. Angle (steer) the box toward the patient's feet.
- Use a heel-toe tilt of the transducer toward the patient's feet to create an adequate color angle to flow within the proximal common carotid artery.
- Invert the color map, if necessary, so that flow within the common carotid artery is displayed as red.
- Optimize the color gain and color scale.
- Locate the color wall filter control. Decrease color wall filter to the lowest setting. Note any color wall motion artifact produced. Obtain a hard-copy image at this setting.
- Increase the color wall filter to the maximum value. Note any loss of actual flow information that occurs. Obtain a hard-copy image at this setting.

OPTION #2

EXPLORE

- Choose a transducer suitable for cardiac imaging such as a 2.5–3.5 MHz sector with Doppler capability. Select an adult cardiac preset.
- Obtain an apical four-chamber view.
- Enter color flow imaging mode, and center the ROI box over the mitral valve inflow.

- Optimize the color gain and color scale.
- Locate the color persistence control. Turn color persistence to the maximum setting, and observe the "smeary" appearance of the color. Now, turn the control to the lowest setting, and observe the grainy appearance of the color display. Finally, increase persistence to the optimal value.
- Locate the color line density control. Increase color line density until the maximum is reached. Observe the changes in the color frame rate. Now, turn the control back to the minimum value. Again, observe the changes in frame rate and the quality of the color display.
- Locate the control for color map selection. Note the current map number (or letter). Select different color maps, and observe the differences in the color flow images. Return to the default color map.

DOCUMENT

- Choose a transducer suitable for cardiac imaging such as a 2.5–3.5 MHz sector with Doppler capability. Select an adult cardiac preset.
- Obtain an apical five-chamber view.
- Select the color flow imaging mode. Center the color ROI box over the left ventricular outflow tract (LVOT) and the aortic valve.
- Optimize the color gain and color scale.
- Locate the color wall filter control. Decrease color wall filter to the lowest setting. Note any color wall motion artifact produced. Acquire a video clip or a hard-copy image at this setting.
- Increase the color wall filter to the maximum value. Note any loss of actual flow information that occurs. Acquire a video clip or a hard-copy image at this setting.

Application Presets

OBJECTIVES

1. To understand the purpose and function of application presets.

2. To appreciate the differences between the default values for various presets.

DISCUSS

In Labs 1 through 16, many parameters of a diagnostic ultrasound system and the methods by which they are applied in clinical practice were considered. In this Lab, *application presets*, which are now available on virtually every ultrasound system, are examined. Application presets are formulated to create a practical, initial starting point for each examination.

Essentially the same scanner controls are manipulated during sonographic examination of the liver, kidneys, heart, carotid arteries, uterus and ovaries, leg veins, neonatal brain, fetus, breast, and thyroid gland. However, the settings of these controls vary significantly, depending on the type of examination. It may be a fluid-filled organ such as the gallbladder or homogeneous tissue such as the spleen. The structures may be stationary or rapidly moving. Often, the sound beam must first pass through the chest wall or the abdominal wall or a full urinary bladder. At times, the sonographer must scan between ribs or through the bone of the skull or image 1 cm beneath the skin surface. In each of these situations, a common set of hardware choices and control settings is available, which will be similar for each occurrence of that particular type of examination. This group of settings becomes the default for that specific application preset.

An ultrasound examination of an adult heart can be considered as an example. Requirements for imaging this organ include scanning between ribs (sector transducer), a relatively low-frequency transducer to penetrate the chest wall, harmonic imaging, high frame rate for B-mode imaging, and color flow imaging. Settings for sector width, persistence, number of focal zones, simultaneous imaging Doppler, color map, color scale, color persistence, and more are required. The heart is a heterogeneous organ which comprises muscular walls and fluid-filled chambers, which necessitates a unique time gain compensation (TGC) curve.

As another example, consider a gynecologic examination. The transducer must provide a medium-sized field of view (FOV) (curvilinear array), and the sound beam must penetrate the abdominal wall, including fat layers (influences the choice of transmit frequency). The beam path includes the full urinary bladder, where very little attenuation occurs. The organs of interest lie deep within the pelvis, so excellent detail at a deep scan depth (focal depth) is required. A high frame rate is not required (allowing increased frame averaging and multiple transmit foci). A wide FOV is needed near the transducer to evaluate the anterior bladder wall (a sector would not be the ideal choice). For this examination, the choice of transducer, TGC, transmit frequency, persistence, number of focal zones, color settings, and others would be very different from those for the examination of the heart described above.

Default values for each application preset are installed at the time of manufacture. Typically, an ultrasound machine is pre-programmed with a generic listing of common examinations with corresponding subsets. Default values for each preset represent typical values for each control, tailored to each type of examination. Most ultrasound systems allow user-programmable application presets. For example, if the sonographer prefers to begin an abdominal examination with a different display depth, he or she can create a new preset (with a different name) employing the new depth setting. Multiple sonographers can each configure his or her own presets, as desired.

Within each type of examination, control settings vary from patient to patient on the basis of age, size, weight, body habitus, and disease process. Therefore, the application preset is only a starting point. The sonographer must either confirm the correct settings or make adjustments in the controls, as necessary, to produce the optimal image. Often, these controls must be adjusted frequently as the transducer is moved into different scan planes during the course of the actual examination.

Typically, the examination preset selection control (Figures L17-1 and L17-2) generates a hierarchical drop-down menu listing the top level of examination

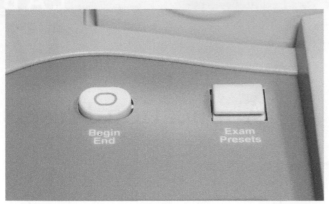

FIGURE L17-1 System controls for the selection of new examination and examination presets.

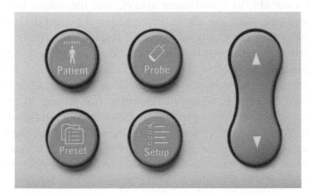

FIGURE L17-2 System controls for the selection of new examination and examination presets from a different manufacturer.

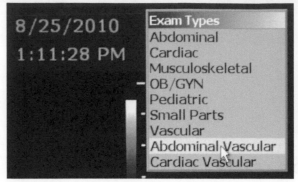

FIGURE L17-3 Top level drop-down menu for general preset selection.

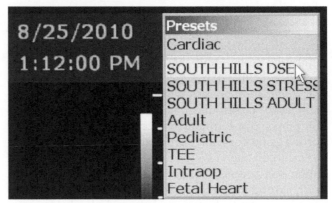

FIGURE L17-4 Secondary menu listing the subset of examination types under the selected main category. Note that the top three listings in capital letters represent user-generated custom application presets.

presets. The general examination type is then selected from a list of available examination presets (Figure L17-3). After selection of the top level examination category, a secondary menu lists the subset of examination types (Figure L17-4).

OPTION #1

EXPLORE

- Choose a transducer suitable for abdominal imaging such as a 3–5 MHz curvilinear array. Select an examination preset for abdominal imaging.
- Obtain a sagittal image of the right hepatic lobe and the right kidney.
- Without adjusting any controls, note the default values for the following:
  - Output power
  - Dynamic range
  - Gray-scale map
  - Number of focal zones
  - Persistence or frame averaging
  - Harmonic imaging on or off
  - Display depth
- Again, without adjusting any controls, activate the color flow imaging.
- Note the preset values for the following:
  - Color velocity scale
  - Color gain
  - Color persistence
  - Color map
  - Color region-of-interest (ROI) box size

DOCUMENT

Create a table to record the default values. The worksheet should contain 7 columns and 10 rows (not including the row for column headings).

The table should look something like this:

Preset Name	# Focal Zones	Display Depth	Transmit Frequency	2D-Dimensional Persistence	Color Scale	Color Persistence

Select five different general preset categories. For each category, choose two subcategories. For example, choose the "abdomen" heading, which may contain four or five subcategories. A different probe may be required for certain categories. If that is the case, select the appropriate transducer from one category to the next.

Select two of the subcategories under each general category, such as "liver" and "aorta" (under abdomen). Record the default values for each control listed in the table. After recording the values for the four B-mode controls, activate the color flow imaging mode, and record the values for the two color controls. When you are finished, you should have characterized 10 application presets. Compare the values for the different presets, and consider the specific requirements of each type of examination, which would affect the specific control values. For example, what is the default value for B-mode transmit frequency for a renal examination compared with B-mode transmit frequency for a gynecologic examination? What is the reason for the difference?

OPTION #2

EXPLORE

- Choose a transducer suitable for adult cardiac imaging such as a 2.5–3.5 MHz sector. Select an examination preset for adult cardiac imaging.

- Obtain a sagittal long axis view of the heart.
- Without adjusting any controls, note the default values for the following:
  - Sector display width
  - Output power
  - Dynamic range
  - Gray-scale map
  - Number of focal zones
  - Persistence or frame averaging
  - Harmonic imaging on or off
  - Display depth
- Again, without adjusting any controls, activate color flow imaging.
- Note the preset values for the following:
  - Color velocity scale
  - Color gain
  - Color persistence
  - Color map
  - Color ROI box size

DOCUMENT

Create a table to record the default values. The worksheet should contain 7 columns and 10 rows (not including the row for column headings).

The table should look something like this:

Preset Name	# Focal Zones	Display Depth	Transmit Frequency	B-mode Persistence	Color Scale	Color Persistence

Select the cardiac general preset category. For each subcategory listed under the cardiac category, record the default values for each control listed on the table. After recording the values for the four 2D controls, activate the color flow imaging mode, and record the values for the two color controls. When you are finished, you should have a row of data for each cardiac subcategory.

Next, choose two more general categories such as "abdomen" and "vascular." A different probe may be required for certain categories. If that is the case, select the appropriate transducer from one category to the next.

Choose two subcategories under each of those general headings, and record the preset control values. Compare the values for the different presets and think about what specific requirements of each type of examination result in the selection of those specific control values. For example, what is the default value for B-mode transmit frequency for an adult cardiac examination compared with B-mode transmit frequency for a pediatric cardiac examination? What is the reason for the difference?

Tissue-Mimicking Phantoms

OBJECTIVES

To conduct performance testing of B-mode scanners using tissue-mimicking (TM) phantoms.

MATERIALS

TM phantoms (CIRS Model 40 and Gammex-RMI Model 403).

DISCUSS

The objective assessment of the performance of a B-mode scanner is necessary to ensure optimal image quality. Quality control programs using *tissue-mimicking (TM) phantoms* enable routine monitoring of scanner performance. Sonographers should be knowledgeable about the test methods that use TM phantoms.

EXPLORE AND DOCUMENT

- Select a transducer with a 3.5–5 MHz center frequency.
- Select the examination preset for the abdomen (liver), or apply the operator controls as indicated:

Parameter	Setting
Power	50%
Scan range (cm)	13–15
Number transmit focal zone(s)	2
Depth of transmit focal zone(s) (cm)	5, 10
Receiver gain	50% (adjust)
Dynamic range (dB)	65–75
TGC sliders	Adjust
Frame rate (fps)	15–20
Edge enhancement	Mid-range
Persistence	Mid-range
Gray-scale map	Near linear

cm, centimeter; *dB*, decibel; *TGC*, time gain compensation; *fps*, frames per second.

- Scan the dead zone target group in the Model 403 TM phantom. Use a single transmit focal zone at a depth of 1 to 3 cm. Freeze the image.
- Observe the depth of the rod closest to the phantom surface that can be visualized (see Figure 18-3, p. 78).

- On the data sheet, record the depth of the dead zone.
- Scan the vertical rod group in the Model 403 TM phantom. Use multiple transmit focal zones throughout the scan range. Freeze the image.
- Using electronic calipers, measure the separation between the vertical rods at the extremes of the field of view (FOV) (see Figure 18-4, p. 78).
- Record the known distance between the vertical rods and the measured distance between these rods on the data sheet.
- Scan the horizontal rod group at a depth of 12 cm in the Model 403 TM phantom. Adjust the single transmit focal zone depth to 12 cm, or use multiple transmit focal zones throughout the scan range. Freeze the image.
- Using electronic calipers, measure the separation between horizontal rods at a depth of 12 cm (see Figure 18-5, p. 79).
- On the data sheet, record the known distance between the horizontal rods and the measured distance between these rods.
- Scan the lateral resolution group at a depth of 6 cm in the Model 40 TM phantom. Adjust the single transmit focal zone depth to 6 cm. Freeze the image.
- The smallest distance between any two separable rods is the lateral resolution (see Figure 18-6, p. 79).
- On the data sheet, record the lateral resolution and the depth of the rod group.
- Scan the lateral resolution group at a depth of 10 cm in the Model 40 TM phantom. Adjust the single transmit focal zone depth to 10 cm. Freeze the image.
- On the data sheet, record the lateral resolution and depth of the rod group.
- Scan the axial resolution group at a depth of 8 cm in the Model 403 TM phantom. Adjust the single transmit focal zone depth to 8 cm. Freeze the image.
- Axial resolution is the smallest distance between any two rods that can be visualized as separate entities (see Figure 18-8, p. 80).
- On the data sheet, record the axial resolution and the depth of the rod group.

- Scan the axial resolution group at a depth of 14 cm in the Model 403 TM phantom. Adjust the single transmit focal zone depth to 14 cm. Freeze the image.
- On the data sheet, record the axial resolution and depth of the rod group.
- Scan a region of the Model 403 TM phantom that is relatively free of simulated cysts and rods. Use multiple transmit focal zones throughout the scan range. Set output power to maximum, receiver gain to high, and reject control to off or low. Freeze the image.
- Measure the maximum depth at which parenchyma scatterers are visualized (see Figure 18-9, p. 80).
- On the data sheet, record the sensitivity as the depth of penetration.
- Inspect the region of the image corresponding to uniform TM material for artifacts and signal loss. At each depth, the brightness should be relatively constant across the FOV. Also, a one-to-one matching between the rods in the phantom and in the image should be preserved.
- On the data sheet, indicate the presence or absence of artifacts (Table L18-1).

EXPLORE AND DOCUMENT

- Select a transducer with an 8–15 MHz center frequency.
- Select the examination preset for the breast, or apply the operator controls as indicated:

Parameter	Setting
Power	50%
Scan range (cm)	5
Number transmit focal zone(s)	1
Depth of transmit focal zone(s) (cm)	2–3
Receiver gain	50% (adjust)
Dynamic range (dB)	65–75
TGC sliders	Adjust
Frame rate (fps)	15–20
Edge enhancement	Sharp
Persistence	Mid-range
Gray-scale map	Near linear

cm, centimeter; *dB*, decibel; *TGC*, time gain compensation; *fps*, frames per second.

- Scan the dead zone target group in the Model 403 TM phantom. Freeze the image.
- Observe the depth of the rod closest to the phantom surface that can be visualized.
- On the data sheet, record the depth of the dead zone.
- Scan the vertical rod group in the Model 403 TM phantom. Use multiple transmit focal zones throughout the scan range. Freeze the image.
- Using electronic calipers, measure the separation between vertical rods at the extremes of the FOV.
- On the data sheet, record the known distance between the vertical rods and the measured distance between these rods.

TABLE L18-1	Tissue-Mimicking Phantom Lab Data Sheet	
Descriptor	**Liver**	**Breast**
Transducer		
Center frequency (MHz)		
Model 403 S/N		NA
Model 40 S/N		NA
Dead zone (mm)		
Vertical rod separation (mm)		
Measured vertical distance (mm)		
Horizontal rod separation (mm)		
Measured horizontal distance (mm)		
Depth of lateral rod group (cm)		
Lateral resolution (mm)		
Depth of lateral rod group (cm)		NA
Lateral resolution (mm)		NA
Depth of axial rod group (cm)		
Axial resolution (mm)		
Depth of axial rod group (cm)		NA
Axial resolution (mm)		NA
Depth of penetration (cm)		
Artifacts present?		

MHz, megahertz; *mm*, millimeter; *cm*, centimeter; *NA*, not applicable.

- Scan the horizontal rod group at a depth of 2 cm in the Model 403 TM phantom. Adjust the single transmit focal zone depth to 2 cm. Freeze the image.
- Using electronic calipers, measure the separation between horizontal rods at a depth of 2 cm.
- On the data sheet, record the known distance between the horizontal rods and the measured distance between these rods.
- Scan the lateral resolution group at a depth of 2.5 cm in the Model 40 TM phantom. Adjust the single transmit focal zone depth to 2.5 cm. Freeze the image.
- On the data sheet, record the lateral resolution and depth of the rod group.
- Scan the axial resolution group at a depth of 3 cm in the Model 403 TM phantom. Adjust the single transmit focal zone depth to 3 cm. Freeze the image.
- On the data sheet, record the axial resolution and depth of the rod group.
- Scan a region of the Model 403 TM phantom that is relatively free of simulated cysts and rods. Set output power to maximum, receiver gain to high, and reject control to off or low. Use multiple transmit focal zones throughout the scan range. Freeze the image.
- Measure the maximum depth at which parenchyma scatterers are visualized.
- On the data sheet, record the sensitivity as the depth of penetration.
- Inspect the region of the image corresponding to uniform TM material for artifacts and signal loss.
- On the data sheet, indicate the presence or absence of artifacts (Table L18-1).

Review Questions

1. Which adjustment can increase the frame rate in B-mode imaging?
   A. Increasing the number of scan lines
   B. Increasing the number of transmit focal zones
   C. Decreasing the scan range
   D. Decreasing power

2. What is the wavelength of an ultrasonic wave in soft tissue generated by a 7-MHz transducer?
   A. 0.22 cm
   B. 0.22 mm
   C. 0.51 mm
   D. 0.51 cm

3. Which adjustment can improve the axial resolution in B-mode imaging?
   A. Decreasing the number of scan lines
   B. Decreasing the number of transmit focal zones
   C. Increasing the operating frequency
   D. Increasing power

4. What term describes the region of increased molecular density induced by sound propagation in a medium?
   A. Compression
   B. Focal
   C. Fresnel
   D. Rarefaction

5. What is the frequency of the ultrasound wave?
   A. Speed of vibrating particles in a medium
   B. Amount of time required to complete one cycle
   C. Acoustic velocity multiplied by wavelength
   D. Number of pressure oscillations per unit time

6. Which adjustment can improve the lateral resolution of the B-mode image?
   A. Decreasing the number of scan lines
   B. Increasing the number of transmit focal zones
   C. Decreasing the operating frequency
   D. Increasing power

7. What property of the interface is represented by the pixel value in the digital B-mode image matrix?
   A. Location
   B. Reflectivity
   C. Size
   D. Velocity

8. What is the wavelength of the ultrasound wave?
   A. Distance between successive compression zones
   B. Distance required to complete one cycle
   C. Acoustic velocity divided by frequency
   D. All of the above

9. What property of the medium provides a measure of the resistance to ultrasound transmitted through the medium?
   A. Acoustic impedance
   B. Bulk modulus
   C. Dielectric constant
   D. Index of refraction

10. What is the frequency of the ultrasound wave that has a wavelength of 0.15 mm in soft tissue?
    A. 10 MHz
    B. 8 MHz
    C. 4 MHz
    D. 2 MHz

11. Which tissue type has the lowest acoustic velocity?
    A. Bone
    B. Fat
    C. Muscle
    D. Soft tissue

12. Which focusing technique increases the time necessary to collect the echo data along a single scan line in B-mode imaging?
    A. Apodization
    B. Aperture
    C. Dynamic receive focusing
    D. Multiple zone transmit focusing

13. What is produced by the absorption of ultrasound wave energy by soft tissue?
    A. Heat
    B. Light
    C. Lower frequency sound waves
    D. X-rays

14. What term describes the fraction of time that a transducer is actively generating ultrasound energy?
    A. De-rating factor
    B. Duty factor
    C. Pulse repetition period
    D. Q-value

15. Which tissue type has the highest rate of attenuation?
    A. Fat
    B. Lung
    C. Muscle
    D. Soft tissue

16. Which signal processing technique determines the area (or relative magnitude) of the enveloped signal?
    A. Compression
    B. Differentiation
    C. Integration
    D. Rectification

17. What does a hydrophone measure?
    A. Acoustic pressure
    B. Attenuation coefficient of tissue
    C. Time delay between echoes in B-mode imaging
    D. Velocity of a moving reflector

18. How does scan line density vary as a function of depth for B-mode imaging using the sector image format?
    A. Highest near the transducer
    B. Lowest near the transducer
    C. Highest in the transmit focal zone
    D. Constant for all scan depths

19. What is the fractional reduction in ultrasound intensity if a 3-dB loss has occurred?
    A. 0.1
    B. 0.25
    C. 0.5
    D. 0.75

20. Which operator control adjusts the intensity of the transmitted pulse in B-mode imaging?
    A. Receiver Gain
    B. Depth of scanning
    C. Power (decibel; dB)
    D. Time gain compensation (TGC)

21. What is the period of an ultrasound wave whose frequency is 4 MHz?
    A. 0.004 s
    B. 4×10^6 s
    C. 3.8×10^{-4} s
    D. 2.5×10^{-7} s

22. What parameter is unchanged when an ultrasound wave moves from fat into soft tissue?
    A. Wavelength
    B. Acoustic velocity
    C. Frequency
    D. Acoustic impedance

23. What term describes the reflection of ultrasound at large, smooth interfaces?
    A. Specular
    B. Diffuse
    C. Nonspecular
    D. Scattering

24. What method allows a determination of interface location by measuring the elapsed time between the transmitted pulsed ultrasound wave and the detected echo from that interface?
    A. Autocorrelation
    B. Echo ranging
    C. Fast Fourier transform
    D. Pulse inversion

25. How can the accuracy of the analog-to-digital conversion of the received signal be improved?
    A. Increase clock frequency
    B. Increase the number of bits
    C. Increase the voltage range of signals
    D. Increase pulse repetition frequency

26. Which signal-processing technique attempts to correct for attenuation of the ultrasound beam along the beam path from the transducer to the reflector and back to the transducer?
    A. Apodization
    B. Interpolation

C. Low pass filtering
D. Time gain compensation

27. Which method is used to isolate the harmonic frequency component in tissue harmonic imaging?
    A. Autocorrelation
    B. Pulse inversion
    C. Quadrature detection
    D. Time domain

28. Doppler shift frequency depends on all the following factors *except*:
    A. Acoustic velocity of soft tissue
    B. Angle of incidence
    C. Reflection coefficient
    D. Transmitter frequency

29. Which method determines the spectral waveform in pulsed wave Doppler?
    A. Autocorrelation
    B. Fast Fourier transform
    C. Transmit pulse inversion
    D. Time domain

30. What is the maximum temperature rise in tissue if the thermal index is 2?
    A. 0.5°C
    B. 2°C
    C. 4°C
    D. Unknown, thermal index cannot predict temperature rise in tissue.

31. If reflectors at the same depth produce echoes of varying amplitude, but the induced signals are depicted with nearly the same gray level in the image, which control is most likely to separate the displayed brightness of signal levels?
    A. Gray-scale map
    B. Persistence
    C. Receiver gain
    D. Time gain compensation

32. What assumption must be met for the proper summation of the echo-induced signals from multiple elements in the receive beam former?
    A. All channel signals must be equal in magnitude
    B. All beam paths from reflector to the respective elements are equal in length
    C. The acoustic velocity is constant along all beam paths to the elements
    D. The echo wavefront strikes each element at the same time

33. Which type of real-time transducer produces a sector format using electronic steering?
    A. Annular phased array
    B. Curvilinear array
    C. Linear array
    D. Phased array

34. What is the capacity of random access memory (RAM)?
    A. Speed of information retrieval
    B. Number of storage locations

C. Address of storage location

D. Number of bits in a storage location

35. What output characteristic determines the Q-value of a transducer?

A. Duty factor

B. Frequency bandwidth

C. Transmitted intensity

D. Pulse repetition frequency

36. What is the dynamic range of a B-mode scanner?

A. Maximum applied receiver gain

B. Maximum transmit power level

C. Ratio of highest signal to lowest signal

D. Highest received signal in the image

37. What is a potential problem in pulsed wave Doppler that imposes a maximum velocity detection limit?

A. Intermittent sampling of moving reflectors

B. Narrow bandwidth of the transmitted pulse

C. Short pulse repetition period

D. Small sampling volume within the vessel

38. Which design feature of the transducer improves the transmission of acoustic energy into tissue?

A. Thin crystal thickness

B. Electrode plating

C. Matching layer

D. Radiofrequency shielding

39. What is the basis for color assignment of a pixel in power Doppler?

A. Number of red blood cells (RBCs)

B. Mean velocity of RBCs

C. Doppler angle

D. Flow direction

40. A strong specular reflector (diaphragm) is disjointed in the B-mode image. Further examination of the image shows that the discontinuity is distal to a mass in the liver. What is the cause of this artifact?

A. Range ambiguity

B. Ghost image

C. Propagation speed error

D. Reverberation

41. What is the purpose of the wall filter applied during the acquisition of the pulsed wave Doppler spectral waveform?

A. Removing low-amplitude signal levels from display

B. Removing high-amplitude signal levels from display

C. Removing low-velocity signals from display

D. Removing high-velocity signals from display

42. What is the highest Doppler shift that can be detected in pulsed wave Doppler without aliasing?

A. One half of pulse repetition frequency

B. Pulse repetition frequency

C. Limit of audible sound or 20 kilohertz (kHz)

D. Transducer center frequency

43. Which imaging mode is based on the nonlinear propagation of ultrasound through tissue?

A. B-mode imaging

B. Power Doppler

C. Elastography

D. Tissue harmonics

44. Which imaging mode is based on the ability of tissue to change shape when a force is applied?

A. Spatial compounding

B. Color Doppler

C. Elastography

D. Tissue harmonics

45. Which type of real-time transducer allows electronic focusing in both in-plane and elevation directions but must be mechanically steered?

A. Linear array

B. Phased array

C. Curvilinear

D. Annular phased array

46. Which of the following factors affects the acoustic velocity in a medium?

A. Bulk modulus of the medium

B. Cross-sectional area of ultrasound beam

C. Thickness of the transducer crystal

D. Frequency bandwidth

47. Which principle of ultrasonic imaging is violated when a mirror image artifact occurs?

A. Sound waves travel along a straight path to and from the reflector

B. Detected echoes originate from the most recent transmitted pulse

C. A narrow beam width limits the sampling volume to a small fraction of the object

D. All echoes originate from the axis of the main beam only

48. Which principle of ultrasonic imaging is violated when a comet tail artifact occurs?

A. Acoustic velocity is a constant 1540 meters per second (m/s)

B. Detected echoes originate from the most recent transmitted pulse

C. A narrow beam width limits the sampling volume to a small fraction of the object

D. Each reflector contributes a single echo when interrogated along a single scan line

49. What is packet size in color Doppler imaging?

A. Number of transmit pulses to form one frame

B. Number of transmit pulses to sample one color line

C. Volume of the sampled region for one color pixel

D. Width of the color field of view

50. What characterizes flow through the lumen with an 85% stenosis?

A. High-velocity jets

B. Flow reversal

C. Eddy flow

D. Turbulence

51. For a linear array transducer, why would five crystals instead of two crystals be excited to form the transmitted beam?
    A. Increased near-field depth
    B. Reduce beam width near the transducer
    C. Increase transmitted frequency
    D. Reduce the frame rate

52. Which of the following B-mode acquisition parameters affects the thermal index?
    A. Frame rate
    B. Scan lines per frame
    C. Transmit power
    D. All of the above

53. Which of the following measurements relies on wave interference?
    A. Acoustic pressure
    B. Doppler shift frequency
    C. Echo ranging
    D. Thermal index

54. What is the dead zone for a B-mode transducer?
    A. Crystal elements within the array, which do not respond to pressure waves
    B. Region within the field of view where echo signals are anechoic
    C. Region near the transducer in which displayed data fail to correlate with objects
    D. Scan range limit for a particular transducer

55. What causes signal enhancement distal to a cyst?
    A. Weak attenuation by cyst
    B. Change in acoustic velocity in cyst
    C. Production of harmonics
    D. Focusing by refraction along curved surface

56. What comparison between coded excitation and the conventional B mode is valid?
    A. Lower intensity peak in the B mode
    B. Longer spatial pulse length in coded excitation
    C. Higher signal to noise level in the B mode
    D. Reduced scan range in coded excitation

57. What is the acoustic impedance in Mrayls for liver when its density is 1060 kg/m^3? Assume the velocity in liver is 1550 m/s and the frequency of sound is 5 MHz.
    A. 0.33
    B. 0.82
    C. 1.64
    D. 8.20

58. Calculate the transmitted angle if an ultrasound beam is directed at a large, smooth interface composed of soft tissue and bone. The angle of incidence is 10 degrees. Assume that the sound beam to be moving from soft tissue to bone.
    A. 2.9
    B. 3.6
    C. 10
    D. 25.9

59. Which performance evaluation would most likely use the SMPTE (Society of Motion Picture and Television Engineers) test pattern?
    A. Velocity measurement in pulsed wave Doppler
    B. Spatial registration in the B mode
    C. Brightness levels depicted on the B-mode monitor
    D. Intensity measurement under free-field conditions

60. Why is a curved, 2-cm-diameter nodule depicted more clearly with spatial compounding?
    A. Autocorrelation detection is applied during signal processing
    B. The nodule is interrogated from multiple angles
    C. High transmitted power is used
    D. High-frequency components from filtering improve spatial resolution

61. Why is lung tissue usually avoided during B-mode scanning?
    A. Comet tail image artifacts are created
    B. High rate of attenuation
    C. Potential for cavitation
    D. The speed of sound in air is 333 m/s

62. Quality control testing with a tissue-mimicking™ phantom yields a vertical distance measurement of 92 mm for a stated separation of 100 mm. What is the most likely cause for this discrepancy?
    A. Velocity calibration for scanner does not match velocity in phantom
    B. Excessive beam width
    C. Low scan line density
    D. None of the above; this is within normal variation

63. Six months ago, the maximum depth of penetration for a 5-MHz linear array transducer was measured to be 8 cm. Using the same instrument settings and a phantom, the maximum depth of penetration is presently measured as 4 cm. No other transducer shows this effect. What could cause this reduction in sensitivity?
    A. Attenuation of the phantom material has increased because of aging of equipment
    B. Separation of the matching layer from the crystal elements in the transducer
    C. Velocity calibration for the scanner does not match the velocity in the phantom
    D. Air is present at the input surface of the phantom

64. Which parameter of image quality is improved if the scan line density is doubled without a change in frame rate?
    A. Axial resolution
    B. Lateral resolution
    C. Sensitivity
    D. Temporal resolution

65. Calculate the Doppler shift in hertz produced by scanning an interface moving at a velocity of 50 cm/s at an angle of 40 degrees with the transducer. The center frequency of the transducer is 3 MHz.
    A. 746
    B. 974
    C. 1492
    D. 1948

66. How many lines of sight are sampled and displayed on the monitor in A mode?
    A. 1
    B. 100
    C. 1000
    D. None of the above; depends on acoustic velocity and scan range

67. If the Doppler angle is changed from 45 degrees to 60 degrees, what is the effect on the observed Doppler shift frequency for a moving interface?
    A. Increases by a factor of 0.7
    B. Decreases by a factor of 0.7
    C. Remains the same
    D. Doppler shift is zero

68. For a linear array transducer, how is the beam directed across the field of view?
    A. Electronic delay lines
    B. Rotating crystal elements
    C. Series of Hanafy lenses
    D. Selective excitation of elements

69. What is the rationale for the 1.5-dimensional transducer?
    A. Focusing in the slice thickness direction
    B. Higher output power
    C. Beam steering throughout a three-dimensional volume
    D. Increased sensitivity

70. What is the intensity loss of a 6-MHz ultrasound beam after it passes through 5 cm of soft tissue?
    A. 5 dB
    B. 6 dB
    C. 21 dB
    D. 99 dB

71. What is the result if the layer of fat at a soft tissue–fat interface is increased in thickness from 1 mm to 2 mm? Assume normal incidence of the ultrasound beam.
    A. The angle of refraction is increased
    B. The reflected sound intensity is increased
    C. The frequency of the sound wave is increased
    D. No change in the reflected sound intensity

72. Which real-time imaging method acquires scan data as the linear transducer is physically moved to compose an image with increased width for the field of view?
    A. Coded excitation
    B. Extended field of view
    C. Tissue harmonic imaging
    D. Elastography

73. What is four-dimensional ultrasound?
    A. Combination of three-dimensional B-mode ultrasound with color Doppler
    B. Display of a sampled three-dimensional volume in real time
    C. Dual B-mode display of two offset scan planes in real time
    D. Dual B-mode display of the field of view with two different transmit frequencies

74. Aliasing is observed in the pulsed wave Doppler spectral waveform. Which of the following responses by the operator is appropriate to eliminate the aliasing artifact?
    A. Decrease the transmitted power
    B. Decrease the Doppler angle
    C. Increase receiver gain
    D. Increase velocity scale

75. What process describes the formation and rapid destruction of microbubbles in tissue by high-intensity ultrasound?
    A. Clutter
    B. Elastography
    C. Cavitation
    D. Scattering

76. What determines the maximum velocity limit for continuous wave Doppler?
    A. Center frequency
    B. Depth of the reflector
    C. Transmit power
    D. None of the above

77. Which scanning mode is least subject to aliasing?
    A. Color Doppler imaging
    B. Combined B-mode and pulsed wave spectral Doppler
    C. Power Doppler imaging
    D. Pulsed wave spectral Doppler

78. Which of the following quality control tests is considered the most sensitive indicator of declining B-mode scanner performance?
    A. Axial resolution
    B. Contrast resolution
    C. Lateral resolution
    D. Maximum depth of penetration

79. Why is the maximum frame rate for color Doppler imaging slower than that for B-mode imaging?
    A. Computer processing of the acquired color scan data requires more time
    B. Multiple transmit pulses are required for each color scan line
    C. Signal-to-noise ratio is lower with color Doppler imaging
    D. Transmit power levels are lower with color Doppler imaging

80. If the scan range for a linear array transducer is decreased from 12 cm to 6 cm and the transmit power is increased by 3 dB, what is the effect on the maximum frame rate?
   A. Increased by a factor of 4
   B. Increase by a factor of 2
   C. Remain unchanged
   D. Decrease by a factor of 2

81. For a linear array, what transmit focusing method is applied to reduce the in-plane beam width?
   A. Curved crystal elements
   B. Changeable lenses
   C. Time delays to excite crystal elements
   D. Variable spatial pulse length

82. What causes a small, circular strong reflector to be depicted as an oval in the B-mode image (elongated in the lateral direction)?
   A. Spatial pulse length larger than reflector
   B. Beam width larger than reflector
   C. High pulse repetition frequency
   D. Comet tail (internal reflections)

83. What interaction causes a change of direction of the sound beam as it moves from one medium into another in which a change occurs in acoustic velocity?
   A. Diffraction
   B. Reflection
   C. Refraction
   D. Scattering

84. How can the sonographer improve penetration and extend the B-mode scan range?
   A. Switch to a lower center frequency
   B. Raise the pulse repetition frequency
   C. Decrease the dynamic range
   D. Increase the receiver gain

85. Which of the following are components of an interface that is most likely to generate the strongest echo?
   A. Fat and soft tissue
   B. Air and soft tissue
   C. Bone and soft tissue
   D. Echo strength does not depend on composition of interface

86. Which of the following will cause an increase in the mechanical index (MI)?
   A. Decrease in acoustic pressure
   B. Decrease in acoustic velocity
   C. Decrease in frequency
   D. Decrease in the duty factor

87. Which mode is most likely to have the highest bandwidth?
   A. Continuous wave Doppler
   B. Pulsed wave Doppler
   C. B mode
   D. All modes have equal bandwidth

88. What adjustment would increase the frame rate in color Doppler imaging?
   A. Reducing pulse repetition frequency
   B. Obtaining a pulse wave spectrum
   C. Reducing the packet size
   D. Increasing the wall filter to a higher frequency

89. What is the function of the digital scan converter in B-mode imaging?
   A. Translating line-by-line acquisition into matrix format for image display
   B. Summation of echo-induced signals from different elements in the array
   C. Digital filtering of signals to enhance boundaries of strong reflectors
   D. Applying variable gain, depending on depth of the reflector

90. A 1-cm diameter mass in the breast is difficult to distinguish in the B-mode image. What adjustment may improve the contrast resolution of the mass?
   A. Increasing the frame rate
   B. Increasing persistence
   C. Decreasing the pulse repetition frequency
   D. Decreasing power

91. If the Doppler shift is 3 kHz at a transmitted frequency of 2 MHz, what is the Doppler shift if the center frequency is raised to 4 MHz?
   A. 0 kHz
   B. 1.5 kHz
   C. 3 kHz
   D. 6 kHz

92. Which transducer has constant scan line density throughout the scan range?
   A. Curvilinear array
   B. Linear array
   C. Phased array
   D. Mechanical sector

93. Which parameter is relatively constant throughout the scan range for a phased array?
   A. Axial resolution
   B. Lateral resolution
   C. Slice thickness
   D. Width of the field of view

94. Which of the following has *no* effect on the mechanical index (MI)?
   A. Transmit power
   B. Degree of focusing
   C. Pulse repletion frequency
   D. Operating frequency

95. What adjustment would improve the depiction of fast moving reflectors in B-mode imaging?
   A. Increasing the operating frequency
   B. Increasing persistence
   C. Decreasing the scan line density
   D. Decreasing the dynamic range

96. What contributes to improved contrast often observed in tissue harmonic imaging compared with fundamental B-mode imaging?
   A. Reflection coefficient is higher at harmonic frequencies

B. Clutter is suppressed at harmonic frequencies

C. Spatial pulse length is shorter at harmonic frequencies

D. Rate of attenuation loss is lower at harmonic frequencies

97. What is a characteristic of the nonlinear propagation of ultrasound?

A. Acoustic velocity is not constant throughout the wave cycle

B. Sinusoidal waveform is distorted

C. Occurs at high intensity

D. All of the above

98. Which mode depicts the motion of reflectors in a graphic display of distance from the transducer with respect to time?

A. A mode

B. Continuous wave Doppler

C. M mode

D. Pulsed wave Doppler

99. Which medium is specified for measurements of the free-field intensity?

A. Alcohol

B. Polyethylene

C. Tissue-mimicking material

D. Water

100. Which intensity descriptor with respect to time yields the lowest numerical value as a characterization of B-mode output?

A. Temporal peak

B. Cycle average

C. Pulse average

D. Temporal average

101. Which adjustment is unlikely to change the displayed thermal index during scanning of soft tissue?

A. Increase in the center frequency

B. Increase in the pulse repetition frequency

C. Increase in transmit power

D. Increase in persistence

102. How many transmit focal zones are possible with one transmit pulse?

A. One

B. Same as the number of crystal elements

C. Variable; depends on type of the array

D. Variable; depends on the transmit power

103. By what factor is the intensity reduced, if the intensity loss is 15 dB?

A. 5

B. 15

C. 32

D. 45

104. Which attribute does *not* affect the total intensity loss along the propagation path to a point of interest in tissue?

A. Acoustic velocity

B. Frequency

C. Tissue type

D. Distance

105. If the time between transmission and reception of the echo is 52 microseconds, how far is the reflector from the transducer?

A. 2 cm

B. 4 cm

C. 8 cm

D. 10 cm

106. Which transducer is most likely to produce grating lobe artifacts?

A. Annular array

B. Linear array

C. Mechanical sector

D. Continuous wave Doppler

107. What detection method is applied in color Doppler imaging?

A. Autocorrelation

B. Demodulation

C. Fast Fourier transform

D. Iterative reconstruction

108. Which intensity descriptor is specified in the American Institute of Ultrasound for Medicine (AIUM) statement on in vivo biologic effects?

A. SPTP (spacial peak temporal peak)

B. SPPA (spacial peak pulse average)

C. SPTA (spacial peak temporal average)

D. SATA (spacial average temporal average)

109. What is the intensity loss in decibels (dB) if the intensity is reduced by a factor of 8?

A. 1 dB

B. 3 dB

C. 9 dB

D. 90 dB

110. What are the units for peak rarefactional pressure?

A. Joules

B. Milliwatts

C. Milliwatts/cm^2

D. Megapascals

111. What is the scientific basis for the statement that fetal exposure to diagnostic medical ultrasound has *not* resulted in adverse effects?

A. Cavitation threshold in blood

B. Epidemiologic studies

C. Experiments with mammals

D. Cell survival studies

112. What parameter denotes the rate at which a transducer is able to transmit acoustical energy into a patient?

A. Intensity

B. Mechanical index

C. Power

D. Thermal index

113. What is the interference pattern produced at the transducer from multiple scatterers within the sampled region?

A. Apodization

B. Speckle

C. Radiofrequency interference

D. Specular reflection

114. What is the reason that a large, smooth, curved, specular reflector is not displayed with uniform brightness in the B-mode image?
  A. Angular reflection from non-normal incidence
  B. Rayleigh scattering redirects the ultrasound energy
  C. Diffusion at the surface causes beam divergence
  D. Refraction of the returning echo

115. What adjustment should be performed to eliminate color bleed?
  A. Decreasing the velocity scale
  B. Increasing the color gain
  C. Increasing the color reject threshold
  D. Decreasing the frame rate

116. Which parameter of image quality is usually enhanced when the B-mode operation is switched to write zoom?
  A. Contrast resolution
  B. Signal-to-noise ratio
  C. Spatial resolution
  D. Artifact reduction

117. At which angle in degrees is the Doppler shift the lowest?
  A. 0
  B. 45
  C. 60
  D. 90

118. Which interaction causes the ultrasound energy to be reflected in all directions when incident on small structures (dimensions less than the wavelength)?
  A. Interference
  B. Diffuse reflection
  C. Refraction
  D. Scattering

119. Which device has the highest duty factor?
  A. B-mode imaging
  B. Color Doppler imaging
  C. Continuous wave Doppler
  D. M-mode imaging

120. Which performance test is *not* conducted with a tissue-mimicking phantom?
  A. Axial resolution
  B. Lateral resolution
  C. Distance accuracy
  D. Intensity at focal zone

121. What term describes the region of reduced molecular density induced by sound propagation in a medium?
  A. Compression
  B. Focal
  C. Fresnel
  D. Rarefaction

122. What frequency is necessary to produce an ultrasound wave with a wavelength of 0.51 mm in soft tissue?
  A. 2 MHz
  B. 3 MHz
  C. 4 MHz
  D. 5 MHz

123. Which signal processing technique removes the negative voltage components of the echo-induced signal?
  A. Demodulation
  B. Enveloping
  C. Integration
  D. Rectification

124. What attribute of red blood cells (RBCs) is depicted in the color-coded pixel display in color Doppler (color flow) imaging?
  A. Maximum velocity
  B. Mean velocity
  C. Spectral distribution of velocities
  D. Amplitude (proportional to the number of RBCs)

125. What is an advantage of power Doppler imaging compared with color Doppler imaging?
  A. Higher frame rates
  B. Higher sensitivity to weak Doppler signals
  C. Accurate measurement of flow volume
  D. Measurement of very fast reflector velocities

126. What does Snell's law predict regarding the incident sound wave at an interface composed by media with differences in acoustic velocity?
  A. Fraction of incident intensity reflected
  B. Change in direction of propagation
  C. Change in wavelength
  D. Frequency composition of the transmitted wave

127. Which of the following is *never* expressed in decibels?
  A. Transmit power
  B. Receiver gain
  C. Operating frequency
  D. Intensity loss

128. Why is aliasing a potential problem in pulsed wave spectral Doppler?
  A. Autocorrelation detection is used
  B. Curved vessels restrict sampling direction
  C. Intermittent sampling of flow
  D. Flow through vessel is not constant during the heart cycle

129. What is responsible for the formation of harmonics in tissue?
  A. High pulse repetition frequency
  B. Acoustic velocity above 1540 m/s in the medium
  C. Nonlinear propagation at high intensity levels
  D. Presence of specular reflectors

130. Which wave parameter is unchanged as ultrasound is transmitted through an interface composed of soft tissue and fat?
  A. Acoustic velocity
  B. Intensity
  C. Frequency
  D. Wavelength

131. Which tissue type has the highest acoustic velocity?
    A. Bone
    B. Fat
    C. Muscle
    D. Soft tissue

132. By what factor is the intensity reduced, if the intensity loss is 6 dB?
    A. 2
    B. 4
    C. 6
    D. 18

133. What affects the lateral resolution along the in-plane direction during B-mode imaging?
    A. Scan line density
    B. Duty factor
    C. Gain setting
    D. Spatial pulse length

134. What may result from excessive frame averaging (or persistence) during B-mode imaging?
    A. Blurring of the edges for stationary structures
    B. Blurring of fast moving structures
    C. More prominent noise
    D. Reduced scan range

135. If the Doppler angle is changed from 45 degrees to 90 degrees, what is the effect on the observed Doppler shift for a moving interface?
    A. Increases by a factor of 0.7
    B. Decreases by a factor of 0.7
    C. Remains the same
    D. Doppler shift is zero

136. Which of the following responses by the operator is appropriate to remove the aliasing artifact in the pulsed wave Doppler spectral waveform?
    A. Increasing the wall filter
    B. Decreasing the Doppler angle
    C. Switching to a lower center frequency
    D. Adjusting the position of the sampling volume

137. If the distance to the reflector is 3 cm, what is the time delay between transmission and reception of the echo?
    A. 1 µs (microsecond)
    B. 13 µs
    C. 39 µs
    D. 78 µs

138. What adjustment will increase the frame rate in color Doppler imaging?
    A. Decreasing the wall filter
    B. Decreasing the width of the color field of view
    C. Decreasing the color packet
    D. Decreasing the color gain

139. What two properties of the medium determine the acoustic impedance?
    A. Density, acoustic velocity
    B. Wavelength, acoustic velocity
    C. Frequency, density
    D. Frequency, acoustic velocity

140. What characterizes blood flow immediately distal to a region with 85% stenosis?
    A. Increased flow volume
    B. Eddy currents
    C. Laminar flow
    D. Plug flow

141. Which parameter describes the ability of the imaging system to resolve objects within the scan plane that are separated in the direction oriented perpendicular to the beam axis?
    A. Axial spatial resolution
    B. Contrast resolution
    C. Lateral spatial resolution
    D. Sensitivity

142. Which of the following is most likely to improve axial spatial resolution in B-mode imaging?
    A. Increasing the threshold for reject control
    B. Changing the transducer transmitted frequency from 3 MHz to 5 MHz
    C. Increasing the pulse duration from 2 cycles to 3 cycles per pulse
    D. Changing the frame rate from 20 Hz to 15 Hz

143. What is the depth of focus for a beam former operating in the receive mode?
    A. A maximum of eight segmented zones along the scan line
    B. All depths along the scan line
    C. Determined by the number of elements in the array
    D. Same as the transmit focal zone

144. What focusing technique improves the ability to focus the beam at a depth near the scan range limit?
    A. Increasing the transmission beam aperture
    B. Decreasing the channel number during reception
    C. Increasing the pulse repetition frequency
    D. Decreasing the pulse repetition frequency

145. Which type of B-mode transducer produces a rectangular field of view?
    A. Annular phased array
    B. Curvilinear array
    C. Linear array
    D. Phased array

146. What term describes the extent of high to low echo-induced signals that can be processed or represented by an ultrasound scanner?
    A. Analog-to-digital conversion
    B. Demodulation
    C. Dynamic range
    D. High pass filter

147. Which of the following are components of an interface that is most likely to generate the strongest echo?
    A. Fat and soft tissue
    B. Bladder wall and urine
    C. Bone and soft tissue
    D. Echo strength does not depend on composition of interface

148. Which parameter does *not* affect the assigned color for a pixel in color Doppler (color flow) imaging?
    A. Color gate
    B. Flow direction
    C. Number of red blood cells (RBCs)
    D. Velocity of the RBCs

149. Which type of processing excludes Doppler shifts from slow-moving structures from the displayed pulsed wave spectral Doppler waveform?
    A. Heterodyne detector
    B. Quadrature phase detector
    C. Spatial smoothing filter
    D. Wall filter

150. How does autoclaving affect a transducer?
    A. Causes the electrical contacts to separate from the piezoelectric material
    B. Destroys the dipoles in the piezoelectric material
    C. Destroys dipole alignment of the piezoelectric material
    D. Vaporizes the backing material

151. Which principle of B-mode imaging is violated when a refraction artifact (position misregistration) occurs?
    A. Acoustic velocity is a constant 1540 meters per second (m/s)
    B. Detected echoes originate from the most recent transmitted pulse
    C. Each reflector contributes a single echo when interrogated by the sound beam
    D. Sound waves travel along a straight path directly to and from the reflector

152. Which principle of ultrasonic imaging is violated when cyst fill-in occurs?
    A. Sound waves travel along a straight path to and from the reflector
    B. A narrow beam width limits the sampling volume to a small fraction of the object
    C. All echoes originate from the axis of the main beam only
    D. Attenuation of sound in tissue is uniform along the beam path

153. What term denotes the number of transmitted pulses used to interrogate one color line of sight in color Doppler imaging?
    A. Color gate
    B. Color persistence
    C. Packet size
    D. Pulse repetition frequency

154. What is the effect on the displayed image of the liver if the dynamic range (compression) control is changed from 75 dB to 40 dB?
    A. Structures become more blurred
    B. Edges are enhanced
    C. Noise is reduced
    D. More emphasis on blacks and whites is seen

155. What term is used to denote the fractional reduction in the measured free-field intensity caused by attenuation in tissue for the calculation of thermal index?
    A. De-rating factor
    B. Duty factor
    C. Kernel
    D. Q-factor

156. What is apodization as applied to the transmitted ultrasound pulse for a multiple element array?
    A. Varying the excitation voltage to each crystal in the group
    B. Varying the center frequency for each crystal in the group
    C. Varying the delay time to each crystal in the group
    D. Apodization is not applied during transmission, only used in signal processing

157. What task does the fast Fourier transform perform in a duplex scanner?
    A. Controls the bandwidth of a transducer
    B. Determines frequency components in a complex Doppler waveform
    C. Calculates the mechanical index in soft tissue
    D. Measures the power output of the transducer

158. Quality control testing with a tissue-mimicking phantom yields a horizontal distance measurement of 61 mm for a stated separation of 60 mm. What is the most likely cause for this discrepancy?
    A. Velocity calibration for scanner does not match the acoustic velocity in the phantom
    B. Internal distance calipers are not calibrated in the horizontal direction
    C. Edge enhancement was applied during signal processing
    D. None of the above; this is within normal variation for ultrasound scanners

159. What is an advantage of the B-mode imaging technique of coded excitation?
    A. Improved penetration
    B. Improved signal-to-noise ratio
    C. Increased power levels with reduced temporal peak intensity
    D. All of the above

160. What is the image processing technique of grayscale mapping?
    A. Adjusts brightness levels on the monitor based on room lighting
    B. Coverts echo signal levels to the digital form
    C. Stores scan data on in a two-dimensional matrix
    D. Translates pixel value to brightness level in the displayed image

161. What is a feature of the two-dimensional transducer?
    A. Electronic beam steering throughout a sample volume
    B. Extremely rapid frame rates (greater than 200 frames per minute)

C. Improved sensitivity throughout the scan range

D. Increased scan range

162. Which real-time imaging method steers scan lines for consecutive frames at different angles and then sums the data collections in the buffer to form a composite image?
    A. Coded excitation
    B. Frequency compounding
    C. Spatial compounding
    D. Tissue harmonic imaging

163. What is speckle?
    A. Echo-induced signals from large, smooth reflectors
    B. Variation in signal at a crystal element from specular reflectors
    C. Interference signal pattern from small scattering centers
    D. Electronic noise from radiofrequency interference

164. For a linear array transducer, which construction component is designed to reduce grading lobes?
    A. Backing material
    B. Radiofrequency shielding
    C. Matching layer
    D. Subdiced elements

165. What is the result when the echo-induced signal from a moving reflector is algebraically added with the reference signal in continuous wave Doppler?
    A. Center frequency
    B. Doppler shift frequency
    C. Second harmonic frequency
    D. One half f the Doppler shift frequency

166. Circular nylon rod (0.1 mm in diameter) is depicted as an ellipsoid in the B-mode scan of a tissue-mimicking phantom. What is the cause for this geometric distortion?
    A. Beam width
    B. High receiver gain
    C. High transmit power
    D. Nonlinear propagation

167. What determines the assignment of reflector position along the beam axis in real-time imaging?
    A. Amplitude of the detected echo
    B. Bandwidth of the detected echo
    C. Shift in frequency between the transmitted pulse and detected echo
    D. Elapsed time between the transmitted pulse and detected echo

168. What adjustment would improve the axial resolution?
    A. Decrease spatial pulse length
    B. Decrease transmitted frequency
    C. Increase pulse repetition frequency
    D. Increase power

169. What is a feature of continuous wave Doppler?
    A. Depth information of moving reflectors
    B. Transmission with wide bandwidth
    C. No velocity limit for moving reflectors
    D. Poor sensitivity to slow flow

170. Which of the following B-mode scanner settings affects the thermal index?
    A. Time gain compensation
    B. Frame rate
    C. Persistence
    D. Gray-scale mapping

171. What does the acoustic output parameter thermal index (TI) indicate?
    A. Maximum temperature rise in tissue
    B. Minutes of exposure time before heating is too great
    C. Likelihood of inducing cavitation
    D. Acoustic power in milliwatts

172. What is the purpose of the matching layer in the transducer?
    A. Insulate the patient from the high temperature crystal
    B. Reduce the transfer of vibrations from the crystal to the patient
    C. Reduce the acoustic impedance mismatch between crystal and tissue
    D. Protect the crystal from mechanical shock

173. In tissue harmonic imaging, where are the harmonic frequencies most likely to be formed?
    A. At the transducer during transmission
    B. Near the transducer
    C. Near the beam axis
    D. Uniformly throughout the ultrasonic field

174. What causes signal reduction distal to a mass?
    A. High attenuation by mass
    B. Change in acoustic velocity in mass
    C. Production of harmonics in the mass
    D. Acoustic impedance mismatch between mass and surrounding tissue

175. The Doppler shift frequency produced by moving arterial blood depends on all the following parameters *except*:
    A. Transducer frequency
    B. Velocity of red blood cells (RBCs)
    C. Number of RBCs
    D. Angle between direction of flow and ultrasound beam

176. What adjustment would increase the frame rate in color Doppler imaging?
    A. Decreasing the pulse repetition frequency
    B. Increasing the wall filter frequency
    C. Increasing the width of the color field of view
    D. Decreasing the packet size

177. What component applies dynamic receive focusing?
    A. Scan converter
    B. Transmitter
    C. Beam former
    D. Demodulator

178. What adjustment would lower the displayed value of the mechanical index?
    A. Decreasing the pulse repetition frequency
    B. Decreasing the width of the field of view
    C. Decreasing the operating frequency
    D. Decreasing the transmit power
179. Why does the formulation for the thermal index assume different models?
    A. Bone is a good absorber of ultrasound
    B. Variations in power levels
    C. Variations in manufacturer design
    D. Patient size
180. What determines the delay time for a particular element (channel) in a beam former operating in transmit mode?
    A. Acoustic velocity in tissue
    B. Depth to the point of focus
    C. Position of the element within the active elements
    D. All of the above
181. Under what condition does Snell's law predict that refraction will *not* occur at an interface?
    A. Media with the same acoustic impedance
    B. Media with the same acoustic velocity
    C. Media with the same density
    D. Media with the same attenuation coefficient
182. What type of sound wave propagates through soft tissue?
    A. Transverse wave
    B. Longitudinal wave
    C. Microwave
    D. Saw-tooth wave
183. What are the units for power?
    A. Joules
    B. Newtons
    C. Pascals
    D. Watts
184. What is the duty factor?
    A. Time for one wave cycle
    B. Time for one transmitted pulse
    C. Fraction of time transducer actively transmitting sound
    D. Fraction of time transducer receiving echoes
185. Which tissue type has the lowest rate of attenuation?
    A. Blood
    B. Calcified plaque
    C. Lung
    D. Soft tissue
186. What is the cause of a comet tail artifact produced by metal?
    A. Multiple internal reflections in metal
    B. Reverberations between metal and transducer
    C. High attenuation by metal
    D. Velocity shift between soft tissue and metal
187. What does the pulsed wave spectral waveform in Figure B-1 indicate?
    A. Aliasing
    B. High speed jets

C. Turbulence
D. Uniform flow velocity

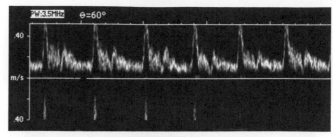

FIGURE B-1

188. What does the pulsed wave spectral waveform in Figure B-2 indicate?
    A. Aliasing
    B. Laminar flow
    C. Flow reversal
    D. Uniform flow velocity

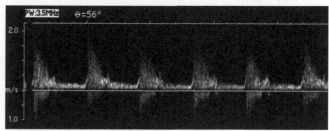

FIGURE B-2

189. What does the B-mode image in Figure B-3 exhibit?
    A. Acceptable image
    B. Improper receive gain
    C. Improper time gain compensation (TGC)
    D. High logarithmic compression

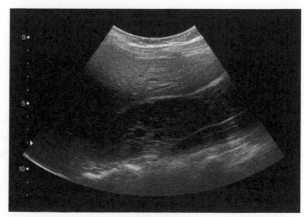

FIGURE B-3

190. What does the B-mode image in Figure B-4 exhibit?
    A. Acceptable image
    B. Improper receive gain

C. Improper time gain compensation (TGC)
D. High logarithmic compression

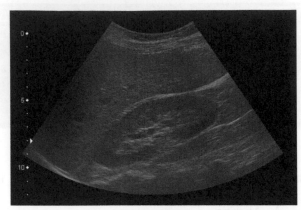

FIGURE B-4

191. What is the approximate intensity loss after a 5 MHz sound wave propagates through 8 cm of soft tissue?
    A. 2.5 dB
    B. 5 dB
    C. 30 dB
    D. 125 dB
192. What determines the slice thickness for a linear array?
    A. Number of crystal elements in the transmitted group
    B. Delay times for the crystal elements in the transmitted group
    C. Fixed focal length lens attached to the crystal array
    D. Width of the elements in the array
193. What is a characteristic of composite ceramic compared with solid piezoelectric transducers?
    A. Lower acoustic impedance
    B. Narrow bandwidth
    C. Formed as thin membranes
    D. Lower intensity output
194. What determines the resonant frequency of a transducer?
    A. Width of the crystal element
    B. Thickness of the crystal element
    C. Voltage of the pulser
    D. Size of the scan head
195. If the Doppler shift frequency is 2 kHz at a center frequency of 2 MHz, what is the Doppler shift frequency if the center frequency is increased to 4 MHz?
    A. 1 kHz
    B. 2 kHz
    C. 4 kHz
    D. 8 kHz
196. What does the reject control eliminate from the B-mode image?
    A. Electronic noise only
    B. Electronic noise and low-amplitude signals
    C. Electronic noise and high-frequency signals
    D. Multiple signals from a single reflector

197. What adjustment improves the mean velocity estimate in color Doppler imaging?
    A. Increasing packet size
    B. Increasing the width of the color field of view
    C. Decreasing color gain
    D. Decreasing color reject
198. How many scan lines typically compose a B-mode image?
    A. 1
    B. 15
    C. 150
    D. 1500
199. What transmit focusing method is used in linear array transducers?
    A. Apodization
    B. Beam aperture
    C. Time delay to excite crystal elements
    D. All of the above
200. How many lines of sight typically compose the M-mode trace?
    A. 0
    B. 1
    C. 100
    D. 300
201. What is the most likely effect on the B-mode frame rate when the number of transmit focal zones is increased?
    A. Increased
    B. Decreased
    C. Unchanged
    D. Number of transmit focal zones is fixed
202. What type of transducer does *not* allow dynamic receive focusing?
    A. Linear array
    B. Phased array
    C. Curvilinear array
    D. Mechanical sector
203. What is the purpose of the backing layer in a B-mode transducer?
    A. Reducing ringing
    B. Reducing the acoustic impedance mismatch with tissue
    C. Adjusting the resonant frequency
    D. Adjusting the focusing depth of the transmitted pulse
204. What is the period of a wave?
    A. Inverse of the frequency
    B. Time for one wave cycle
    C. Wavelength divided by the acoustic velocity
    D. All of the above
205. Which transducer has the highest Q-value?
    A. Continuous wave Doppler
    B. Pulsed wave Doppler
    C. B-mode imaging
    D. Color Doppler
206. Which change in B-mode operation is most likely to increase the potential for cavitation in tissue?
    A. Increase in the pulse repetition frequency

B. Decrease in the pulse repetition frequency

C. Increase in the center frequency

D. Decrease in the center frequency

207. Which type of transducer permits electronic focusing in the elevation direction?

A. Phase array

B. Curvilinear array

C. 1.5-dimensional array

D. Mechanical sector

208. Which of the following will enhance the effect of spatial compounding?

A. Increasing the number of beam steering angles

B. Decreasing the added frames in the buffer

C. Increasing the center frequency

D. Decreasing the pulse repetition frequency

209. What characteristic of the transducer changed if the pulse duration was shortened from 5 cycles to 2.5 cycles?

A. Decreased bandwidth

B. Increased acoustic impedance

C. Increased crystal thickness

D. Decrease Q-value

210. Which signal processing technique corrects the echo-induced signal for attenuation along the propagation path?

A. Dynamic range (compression)

B. Integration

C. Receiver gain

D. Time gain compensation

211. What device measures acoustic pressure under free field conditions?

A. Autocorrelation detector

B. Feedback microbalance

C. Hydrophone

D. Tissue-mimicking phantom

212. If the Doppler shift frequency is 1500 Hz, what is the minimum pulse repetition frequency that the signal can be sampled without aliasing?

A. 750 Hz

B. 1500 Hz

C. 3000 Hz

D. 6000 Hz

213. What is a potential cause for spatial misregistration of a specular reflector in the B-mode image?

A. High transmit power

B. High pulse repetition frequency

C. High receiver gain

D. High rate of attenuation along propagation path

214. What is the piezoelectric effect?

A. Conversion of acoustic energy to electrical energy

B. Transfer of acoustic energy to heat by the attenuating medium

C. Scattering of acoustic energy in a radial symmetric pattern

D. Reduction in ultrasound frequency by the absorbing medium

215. Which characteristic of a tissue-mimicking phantom is most important for the accurate measurement of rod separation along the direction of beam propagation?

A. Acoustic velocity of 1540 m/s

B. Attenuation rate of 0.5 dB/cm-MHz

C. Backscatter properties similar to the liver parenchyma

D. Density of 1 g/cm^3

216. Which of the following will produce the highest scattered intensity from the red blood cells (RBCs)?

A. Double the number of RBCs in the sampled volume

B. Double the center frequency

C. Double the length of the axial gate

D. Double the transmit power

217. What is Huygens' principle?

A. Ultrasonic field calculated by dividing the radiating surface into a series of point sources

B. Calculation of reflection intensity from nonperpendicular incidence

C. Determination of the individual Doppler shift frequencies in the Doppler waveform

D. Determination of bandwidth in a broad bandwidth transducer

218. Which type of transducer is mechanically steered?

A. Linear array

B. Phased array

C. Curvilinear array

D. Annular phased array

219. If the B-mode pulse duration is shortened from 0.8 µs to 0.6 µs, what is the effect on the bandwidth?

A. Bandwidth becomes wider

B. Bandwidth becomes narrower

C. For this small change, the bandwidth remains essentially constant

D. Bandwidth is not dependent on pulse duration

220. What potential interaction or result in tissue is most closely associated with the mechanical index?

A. Temperature rise

B. Cavitation

C. DNA (deoxyribonucleic acid) mutation rate

D. Cell death

221. If an ultrasound wave with an intensity of 5 mW/cm^2 is incident on a specular reflector composed of fat and soft tissue, at what frequency does the reflected wave have the highest intensity?

A. 2 MHz

B. 5 MHz

C. 10 MHz

D. Reflection coefficient is independent of frequency

222. What term describes a region in the B-mode image in which the scattering level is increased compared with the surrounding tissue?

A. Hypoechoic

B. Hyperechoic

C. Clutter

D. Speckle

223. At what size of an interface is scattering likely to occur?

A. Larger than ultrasound beam width

B. Larger than ultrasound wavelength

C. Smaller than ultrasound wavelength

D. Scattering does not depend on the size of the interface

224. What information is presented in the A-mode display?

A. Echo signal strength and depth of origin

B. Reflector distance from transducer as a function of time

C. Reflector physical size and relative depth

D. Two-dimensional image of echo signals composed from multiple scan lines

225. What type of wave causes the displacement of particles in the medium to be perpendicular to the direction of propagation?

A. Longitudinal

B. Transverse

C. Radio

D. Light

226. If the peak pressure amplitude is doubled, what is the change in the peak intensity?

A. Decrease by a factor of 2

B. Increase by a factor of 2

C. Increase by a factor of 4

D. No change

227. Which operating mode produces the highest I(SPTA)?

A. B mode

B. M mode

C. Continuous wave fetal heart monitor

D. Pulsed wave Doppler

228. Which device transforms analog signals into the digital format?

A. ADC (analog-to-digital converter)

B. CPU (central processing unit)

C. RAM (random access memory)

D. USB (universal serial bus)

229. What is a limitation of real-time B-mode compared with static B-mode?

A. Position transmit focal zone

B. Physical extent of the field of view

C. Collection time per frame

D. Reduced dynamic range

230. Which operator control suspends scan data collection and displays a single image for prolonged viewing?

A. Freeze frame

B. Panning

C. Frame averaging

D. Write zoom

231. What is the bit depth of the digital scan converter? (Assume that pixel values range from 0 to 255.)

A. 2

B. 4

C. 8

D. 16

232. The Doppler shift frequency from the red blood cells (RBCs) moving at 50 cm/s is 2000 Hz. The center frequency is 4 MHz, and the Doppler angle is 40 degrees. What is the Doppler shift frequency if the velocity of the RBCs is increased to 100 cm/s?

A. 1000 Hz

B. 2000 Hz

C. 2500 Hz

D. 4000 Hz

233. Which of the following will extend the near field depth of a single element transducer?

A. Increasing the frequency

B. Decreasing the diameter of the crystal

C. Increasing the crystal thickness

D. Decreasing the transmitted bandwidth

234. Inspection of the transducer face demonstrates a pinhole crack in the protective layer. What is the proper response of the sonographer in this situation?

A. Continue scanning

B. Cover the crack with waterproof tape

C. Remove the transducer from service

D. Limit the thermal index to less than 1

235. The ability of the monitor to display all gray levels from black to white has come into question. What is done to evaluate the gray level response of the monitor?

A. Display a grid pattern with equidistance line spacing

B. Measure the luminance at maximum brightness with a photometer

C. Display an SMPTE (Society of Motion Picture and Television Engineers) pattern

D. Scan the uniformity section of a tissue-mimicking phantom

236. Which component has the highest dynamic range?

A. Monitor

B. Receiver

C. Scan converter

D. Printer

237. In what function is mechanical focusing applied for linear and curvilinear arrays?

A. Variable transmit focal zones (number and position)

B. Extends the near-field depth throughout the scan range

C. Establishes the slice thickness at each scan depth

D. Improves the lateral resolution within the scan plane

238. What condition is most likely to cause a side lobe artifact?

A. Operation at low center frequency (2 MHz)

B. High pulse repetition frequency (>3000 Hz)

C. Presence of bowel gas near the scan plane

D. Multiple transmit focal zones

239. What is measured during elastography, which acquires scan data with and without compression (force applied to tissue)?

A. Echo frequency shift
B. Strength of the echo-induced signal
C. Velocity of movement
D. Displacement of the reflector

240. What is the consequence of the partial volume artifact?
A. Decreased penetration
B. Loss of contrast in small lesions
C. Improper application of time gain compensation
D. Overall loss of image brightness

241. Which of the following is NOT true about harmonic frequencies?
A. They are generated from within the body
B. They are integer multiples of the fundamental frequency
C. They are higher in frequency than the transmitted frequency
D. Their intensity is double that of the fundamental frequency

242. All of the following affect the Doppler frequency *except*:
A. Doppler angle
B. Transmit frequency
C. Doppler gain
D. Velocity of blood flow

243. Which of the following relationships is correct?
A. Increased velocity results in decreased kinetic energy
B. Decreased velocity results in increased potential energy
C. Increased velocity results in increased potential energy
D. Decreased velocity results in decreased potential energy

244. Choose the statement that is NOT true about the spatial pulse length (SPL):
A. As the number of cycles in the pulse increases, the SPL increases
B. As the frequency increases, the SPL increases
C. As the SPL increases, the axial resolution increases
D. The SPL is affected by damping

245. Which of the following is the most important advantage of Continuous Wave Doppler?
A. It has no range resolution
B. It has a sending and a receiving transducer
C. It has no upper limit to the Doppler frequency that can be displayed
D. It samples the entire path of the sound beam

246. All of the following affect axial resolution *except*:
A. The transmitted frequency
B. Damping of the transducer element
C. The number of cycles in the pulse
D. It is affected by the beam width at the focal point

247. Which of the following uses phased beam steering as the primary method of scanning the beam through the 2-dimensional image area?
A. Linear Sequenced Array
B. Phased Array Sector

C. Annular array
D. Mechanical Sector

248. A(n) _____ achieves electronic focus by firing concentric ring-shaped elements with slight delays.
A. Mechanical single-element transducer
B. 2-D array
C. Phased Linear array
D. Annular array

249. Which of the following best describes Color Flow Imaging?
A. It is a non-scanned mode
B. It is a scanned mode
C. It has the greatest risk of thermal bioeffects
D. It is both a scanned mode and a non-scanned mode

250. In the picture below, what does the number 27 represent ?
A. The Nyquist Limit in cm/second
B. The transmitted frequency
C. The Nyquist Limit in frequency (kHz)
D. The color wall filter

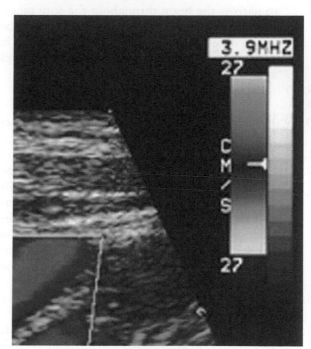

FIGURE B-5

251. In the picture above, what does the number 3.9MHz represent?
A. The Nyquist Limit in cm/second
B. The transmitted frequency
C. The received frequency
D. The Doppler frequency

252. In the picture above, assume the top of the color bar is blue. What is the 4-letter acronym that describes the color relative to the direction of flow?
A. BART
B. BRAT
C. BTRA
D. RABT

1. C. Frame rate is inversely related to the time required to scan the field of view, which is decreased by lower line density, reduced scan range, and fewer of transmit focal zones.

2. B. Determined by the relationship between acoustic velocity, frequency, and wavelength.

3. C. Axial resolution is improved by decreasing the spatial pulse length (higher frequency reduces the distance per cycle).

4. A. The oscillating molecules create regions of high density (compression) and low density (rarefaction).

5. D

6. B. Lateral resolution depends on beam width, near field depth, and the scan line density. High frequency extends the near-field depth and narrows the beam width. Transmit focusing reduces the beam width within the focal zone. Multiple transmit focal zones compose a single scan line to narrow the beam throughout the scan range.

7. B. Signal strength is represented by the pixel value, which is encoded as a gray level for display. The position of the pixel in the matrix depicts the relative location of the reflector.

8. D

9. A

10. A. Determined by the relationship among acoustic velocity, frequency, and wavelength.

11. B

12. D. Multiple zone transmit focusing requires separate pulsed transmission for each focal zone along a scan line, which increases the time required to acquire scan data. Aperture focusing and apodization are applied at transmission and do not cause an increase in scan time. Dynamic receive focusing is applied at reception and does not cause an increase in scan time.

13. A. Ultrasound energy is transferred to soft tissue in the form of heat.

14. B. Duty factor is the ratio of pulse duration to pulse repetition period.

15. B. The presence of air in the lung causes redirection of ultrasound energy.

16. C. The induced radiofrequency signal is converted into a single metric by rectification, enveloping, and finally integration, which sums the area of the enveloped signal.

17. A. The hydrophone is a measurement device with a small diameter piezoelectric crystal that produces an electrical signal whose amplitude is proportional to the acoustic pressure.

18. A. For a sector transducer the width of the field of view becomes broader with depth. Since the number of scan lines is constant for all depths, line density is highest near the transducer where the field of view is narrowest.

19. C. 3 decibels (dB) correspond to a factor of 2. A loss of 3 dB means that the intensity has been reduced by a factor of 2 or is one half or 0.5 of the original intensity.

20. C. Receiver gain and time gain compensation (TGC) are applied during reception and do not affect the transmitted pulse. Scan range sets the time for echo reception following the transmitted pulse. The power setting controls the voltage to excite the piezoelectric elements during transmission.

21. D. The period of the wave equals the inverse of the frequency.

22. C. Fat has lower acoustic velocity and acoustic impedance compared with soft tissue. The rate of pressure oscillations is communicated across an interface. The relationship among acoustic velocity, frequency, and wavelength dictates that wavelength must also decrease in fat.

23. A

24. B. Along the beam axis, the assigned distance is based on the echo ranging principle in which the time of the detected echo is converted into distance by assuming a constant velocity of 1540 meters per second (m/s).

25. B. In the digital format, the number of bits controls the dynamic range and the signal range for each digital step. The accuracy of digitization is improved by increasing the bit depth. Clock frequency affects how fast digitization can occur, but not accuracy. Increased voltage of signals means that digitization must encompass a higher voltage range with the same number of bits, which will not improve signal contrast.

26. D. Time gain compensation (TGC) is a variable amplification technique in which signal gain is based on elapsed time.

27. B. Autocorrelation, time domain, and quadrature detection are Doppler signal processing techniques.

28. C. The reflection coefficient does not appear in the Doppler shift equation.

29. B. The Doppler frequency shifts in the complex Doppler signal are identified by isolating the individual frequency components using fast Fourier transform. Autocorrelation and time domain determine a single metric and the mean velocity, but not the velocity components. Pulse inversion is a tissue harmonic imaging technique.

30. B. The thermal index indicates the maximum temperature rise in degrees centigrade within the ultrasonic field.

31. A. Receiver gain and time gain compensation (TGC) amplifies each signal by the same amount and would not separate their respective signal levels. Persistence averages the signals over time, but again yields average values that are similar. Changing the gray-scale map allows a new translation of signal levels to gray levels so that similar signal levels may be presented with different gray levels.

32. C. Dynamic receive focusing is based on the time for the echo to travel from the point of formation to a specific crystal element. Since the distance from echo formation to each element is different, time of travel will be unique. Distance must be converted into time by assuming a constant acoustic velocity. The time differences that the wavefront strikes the various elements in the receive beam former give rise to the respective timing delays.

33. D

34. B. The capacity of random access memory (RAM) indicates the number of addressable storage locations.

35. B. Q-value is the ratio of the transducer center frequency to the bandwidth. Transducers used in pulse-echo imaging have a broad bandwidth and thus a low Q-value.

36. C. The scanner can respond effectively to signal amplitudes within a specific range, threshold to saturation. Low-amplitude signals slightly above electronic noise can be detected (threshold) and with saturation high-amplitude signals are invariant (all input signals are represented with the same output value).

37. A. Pulsed wave transmission results in discrete sampling of the complex Doppler waveform, which means that the Doppler shift frequencies must be inferred from the limited data available. Beyond the high velocity limit corresponding to a high Doppler shift frequency, the rate of sampling is not sufficient to define the Doppler waveform unambiguously, and aliasing occurs.

38. C. The matching layer reduces the acoustic impedance mismatch between the piezoelectric crystal and the tissue and improves energy transfer from the transducer to the patient.

39. A. Power Doppler presents the amplitude of the Doppler signal, which is most closely associated with the scattering intensity or the number of red blood cells (RBCs). Color coding in Power Doppler is independent of mean flow velocity, flow direction, and Doppler angle.

40. C. The presence of the mass violates the assumption that the acoustic velocity is a constant 1540 meters per second (m/s) along the entire propagation path. Structures distal to the mass are spatially misregistered, since transit time is altered by the mass.

41. C. Slow moving reflectors with low Doppler frequency shifts are eliminated from the display by the wall filter. For example, the vessel wall may cause distracting output if the wall filter is set too low.

42. A. This is a statement of the Nyquist criterion, which requires a minimum of two sampling points within a cycle in order to determine the frequency unambiguously. The pulse repetition frequency (PRF) is the rate of sampling. One half of the PRF yields the maximum Doppler shift frequency that can be detected without aliasing.

43. D. Nonlinear propagation at relatively high intensity generates harmonics along the propagation path. Tissue harmonic imaging isolates the harmonics from the fundamental frequency, both of which are present in echoes, to reduce clutter and improve contrast.

44. C. The application of a force will cause alteration in the shape of an object. The amount of deformation is indicated by a change in echo position obtained for transmit pulses with compression applied and no compression applied. Large movement or small movement denotes elastic or stiff structures.

45. D. Delay time excitation of annular rings focuses the beam in elevation and in-plane directions simultaneously but does not allow beam steering. Beam scanning is accomplished by mechanical means. Linear array, phased array, and curvilinear array all employ mechanical focusing in the elevation direction.

46. A. Acoustic velocity is dictated by the properties of the medium (bulk modulus and density) and not by the characteristics of the ultrasound beam.

47. A. The presence of a strong reflector along the propagation path causes additional echoes to be generated by an object, and these echoes do not travel a direct path to the transducer.

48. D. Multiple internal reflections occur within the object generating a series of echoes from one interrogation transmit pulse.

49. B

50. A. The restricted lumen causes an increase in velocity to maintain flow rate.

51. A. Beam aperture affects near-field depth and is method for transmit focusing. Very close to the transducer beam the five-element transmitted pulse would have greater beam width than that generated with the two-element transmitted pulse. However, at increased depth, the five-element transmitted pulse would have a narrower beam width. Frame rate and center frequency are not dependent on the number of excited crystals in a single transmit pulse.

52. D. The thermal index primarily depends on the ultrasound energy transmitted into the patient.

Scan lines per frame and frame rate affect the pulse repetition frequency. Transmit power altars the intensity of the transmitted pulse.

53. B. The Doppler shift frequency is detected by demodulation of the reference signal combined with the echo-induced radiofrequency signal to form the beat frequency.

54. C

55. A. Weak attenuation by the cyst results in a small loss of intensity compared with that associated with the adjacent soft tissue. Since the soft tissue distal to the cyst is interrogated with higher intensity that the adjacent soft tissue at that same depth but not in the path of the cyst, signal enhancement occurs.

56. B. Coded excitation employs a long series of transmit pulses to increase the overall time-averaged intensity, but with reduced peak intensity. The relatively high total transmitted energy improves both penetration and signal-to-noise ratio.

57. C. Acoustic impedance equals the product of the acoustic velocity and the density and is independent of frequency.

58. D. Snell's law predicts the angle of transmission based on the incident angle and the ratio of the acoustic velocities in the two media.

59. C. The SMPTE (the Society of Motion Picture and Television Engineers) video test pattern is used in the performance evaluation of monitors and hard-copy imaging devices.

60. B. Spatial compounding interrogates a curved structure from multiple angles, and it can produce higher echo intensity when the direction of propagation is perpendicular to the curve surface of the nodule.

61. B. The high rate of attenuation limits penetration.

62. A. Spatial registration of structures in the vertical direction is based on echo ranging and, thus, the velocity calibration of the B-mode scanner.

63. B. The loss in sensitivity in this case is associated with the transducer itself. The separation of the matching layer from the crystal elements affects the transmission of energy into the phantom and, thus, can reduce the sensitivity.

64. B. Lateral resolution is improved by increased scan line density. In this case, the pulse repetition frequency must be increased to maintain the frame rate with this higher line density.

65. C. Calculated from the Doppler shift equation, which depends on center frequency, velocity of the moving reflector, cosine of the Doppler angle, and acoustic velocity in soft tissue.

66. A. A-mode samples along one line of sight only, which is refreshed at the pulse repetition frequency.

67. B. Doppler shift frequency depends on the cosine of the Doppler angle. As the Doppler angle is increased, the Doppler shift frequency becomes lower in frequency.

68. D. For a linear array, selective excitation of crystal elements establishes the beam direction.

69. A. Multiple rows of crystal elements in the 1.5D transducer allows focusing in the direction of the slice thickness.

70. C. The rate of attenuation in soft tissue is approximately 0.7 dB/cm-MHz. For 6-MHz ultrasound, the rate of attenuation is 4.2 dB/cm; and after passing through a thickness of 5 cm, the reduction in intensity is 21 dB.

71. D. The reflection coefficient does not depend on the thickness of the media that compose the interface, only the mismatch in their respective acoustic impedances.

72. B

73. B

74. D. Receiver gain and transmit power do not affect the Doppler shift frequency. Decreasing the Doppler angle will make aliasing more pronounced. Increasing the velocity scale expands the frequency range to present moving reflectors without aliasing.

75. C

76. D. Continuous wave Doppler has no velocity limit.

77. C. Power Doppler depicts the strength of the signal from the moving reflectors without assessment of the frequency shift.

78. D. The maximum depth of penetration is considered the best indicator of a change in scanner performance, since this quality control test monitors the signal-to-noise ratio.

79. B. A proper assessment of motion requires multiple samplings repeated over a time interval. The packet size denotes the number of transmit pulses used to interrogate each color line of sight.

80. B. Reduced scan range enables frame formation to occur in a shorter time (less time is denoted to listen for echoes). Transmit power does not affect frame rate.

81. C. The distance from the crystal element to the point of focus determines the time of travel for the ultrasound wave generated by that crystal element. Since the excited crystals in the transmit aperture do not have the same distance to the focal point, the time of excitation for each crystal must be staggered to arrive simultaneously.

82. B. A reflector smaller than the beam width produces a signal whenever the reflector lies within the sampling volume of the ultrasound beam. The spatial registration of the reflector will extend to nearby scan lines whose beam width includes the reflector. Consequently, the small reflector will be presented with increased width in the lateral direction.

83. C. This physical phenomenon is described by Snell's law.

84. A. Penetration is highly dependent on frequency.
85. B. The acoustic impedance mismatch is greatest for air and soft tissue.
86. C. The mechanical index is inversely proportional to the square root of frequency.
87. C. Continuous wave Doppler and pulsed wave Doppler have longer transmission time than B-mode imaging and thus have a narrower bandwidth.
88. C. The acquisition time for color information depends on the packet size (the number of transmit pulses along a color line of sight). By reducing the packet size, frame rate is increased.
89. A. Digital imaging is based on a matrix format of pixels. The pixels are arranged in rows and columns, but the sampling by beam direction does not necessarily conform to this geometric format. Also, multiple scan lines are required to sample the field of view. The scan converter is essentially computer memory, which holds the scan data until they are read for image display.
90. B. The addition of frames by persistence control reduces acoustic noise and improves contrast resolution. Reduced power lowers the signal-to-noise ratio. Frame rate, pulse repletion frequency, and persistence all affect the temporal resolution.
91. D. The Doppler shift frequency is directly proportional to the center frequency. Doubling the center frequency also doubles the Doppler shift frequency.
92. B. Scan line density is the number of scan lines divided by the width of the field of view. For the linear array, the width of the field of view is constant for all depths, and therefore, the scan line density is constant within the field of view. The width of the field of view increases with depth for the curvilinear array, phased array, and mechanical sector transducers.
93. A. Axial resolution depends primarily on spatial pulse length, which is established at transmission and is essentially constant along the scan line.
94. C. The mechanical index is defined as peak negative pressure divided by the square root of frequency. Transmit power and degree of focusing affect the peak negative pressure within the ultrasonic field. Pulse repetition frequency is directly proportional to the temporal averaged intensity but has no effect on the maximum intensity.
95. C. Temporal resolution—the ability to depict movement—depends on frame rate. The reduction of scan lines in a B-mode frame decreases the time to compose the frame and thus allows faster frame rates.
96. B. Clutter is generated most prominently at the fundamental frequency (e.g., fat near the transducer where only the fundamental frequency is present). Tissue harmonic imaging suppresses all signals at the fundamental frequency, and thus, clutter is reduced and contrast is improved.
97. D. At relatively high intensity, variable acoustic velocity within the wave cycle causes distortion of the sinusoidal waveform.
98. C. The view for M-mode imaging is along a single axis, which depicts reflector distance from the transducer as a function of time. To be shown, the motion of the reflector must remain within the sampling volume of the ultrasound beam.
99. D. Free-field conditions establish water as the medium. Water allows easy placement of the hydrophone and is weakly attenuating. Conversion of measured pressure or intensity to soft tissue requires a derating factor.
100. D. Temporal average intensity is obtained by including both the active transmission and the passive listen in the time parameter for averaging. The other intensity descriptors only consider some aspects of active transmission.
101. D. Persistence is a processing technique that adds the acquired frames together for display but does not change the rate of data collection. Transmit power and pulse repetition frequency affect the energy transmitted into tissue. Energy transfer to tissue increases with frequency.
102. A. In a multiple-element array, several crystals participate in the formation of the transmitted pulse, but focusing can be to a single depth only.
103. C. For every 3 dB, the intensity is reduced by a factor of 2. A 15-dB reduction corresponds to five factors of 2, or 2^5, or 32.
104. A. The rate of attenuation loss depends on tissue type and frequency. Total intensity loss is proportional to the distance of travel.
105. B. Each 1 cm in depth requires a total transit time of 13 microseconds (μs). An echo time of 52 μs corresponds to 4 times 13 μs or a distance of 4 cm.
106. B. Grating lobes are produced by the regular spacing of crystal elements across the aperture of the linear array.
107. A. Doppler imaging uses the fast technique of autocorrelation detection to maintain frame rate.
108. C. The threshold for thermal effects is stated to be 100 mW/cm^2 SPTA (spatial peak temporal average) for unfocused beams and 1 W/cm^2 SPTA for focused beams.
109. C. For every 3 dB, the intensity is reduced by a factor of 2. A reduction by a factor of 8 corresponds to 2^3, or 3 times 3 dB = 9 dB in decibel notation.
110. D
111. B. For any agent in which the damage is expected to be subtle, delayed, or infrequent, studies of large populations is essential to identify the

risk. Results of epidemiologic studies have been generally negative.

112. C. Power denotes the energy generated over the aperture. The thermal index is determined from the transducer power but also depends on how that energy is distributed in the ultrasonic field and the conversion of ultrasound energy to heat. The mechanical index is derived from the peak negative pressure. Intensity indicates the spatial distribution of the power and is expressed in units of W/cm^2.

113. B. Small scatterers cannot be resolved as individual entities in the B-mode image. Echoes from multiple scatterers reach the transducer simultaneously and the sum of their signals sum gives rise to speckle.

114. A. For a particular sampling direction, the angle of incidence varies across the curved surface. Often, the echo is generated with a large angle of reflection, whose path does not intercept the transducer.

115. C. Movement of tissue next to flowing blood is falsely assigned a color. Color gain is set too high, or color reject of signals is set too low.

116. C. With write zoom activated, a small, selected region as a subset of the main field of view is displayed. Since the reduced field of view is shown with a high number of pixels, spatial resolution is generally improved.

117. D. The cosine of 90° is zero.

118. D

119. C. The duty factor for continuous emission is 1.

120. D. Tissue-mimicking phantoms cannot measure intensity levels. The placement of small rods within the tissue-mimicking material allows the assessment of lateral resolution, axial resolution, and distance accuracy.

121. D. The oscillating molecules create regions of high density (compression) and low density (rarefaction).

122. B. Determined by the relationship between acoustic velocity, frequency, and wavelength.

123. D. The induced radiofrequency signal is converted into a single metric by rectification, which removes the negative components, followed by enveloping and integration.

124. B. Autocorrelation employed in Doppler imaging yields signal strength and mean velocity. For the color Doppler mode, mean velocity is encoded in color.

125. B. The signal is summed independent of Doppler angle, which improves the signal-to-noise ratio and allows the presentation of low-volume flow.

126. B. Snell's law predicts the angle of transmission based on the incident angle and the ratio of the acoustic velocities in the two media.

127. C. Operating frequency is always expressed in megahertz.

128. C. Pulsed wave transmission results in discrete sampling of the complex Doppler waveform, which means that the Doppler shift frequencies must be inferred from the limited data available. Above the velocity limit corresponding to a high Doppler shift frequency, the rate of sampling is not sufficient to define the Doppler waveform unambiguously, and aliasing occurs.

129. C. Nonlinear propagation at relatively high intensity generates harmonics along the propagation path. Harmonics are formed near the beam axis but displaced from the transducer.

130. C. Fat has lower acoustic velocity and acoustic impedance compared with soft tissue. Frequency is unchanged across an interface. The relationship between acoustic velocity, frequency, and wavelength dictates that wavelength in fat must decrease.

131. A. The speed of sound in a medium equals the square root of the bulk modulus divided by density. The relative high bulk modulus of bone produces an acoustic velocity of 4080 m/s.

132. B. For every 3 dB, the intensity is reduced by a factor of 2. A 6-dB reduction corresponds to two factors of 2, or 2^2, or 4.

133. A. Lateral resolution depends on beam width, near-field depth, and scan line density. Interrogation of the reflector with a series of narrow beams distributed along the surface yields improved definition of the reflector in the image. Interpolation between adjacent scan lines separated by small distances assigns values to unsampled pixels.

134. B. Since multiple frames, separated in time, are combined together to form the displayed image, motion of the reflectors during the averaging period results in blurring.

135. D. When the Doppler angle is 90 degrees, the Doppler shift frequency is zero.

136. C. The Doppler shift frequency is proportional to the transmit frequency. Reducing the center frequency will lower the Doppler shift frequency, and if this results in the pulse repetition frequency being greater than one half of the Doppler shift frequency, aliasing will be eliminated. Decreasing the Doppler angle will make aliasing more pronounced. Increasing the wall filter eliminates low velocity components from the display. Sampling position is dictated by anatomy and not by the presence of aliasing.

137. C. Each 1 cm in depth requires a total transit time of 13 microseconds (μs). For a depth of 3 cm, an echo time of 39 μs is required.

138. B. Acquisition time for color information depends on packet size (the number of transmit pulses along a color line of sight), scan range, color

line density, and the width of the color field of view. By reducing the width of the color field of view while maintaining the color line density, frame rate is increased.

139. A

140. B. Eddy flow is the localized slow rotation of blood layers distal to an obstruction. The rotation creates regions of reversed flow.

141. C. Lateral resolution depends primarily on beam width, but near-field depth and scan line density also influence spatial detail.

142. B. Increasing the transmitted frequency reduces the wavelength and the spatial pulse length and thus, improves axial resolution.

143. B. Dynamic receive focusing is based on the timed summation of received signals. The delay times for the respective crystal elements are defined by the depth of sampling (via echo ranging). Dynamic receive focusing is applied to all depths along the scan line by varying the delay times according to depth.

144. A. Widening the aperture extends the near-field depth and narrows the beam width far from the transducer. More channels and higher frequency (if penetration is sufficient for the depth of interest) would improve focusing. The pulse repetition frequency does not affect transmit focusing.

145. C. Linear arrays with parallel scan lines produces a rectangular filed of view whose width is equal to the physical length of the array.

146. C. Dynamic range is expressed quantitatively as the ratio of the highest signal to the lowest signal that can be detected by the scanner.

147. C. The acoustic impedance mismatch between the media that compose the interface determines the intensity reflection coefficient for specular reflectors.

148. C. Color assignment is based on mean velocity of flow and flow direction. The color gate establishes the size of the color pixel over which the averaging of flow velocities occurs. The strength of the Doppler signal is not displayed in color Doppler (color flow) imaging.

149. D. Slow moving reflectors with low Doppler frequency shifts are eliminated from the display by the wall filter.

150. C. The dipoles are free to reorient when the piezoelectric material is raised to temperature above the Curie temperature.

151. D. Refraction changes the propagation path, and consequently, reflectors encountered by this altered path are spatially registered as if they were located along a straight-line path defined by the sampling direction.

152. B. The ultrasound beam extends laterally in the scan plane beyond the cyst. All reflectors within the sampling volume contribute to the signal at that image location. The cyst, which occupies a small portion of the sampling volume, contributes little or no signal, but this is averaged with signals from other nearby structures causing fill-in.

153. C

154. D. Lower dynamic range restricts the gray levels to a smaller range of echo signals. Low and high signals are displayed as black and white, respectively. The 40-dB setting produces images with high contrast.

155. A. Intensity for a transducer under certain operating conditions is measured in water with a hydrophone. To apply these measurements to tissue for the determination of temperature rise, a correction must be made for the increased attenuation by tissue. This derating factor is usually assumed to be 0.3 dB/cm-MHz.

156. A. Apodization adjusts the strength of the interference pattern for each crystal based on the relative importance of the position of the crystal in the transmit group.

157. B. Fast Fourier transform determines the individual Doppler shift frequencies that are present within the sampling volume.

158. D. Control limits for horizontal distance accuracy is usually 3 mm or 3%, whichever is less restrictive.

159. D. In coded excitation, the transmitted ultrasound energy is distributed over a long transmission duration. Even though the peak intensity is less than that in conventional B-mode imaging, higher cumulative energy results in increased signal-to-noise ratio, increased penetration, or both.

160. D. Each pixel is displayed uniformly as a particular shade of gray as governed by the pixel value and the gray-scale map. The gray-scale map can be selected by the operator, depending on the range of pixel values that need to be differentiated as distinct shades of gray. That is, most of the brightness levels can be distributed over the low signals or high signals as appropriate for the clinical application.

161. A. The two-dimensional array of crystal elements allows beam steering in many different directions on the basis of element selection and time delays.

162. C. Spatial compounding changes the relative beam direction with respect to an interface to maximize reflectivity. Acquiring multiple beam angles and averaging the scan data improve the definition of the curved boundaries throughout the field of view.

163. C. Speckle is the interference pattern incident on the transducer produced by numerous scatterers.

164. D. Grading lobes are produced by the regular spacing of crystal elements across the array.

By reducing the spacing between elements, grading lobes are directed away from the main beam at lower intensity.

165. B. The beat frequency, which is the difference between the transmitted frequency and received frequency (the Doppler shift frequency), is obtained.

166. A. The rod will be presented with increased width in the lateral direction. A reflector smaller than the beam width produces a signal whenever the reflector lies within the sampling volume of the ultrasound beam. The spatial registration of the rod will extent to nearby scan lines whose beam width includes the rod.

167. D. Spatial assignment along the direction of propagation is based on the echo ranging principle.

168. A. Axial resolution is improved by decreasing the spatial pulse length (higher frequency reduces the distance per cycle, or less ringing reduces the number of cycles in the transmitted pulse).

169. C. Since sampling is not intermittent, continuous wave Doppler is not subject to aliasing and the maximum velocity limit imposed by aliasing. Continuous sampling prohibits depth information to be assigned to the moving reflectors. Slow flow with a very small Doppler shift frequency is most likely to be detected when sampling is conducted over several wave cycles.

170. B. A higher frame rate would most likely increase the pulse repetition frequency, which would result in the transmission of more ultrasonic energy into the patient. Time gain compensation (TGC), persistence, and gray-scale mapping are processing techniques that do not affect energy transmission.

171. A. The thermal index indicates the highest temperature rise in degrees Celsius at any point within the ultrasonic field.

172. C. The matching layer reduces the acoustic impedance mismatch between the piezoelectric crystal and the tissue to improve energy transfer into the patient from the transducer.

173. C. The production of harmonics depends on intensity. High-intensity regions in the ultrasonic field are most likely to be near the beam axis.

174. A. Strong attenuation by the mass results in a major loss of intensity compared with that associated with the adjacent soft tissue. Since the soft tissue distal to the cyst is interrogated with lower intensity that the adjacent soft tissue at that same depth but not in the path of the mass, signal reduction occurs.

175. C. The number of scatterers does not appear in the Doppler shift equation.

176. D. The acquisition time for color information depends on packet size (the number of transmit pulses along a color line of sight), scan range, color line density, and the width of the color field of view. By reducing the packet size while maintaining the pulse repetition frequency, frame rate is increased.

177. C. Dynamic receive focusing is applied during reception by the receive beam former.

178. D. Decreasing the transmit power will reduce the peak negative pressure and thus the mechanical index.

179. A. The location of bone within the ultrasonic field has a major impact on the absorption of ultrasound energy and the production of heat.

180. D. Transmit focusing is based on the time for the sound to travel from a specific crystal element to the point of interest. Since the distance from each element to the focal zone is different, the time of travel will be unique. Distance must be converted into time by assuming a constant acoustic velocity. The differences in the times that the wavefronts from the various crystals reach the focal zone give rise to the respective timing delays.

181. B. Snell's law predicts the angle of transmission based on the incident angle and the ratio of the acoustic velocities in the two media.

182. B

183. D

184. C. In many operation modes, the ultrasound beam is pulsed so that active transmission occurs during a small fraction of the time. The duty factor is calculated as the ratio of the pulse duration to the pulse repetition period.

185. A. Blood with relatively few scattering centers is weakly attenuating.

186. A. The large acoustic impedance mismatch between soft tissue and metal creates a situation in which multiple internal reflections occur back and forth within the metal.

187. A

188. C

189. C

190. D

191. C. The rate of attenuation in soft tissue is approximately 0.7 dB/cm-MHz. For 5-MHz ultrasound, the rate of attenuation is 3.5 dB/cm, and after it passes through a thickness of 8 cm, the reduction in intensity is 28 dB.

192. C. Linear arrays have a fixed mechanical focus in the elevation direction.

193. A. The characteristics of composite ceramic materials include lower acoustic impedance, broader bandwidth, and higher sensitivity compared with solid piezoelectric crystals.

194. B. To create constructive interference between the two surfaces necessary for resonance, the distance from one surface to the other must equal

one half of the wavelength. At high center frequency, these crystals are very thin.

195. C. The Doppler shift frequency is directly proportional to the center frequency. Doubling the center frequency also doubles the Doppler shift frequency.

196. B. Reject control eliminates all signals and noise below a threshold value.

197. A. Autocorrelation detection compares signals from successive wavetrains and relies on changes in echo signals to estimate the mean velocity. Noise variations in Doppler processing lead to inaccuracy in the estimation of velocity. A large packet size includes more wavetrains in the analysis and reduces error caused by fluctuating signals.

198. C. The number of scan lines used to compose an image is a compromise between spatial resolution and frame rate. A desire for faster frame rate usually means a reduction in the number of scan lines and poorer spatial detail. The inverse is also true—more scan lines per frame slows the frame rate.

199. D. Transmit focusing reduces the beam width within the focal zone. Constructive interference within the focal zone for the wavefronts from the various crystals gives rise to the respective timing delays. The beam aperture affects the width and the near-field depth of the ultrasonic field. Near the transducer, a small aperture is used (few crystals make up the transmit group). The beam aperture becomes larger as the region of interest extends from the transducer. Apodization adjusts the strength of the interference pattern for each crystal based on the relative importance of the crystal position in the transmit group.

200. B. The view for M-mode imaging is along a single axis and depicts reflector distance from the transducer as a function of time.

201. B. Multiple-zone transmit focusing requires separate pulsed transmission for each focal zone along a scan line, which increases the time required to acquire scan data, resulting in a slower frame rate (if the pulse repetition frequency is unchanged).

202. D. Single element transducers cannot apply dynamic receive focusing.

203. A. Reduced ringing shortens the pulse duration, resulting in broad bandwidth and more efficient energy transmission.

204. D

205. A. Q-value is the ratio of the center frequency to the bandwidth. Continuous wave transducers have a narrow bandwidth and large Q-values.

206. D. The probability for cavitation is inversely proportional to the square root of frequency.

207. C. The 1.5D array has five to seven rows of crystals along the transducer width to enable electronic focusing in the elevation direction.

208. A. Increasing the number of samplings from multiple directions across the field of view causes each reflector to be interrogated at different angles, improving the likelihood for a more favorable reflection angle.

209. D. Q-value decreases as pulse duration becomes shorter. Crystal thickness regulates resonant frequency. Increased acoustic impedance will create a more pronounced mismatch with tissue and inhibit the transmission of energy into the patient (more ringing). A short pulse duration requires a wide frequency range to compose the transmitted pulse.

210. D. Intensity reduction by attenuation is proportional to the distance traveled by the transmitted pulse and the echo. The time of the received echo indicates the length of the propagation path. To compensate for attenuation, time-dependent gain is applied to increase the amplitude of the induced signal.

211. C. A hydrophone is a small-diameter piezoelectric element mounted on a probe, which is placed at various points in the ultrasonic field to measure acoustical pressure at each location.

212. C. Two transmit pulses per cycle are necessary to define the Doppler shift frequency unambiguously. The maximum Doppler shift frequency that can be detected without aliasing is one half of the pulse repetition frequency.

213. B. Range ambiguity artifact occurs when the pulse repetition frequency is high and the delay time for the echo exceeds the time interval between transmitted pulses. The measured echo time is erroneously assigned on the basis of the most recent transmitted pulse, and the reflector is incorrectly placed closer to the transducer in the image. A high attenuation rate and receiver gain affect the displayed brightness of reflectors, but not their position. High power improves signal-to-noise ratio and penetration.

214. A

215. A. Along the beam axis, the assigned distance is based on the echo ranging principle, in which the time of the detected echo is converted into distance by assuming a constant velocity of 1540 m/s. If the tissue-mimicking material has a velocity faster than 1540 m/s, the rod separation will be shorter than the true value. If the tissue-mimicking material has a velocity slower than 1540 m/s, the rod separation will be longer than the true value.

216. B. Red blood cells (RBCs) are Rayleigh scatterers that exhibit a very strong frequency dependence (f^2 to f^6, usually assumed f^4). Doubling the center frequency will increase the scattered intensity by a factor of 16. The intensity of the scattered sound is proportional to the number of RBCs within the sampled volume. Doubling the volume or the concentration increases the scattered intensity by a factor of 2. Doubling the power will also increase the scattered intensity by a factor of 2.

217. A. At any location in the ultrasonic field, intensity can be calculated by adding the contributions from point sources distributed across the transducer surface.

218. D. In an annular array, ring-shaped elements, arranged concentrically, surround a central circular element. This configuration allows multiple transmit focal zones, dynamic receive focusing, and dynamic aperture. However, electronic steering is not possible, and beam direction must be steered by mechanical means.

219. A. Bandwidth is inversely related to the pulse duration. a shortened pulse duration (reduced number of cycles in the transmitted pulse) produces higher bandwidths.

220. B. The mechanical index is directly proportional to the peak rarefactional pressure and inversely proportional to the square root of frequency. These parameters have been demonstrated to affect cavitation.

221. C. The reflection coefficient only depends on the acoustic impedances of the media that compose the interface.

222. B. Relative comparisons of scattered intensity in nearby regions are described as hyperechoic (increased levels) or hypoechoic (decreased levels). A region with no signals is described as anechoic.

223. D. The intensity of scattered ultrasound depends on the number of scatterers per volume, size of the scatterers, acoustic impedance, and frequency.

224. A. The amplitude mode indicates the echo strength by the height of the voltage spike on the monitor, and the displacement along the horizontal axis represents depth of the reflector. One line of sight is repeatedly sampled at the pulse repetition frequency.

225. B. Transverse waves propagate through solid materials such as bone but are not effectively transmitted through soft tissue.

226. C. Intensity is directly proportional to the square of pressure.

227. D. In pulsed wave Doppler, the sampling direction is fixed, and a high pulse repetition frequency is applied to prevent aliasing. Since the same tissue is repeatedly sampled, the temporal averaged intensity is high. M-mode imaging also operates with a fixed scan line, but the pulse repetition frequency is much lower (<500 Hz). The sampling direction in B-mode imaging is repeatedly changed to sample throughout the field of view. Continuous wave fetal heart monitors produce a low power output.

228. A. The analog-to-digital converter (ADC) changes continuously variable analog signals into discrete steps of 0s and 1s.

229. B. Autoscanning of the ultrasound beam by electronic sequencing or steering is limited by the physical length of the array, the beam angle, or both such that the width of the field of view is reduced in size compared with static B-mode imaging. Extended field-of-view imaging is one approach to address this limitation of real-time B-mode imaging.

230. A. Freeze frame suspends ultrasound transmission and displays the last frame acquired. Write zoom and panning are acquisition techniques that use a portion of the total field of view for the transducer. Frame averaging holds scan data in a buffer and combines them with the most recently acquired data to update the display in real time.

231. C. The number of numerical combinations that can be symbolized by a collection of binary digits is given by 2^n, where n is the number of bits. In this example, which is the common configuration of B-mode scanners, 8 bits are necessary to represent 256 different pixel values (0 to 255).

232. D. The Doppler shift frequency is directly proportion to the reflector velocity. If the center frequency and the Doppler angle are unchanged, doubling the velocity also doubles the Doppler shift frequency.

233. A. Near-field depth is directly proportional to frequency and the square of the crystal diameter and inversely proportional to acoustic velocity. The acoustic velocity of soft tissue is fixed by tissue properties so that the manufacturer must rely on frequency and crystal size to alter the ultrasonic field.

234. C. Any break in the integrity of the casing will allow moisture to penetrate the crystal electronics. This poses an electrical hazard to the operator and most likely will cause extensive damage to the transducer. The sonographer has the responsibility to routinely inspect the transducer for cracks and delamination and remove the transducer from service if any damage is found.

235. C. The SMPTE (Society of Motion Picture and Television Engineers) test pattern has been designed to evaluate the performance of monitors and hard copy devices. Boxes with varying brightness levels are presented in 11 steps from 0% to 100% in increments of 10%. All 11 steps should be clearly distinguished and should range from black to white. Contrast and spatial distortion are also evaluated using the SMPTE test pattern.

236. B. The range of echo-induced signals can extend over a range of 100 to 150 dB. All other components in the system have a lower dynamic range, particularly output devices.

237. C. An acoustic lens in front of each crystal in the array narrows the ultrasound beam in the elevation direction. Mechanical focusing fixes the focal zone to one specific depth, where slice thickness is the smallest within the field of view. Outside the focal zone, slice thickness is increased.

238. C. Side lobes are emitted at an angle to the main beam (may be in or out of the scan plane) but are at reduced intensity. A strong reflector encountered along the path of the side lobe will be incorrectly positioned along the scan line direction. Bowel gas or metal are most often responsible for side lobe artifacts, since the large fractional reflection is necessary to generate a detected echo from the weak-intensity side lobe.

239. D. Elastography depicts the relative tissue displacement between precompression and compression by examining the A-mode wavetrains. The echo patterns in short time segments with compression are shifted to match the precompression signal pattern. The time shift yields the displacement, which denotes the strain in response to the stress.

240. B. At each location in the image, the ultrasound beam extends laterally in the scan plane and perpendicular to the scan plane (slice thickness). All reflectors within the sampling volume contribute to the signal at that image location. Large objects within the scan plane solely contribute to the echo signal. A focal lesion that occupies a small portion of the sampling volume contributes a signal, but the signal is partially masked by signals from other nearby structures. Contrast is reduced, since the composite echo signal is not purely from the focal lesion.

241. D. The intensity of the second harmonic is *less* than the fundamental frequency by a magnitude of 100 or more.

242. C. All the choices listed except "C" are part of the Doppler equation, and thus affect the Doppler frequency.

243. B. As velocity of blood decreases, the kinetic energy decreases and the potential energy increases.

244. B. The spatial pulse length is equal to the number of cycles in the pulse multiplied by the wavelength. Increasing the frequency results in a simultaneous decrease in the wavelength, with resultant decrease in the spatial pulse length. Keep in mind that "axial resolution increases" (in choice C) means that axial resolution is poorer.

245. C. Although all four statements are true of CW Doppler, the most important advantage of CW Doppler is it's ability to accurately display high velocities with essentially no upper limit for clinical applications.

246. D. Beam width affects lateral resolution, but not axial resolution.

247. B. Because of the small footprint of a phased array sector transducer, the beam must be electronically steered to the left and right to create the characteristic wedge-shaped sector image.

248. D. The annular array is the only transducer type with concentric ring-shaped elements. Phasing is used to achieve variable focus.

249. D. Color flow imaging uses a combination of scanned and non-scanned technologies. Each color line requires multiple pulses along the same beam path (non-scanned mode). Subsequent lines of color information are obtained by transmitting additional pulse groups or "packets" along successive beam paths (scanned mode).

250. A. The number 27 (+ or -) represents the Nyquist limit of the mean velocity in centimeters per second.

251. B. The 3.9 MHz represents the transmitted frequency for color flow imaging, which is different from the B-mode imaging frequency.

252. D. "Red Away, Blue Towards". Although "Blue Towards, Red Away" (C) would also technically be correct, the two acronyms in common use are "BART" or "RABT".

3D ultrasound An imaging mode in which spatial relationships of structures within a scanned volume are represented in three dimensions. The display of tomographic data is by a surface-rendered image, volume-rendered image, or multiple format planes.

4D ultrasound An imaging mode in which three-dimensional echo data of the sampled volume is displayed in real time.

absorption The process whereby ultrasound energy is dissipated to a medium by conversion to other energy forms, primarily heat. Intensity loss from absorption exhibits an exponential decrease and is the major factor in the total attenuation of the beam.

acoustic impedance A measure of the resistance of a medium to the transmission of sound. Acoustic impedance is expressed as the product of acoustic velocity and the density of the medium.

acoustic velocity The speed at which sound propagates through a medium. The average velocity of sound in soft tissue is 1540 meters per second (m/s).

aliasing An artifact in pulsed wave Doppler, in which Doppler shift frequency is incorrectly interpreted as a lower frequency. Aliasing is caused by the intermittent sampling of moving reflectors.

A-mode Type of scanning mode in which the amplitude of the signal is plotted against the depth of the interface. The signal strength of the detected echo is represented by the height of the vertical deflection of the trace.

amplification A technique in signal processing where all signals are increased by the same amount.

amplitude Normally refers to the particle displacement, particle velocity, or acoustic pressure of a sound wave. Amplitude also indicates the strength of the detected echo or the voltage induced in a crystal by a pressure wave.

analog A continuously variable signal, as opposed to discrete values.

analog-to-digital converter (ADC) A device that translates continuously variable signals (analog) into discrete values (digital). The digital form can then be manipulated and stored by computers.

anechoic Description of a region in an image that is void of signal.

angle of incidence The angle at which the sound beam strikes the interface. The angle is defined with respect to a line drawn perpendicular to the interface.

angle of reflection The angle at which the sound beam is reflected from the interface. The angle is defined with respect to perpindicular to the interface.

annular phased array Type of transducer in which the crystal arrangement consists of a central disc surrounded by concentric rings. Electronic focusing narrows the beam width for both in-plane and out-of-plane directions. Sampling along different lines of sight is achieved by the mechanical movement of the crystal array.

aperture The physical extent of the piezoelectric element(s) activated to form a transmitted beam.

apodization A technique applied during transmission and reception to reduce secondary lobes and enhance beam formation. During transmission, the excitation voltage is varied for each crystal element across the aperture of a multiple-element array. During reception the applied gain is varied for each crystal element in the array.

artifact A structure in the image that does not provide a true representation of the scanned object. Artifacts are created by the inherent nature of sound interactions (e.g., reflection, refraction, and attenuation) or by equipment malfunction or by improper operation of the equipment.

asynchronous scanner In Doppler imaging, flow data and gray-scale scan data are acquired independently (separate and distinct transmission for each).

attenuation The decrease in intensity via scattering and absorption as a sound beam travels through a medium.

autocorrelation A signal processing technique in Doppler imaging whereby a series of echoes from the same reflector (red blood cell group) are compared to assess motion. This is a very fast data collection method by which the mean frequency and amplitude of the Doppler signal are measured.

axial resolution The ability to resolve, as separate entities, objects located near each other along the axis of propagation. Axial resolution depends primarily on spatial pulse length.

backing material The material placed behind the crystal in the transducer to control the ringing of the crystal. In B-mode imaging, the acoustic impedance of the backing material is nearly the same as that for the crystal to dampen ringing.

bandwidth A parameter that describes the spread of frequency components in a wave (e.g., transmitted pulse).

baseline In pulsed-wave spectral Doppler scanning, a control that shifts the center point of the velocity scale to vary the range of velocities displayed in the forward and reverse directions.

beam cross-sectional area The area on the surface of a plane perpendicular to the beam axis consisting of all points at which the intensity is greater than 25% of the maximum intensity.

beam formation (reception) Echo-induced signals from multiple crystal elements are delayed in time and then summed to maximize the net signal associated with the reflector.

beam formation (transmission) Timed sequence of excitation pulses applied to crystal elements across the aperture to enable focusing of the ultrasound beam, steering of the ultrasound beam, or both.

beam width The lateral extent of the beam perpendicular to beam propagation. Beam width (in-plane and elevation) varies along the beam axis.

beat frequency A phenomenon caused by wave interference in which waves of different frequencies, when added together, produce rhythmic cycles or beats. In pulsed wave spectral Doppler scanning, the transmitted waveform and the received signals are combined to yield the beat frequency (Doppler shift frequency), which indicates the presence of motion.

bilinear interpolation A scan conversion method to assign echo amplitude to a pixel, which is not interrogated by a scan line. The interpolation is performed in axial and angular directions.

broadband transducer A transducer with a wide frequency distribution. The fractional bandwidth is ≥15%.

bulk modulus A physical parameter that quantifies the fractional change in volume when a pressure is applied to material.

cavitation Dynamic behavior of microbubbles in the medium exposed to an ultrasonic beam. Two types of cavitation are possible: stable and transient.

center frequency The dominant frequency in the transmitted pulse (highest magnitude in a graph of frequency components).

channel A communication pathway between a crystal element and the transmitter or summing circuit in the beam former. The total number of channels limits the number of crystal elements that participate in beam formation.

cine loop Multiple frames of a real-time acquisition stored in computer memory for playback.

clutter Spurious echo signals originating outside the main beam caused by side lobes, grating lobes, and scattering.

coded excitation Frequency modulation or binary encoding of the transmitted pulse to improve signal-to-noise ratio. On reception, the echo wavetrain must be manipulated mathematically (deconvoluted) to identify individual reflectors.

color aliasing An artifact in Doppler imaging, in which the Doppler shift frequency above the Nyquist limit is depicted by colors associated with slower flow.

color bleed An extension of color beyond the region of flow in Doppler imaging.

color flash Sudden burst of color associated with tissue movement in Doppler imaging.

color flow imaging A real-time imaging modality in which flow information encoded in color is superimposed on a gray-scale image depicting stationary structures.

color gain Doppler imaging control that adjusts the amplification of the Doppler signal.

color gate Doppler imaging control that sets the axial length of the color sampling volume.

color map Assignment of various shades or brightness of color to depict different velocities while maintaining directional information.

color M-mode The presentation of the color Doppler image in conjunction with the M-mode trace. The sampling direction for the M-mode trace is shown on the color Doppler image.

color noise Random variations in signal detection cause areas with no flow to be color encoded in Doppler imaging.

color persistence Frame averaging in Doppler imaging.

color reject Doppler imaging control that sets the minimum signal strength for the display of color Doppler signals.

color threshold Doppler imaging control that sets the lower velocity limit for the display of moving reflectors.

combined Doppler mode The presentation of the color flow image in conjunction with the time display of the pulsed wave spectral analysis.

comet tail artifact An artifact created from small, highly reflective interfaces. Multiple internal reflections are ultimately detected and are mapped in the image extending distally from the reflector.

compressibility The ease with which a medium can be reduced in volume. The velocity of sound in a medium is inversely proportional to the square root of the compressibility of the medium.

compression (wave propagation) A high-pressure region or a region of increased density of particles created by the action of the sound wave.

constructive interference A process whereby two waves algebraically add together to produce a wave with greater amplitude than either of the original waves.

contrast enhancement An image processing technique that changes the association between pixel values and gray levels to display pixels with similar signal levels as different shades of gray.

contrast resolution The ability to resolve two objects with similar reflective properties (signal levels) as separate entities.

converse piezoelectric effect A property of piezoelectric materials whereby an electric stimulus causes the dipolar material to expand and contract, producing a pressure wave (sound wave). This property permits a material to be used as a transmitter of ultrasound.

curvilinear array Multiple crystal elements arranged linearly on a curved surface. The width of the field of view extends beyond the physical dimension of the row of crystal elements.

cycle A sequence of events recurring at regular intervals in time or space. For example, particle density varies from a maximum in the compression zone to a minimum in the rarefaction zone and back to a maximum in the successive compression zone to complete one cycle.

damping The process to reduce ringing so that pulse duration is decreased following crystal excitation. Damping is affected by the backing material and is quantified by the Q-value of the transducer.

dead zone The distance from the face of the transducer to the closest identifiable echo.

decibel Unit to express relative intensity.

delay gain A control to set the depth at which the time gain compensation is first applied.

demodulation (signal isolation) Waves that have undergone interference are subsequently manipulated to isolate a signal. This procedure is often used in Doppler ultrasound, in which the sum of the reference and received signals produce oscillations that vary in strength at the Doppler shift frequency.

demodulation (signal processing) The technique of enveloping the radiofrequency signal by ignoring the rapid oscillations and retaining the maximum amplitude of each cycle.

density A physical parameter that describes the mass per unit volume of a medium.

depth of field Length of the focal zone for a focused transducer.

derating factor Fractional reduction in intensity or pressure caused by attenuation.

destructive interference A process whereby waves add together algebraically to give a resultant wave of lower amplitude than either of the original waves.

diffraction The spreading out of the beam that results from the beam passing through a small aperture.

diffuse reflection The reflection of an ultrasound beam in multiple directions from a large rough-surfaced object.

dipole Positively and negatively charged regions on a molecule.

dispersion The dependence of the velocity of sound or other physical parameter on the frequency of the sound.

distortion A parameter of image quality that describes the lack of adherence to actual geometric relationships.

divergence The spreading out of a beam from a source of small physical dimensions, diffraction, or scattering. Divergence reduces beam intensity.

Doppler angle The angle between the beam axis and the direction of travel for the moving reflector.

Doppler effect Relative motion between the sound source and sound receiver causes a change in the observed frequency.

Doppler imaging Moving reflectors encoded in color and stationary reflectors encoded in shades of gray are depicted throughout the field of view in real time.

Doppler shift frequency The change in frequency between the transmitted frequency (f) and received frequency by reflection from an interface moving with velocity (v) at an angle (θ) to sound propagation:

$$\text{Doppler shift} = \frac{2f\,v\cos\theta}{c}$$

where c is the velocity of sound in the medium.

Doppler spectral waveform The time display of the velocity distribution present in the Doppler signal.

duplex scanner Instrument that combines real-time imaging with spectral Doppler scanning

duty factor The fraction of the time the transducer is actively producing the ultrasound beam. Duty factor equals pulse duration divided by pulse repetition period.

dwell time The time required to interrogate one line of sight.

dynamic range A measure of the spread of signal magnitudes that can be represented or processed by a device.

dynamic receive focusing An electronic focusing method that uses continuously variable delay lines to sweep the receive focal zone through all depths during the reception of returning echoes.

echo-ranging A technique to determine the distance of an object from the transducer that relies on the measured time delay from pulse transmission to echo detection.

echo wavetrain The succession of echoes detected along a line of sight following the transmitted pulse.

edge enhancement A filtering technique to make the boundaries of structures more distinct.

elastography An imaging modality that depicts the resistance of tissue to a change in shape when force is applied.

electronic focusing Electronic delay lines connected to individual crystals of a multiple-element transducer are adjusted to cause the ultrasonic wavefronts to reach the point of interest in phase (focus) and to reinforce the induced signals on reception of the echo.

endosonography Specialized real-time imaging with small probes that can be inserted into various body cavities (e.g., endovaginal and endorectal).

enhancement An image artifact caused by unequal attenuation along scan lines. Reflectors distal to a low-attenuating object appear with greater signal level than do identical reflectors located in the neighboring region.

ensemble length The number of transmit pulses that sample a color line of sight in Doppler imaging. Also called *packet size*.

enveloping Signal processing in which the boundary of the peaks of the rectified radiofrequency signal is encircled.

extended field of view Imaging method to enlarge the field of view of a real-time transducer. As a transducer is moved across the patient, successive frames are combined to form a panoramic image.

far-field The region beyond the near-field for a nonfocused transducer in which the ultrasound beam diverges rapidly. Also called *Fraunhofer zone*.

far gain The time gain compensation control that sets maximum amplification near the limit of the scan range.

fast Fourier transform (FFT) Mathematic algorithm that separates a waveform into the various frequency components. Spectral analysis of the complex Doppler signal identifies the Doppler shift frequencies and their relative importance.

field of view (FOV) The physical region probed by the ultrasound beam that corresponds to the image.

focal length The distance from the front face of the transducer to the focal point.

focal point The point along the beam axis with minimum width and maximum intensity for a focused transducer.

focal zone For a focused transducer, the region defined by the pressure amplitude that is within 3 decibels (dB) of the maximum pressure amplitude of the transmitted beam. The focal zone corresponds to the region of minimum beam width.

focusing A process whereby the beam width is reduced by mechanical or electronic means.

footprint The active piezoelectric area of a transducer that transmits ultrasound waves.

fractional bandwidth The spread of frequency components in a transmitted wave expressed as a fraction of the center frequency.

frame rate In B-mode imaging, the number of images acquired per second. Also describes the refresh rate of a display.

free-field measurements Performed in water without reflectors or other disturbances to the ultrasonic field.

freeze frame A single image acquired during real-time scanning that is designated for display.

frequency The number of wave cycles passing a given point in a given increment of time. The unit is cycles/second or hertz. Frequency is the inverse of period.

frequency compounding Frequency components in the echo signal are processed separately and then recombined in a single image to improve penetration, resolution, or tissue texture.

gain B-mode control which amplifies all received signals equally.

ghosting artifact An artifact whereby an object located distal to refractive structures is replicated multiple times in the image.

grating lobes Secondary intensity lobes created by the regular spacing of crystal elements.

gray-scale mapping The translation of pixel signal values to gray levels for display.

half-value layer (HVL) The amount of material required to reduce the intensity by half of its original value. A half-value layer results in a 3-decibel (dB) reduction in intensity.

harmonic frequencies Frequencies which are integer multiples of the fundamental frequency.

hertz The unit of frequency that expresses the number of cycles per second.

high-PRF mode A method to reduce aliasing by increasing the pulse repetition frequency above the constraint imposed by echo ranging, but with some ambiguity in depth position.

horizontal distance Measurement of distance in the direction perpendicular to the central axis of the beam.

Huygens' principle The division of a large sound source into a collection of small radiating sources. Each small individual source creates a distinctive beam pattern, which interferes with those from other sources to form a complex beam pattern.

hydrophone A device to measure pressure variations in the ultrasonic field.

hyperechoic Description of a region in an image that is relatively high in signal compared with the surrounding area.

hypoechoic Description of a region in an image that is relatively low in signal compared with the surrounding area.

infrasound Low-frequency (<20 hertz [Hz]) mechanical waves that the human ear cannot detect.

integration A signal processing technique in which the area under the enveloped signal is measured. The area corresponds to the signal strength of the returning echo.

intensity A physical parameter that describes the amount of energy flowing through the cross-sectional area of a beam each second.

intensity descriptors Parameters used to specify the intensity of the ultrasonic field with respect to space and time.

intensity reflection coefficient The fraction of beam intensity reflected from an acoustic interface, given as

$$\alpha_R = \left(\frac{Z_2 - Z_1}{Z_2 + Z_1}\right)^2$$

where Z_1 and Z_2 are the acoustic impedances of the media that compose the interface.

Inter-element coupling The vibration or electrical stimulation of one crystal element in an array affecting adjacent crystal elements.

interface The junction of two media with different acoustic properties.

interference The superposition or algebraic summation of waves. Constructive or destructive interference can occur.

lateral resolution The ability to resolve, as separate entities, two adjacent objects that lie perpendicular to the beam axis. Lateral resolution depends on beam width.

length focusing (in-plane) Electronic focusing of a multiple-element array to reduce in-plane beam width. This type of focusing is accomplished electronically.

linear array A multiple-element transducer in which the crystal elements are positioned next to one another in a row. Selective activation of crystal elements determines the direction of sampling. The image format is rectangular.

line density The number of scan lines per linear distance or angular degree within the field of view.

line of sight The sampling direction of the sound beam. Multiple lines of sight are necessary to compose a B-mode image.

log compression In the scan converter, signals throughout the dynamic range are assigned discrete digital values according to a logarithmic scale.

longitudinal wave A wave in which the particle motion is along the same direction as the propagation of the wave energy (direction of travel of the wave).

matching layer A layer of material placed next to the radiating surface of the crystal in the transducer to facilitate the transmission of sound energy into the patient.

matrix size The number of rows and columns of pixels that compose the image.

maximum depth of visualization The maximum depth at which scatterers are perceived.

maximum velocity waveform The time display of the highest velocity component of the Doppler signal.

mean frequency The average of all Doppler shift frequencies in the Doppler signal.

mechanical focusing The method of focusing using an acoustic lens or a curved crystal.

mechanical index A parameter that describes the acoustic output in terms of the likelihood of cavitation, predicted by the ratio of the peak rarefactional pressure to the square root of the frequency.

megarayls Unit of acoustic impedance, which equals 10^6 kilogram per meters squared–second (kg/m^2-s).

mirror-image artifact An artifact in which an object is duplicated in the image. The incorrect placement of the object occurs distal to the strong reflector in the image.

misregistration The improper placement of a reflector in the image such that the geometric relationships of the structures are misrepresented.

M-mode scanning A scanning technique that depicts the reflector position with respect to time in a two-dimensional display.

multiple-path artifact An image artifact that occurs when the beam strikes multiple interfaces before returning to the transducer. The reflector is placed at the incorrect location with improper brightness.

narrowband transducer A transducer with a narrow frequency spectrum. The fractional bandwidth is less than 15%.

near-field For the nonfocused transducer, the region that extends from the front face to the beginning of divergence.

near-gain A time gain compensation control that sets amplification in the region close to the transducer.

noise Random variations in measured echo signals, which do not correspond to reflectivity.

nonfocused transducer A transducer with no mechanical or electronic focusing. The beam width is normally the same dimension as the crystal in the near-field with rapid divergence in the far-field.

nonlinear propagation At high intensity, the sound wave is distorted from the sinusoidal shape with the introduction of additional frequency components (harmonics).

nonspecular reflector An interface with small physical dimensions (i.e., a wavelength or less in size). Also called *scattering*.

Nyquist limit The minimum rate the Doppler signal that can be sampled without aliasing.

output display standard (ODS) The effect of current operating parameters on acoustic output expressed as the thermal index (TI) and the mechanical index (MI).

packet size The number of transmit pulses used to sample a color line of sight in Doppler imaging. Also called *ensemble length*.

panning Translation of the write zoom field of view within the limits of the field of view imposed by the transducer.

partial volume The assignment of an intermediate signal level when the ultrasonic beam encompasses objects with different reflectivities.

particle displacement The distance traveled by vibrating particles from their unperturbed positions when acted on by a force.

particle velocity The speed at which the particles vibrate back and forth about their unperturbed positions when acted on by a force. The particle velocity induced by a sound wave is not constant.

pascal A unit of acoustic pressure in the meter-kilogram-second system of measurement which corresponds to newton per meter squared (10^5 pascals equals 1 atm).

peak negative pressure The maximum rarefactional pressure produced by the sound wave.

percentage reflection The percentage of the incident beam intensity reflected from an acoustic interface.

percentage transmission The percentage of the incident beam intensity transmitted across an interface.

period The time for one complete wave cycle. Period is the inverse of wave frequency.

persistence A frame-averaging technique to reduce noise.

phantom A test device that mimics the properties of tissue (velocity, attenuation, and scattering) with respect to sound transmission.

phase aberration Loss of signal coherence during beam formation caused by acoustic velocity differences in tissue.

phased array A multiple-element transducer in which the beam is electronically steered and focused by time-delayed excitation of the crystals. The image format is sector.

piezoelectric effect A pressure wave (sound wave) incident on a material with aligned dipolar molecules induces an electric signal. This permits the material to be used as a receiver of sound waves.

pixel A small, square or rectangular picture element in the digital image that represents a portion of the scanned area. A pixel is the smallest spatial component of an image. The value assigned to a pixel denotes the signal strength of the detected echo.

power A measure of the total energy transmitted per unit time summed over the entire cross-sectional area of the beam (intensity multiplied by area). The unit of power is the watt (joule per second).

power (control) B-mode control that varies the excitation voltage applied to transducer elements to adjust the intensity of the transmitted beam.

power Doppler Doppler imaging technique in which the signal strength (not velocity) of moving reflectors at each sampling site is encoded by color.

power map Color assignment in Doppler imaging based on the Doppler signal strength.

power spectrum Graphic representation of the spectral analysis in which the magnitude of each frequency is plotted as a function of frequency.

propagation The transmittal of sound energy to regions remote from the sound source.

propagation error The incorrect assignment of reflector size or position caused by acoustic velocity deviation from 1540 meters per second (m/s) along the beam path. Also called *velocity error*.

pulse average The duration of a single pulse prescribes the time interval over which the intensity is measured.

pulse duration (temporal pulse length) The time interval during which the transmitted pulse is generated. The pulse duration is calculated by multiplying the number of cycles in the pulse by period.

pulse repetition frequency (PRF) The number of transmitted pulsed waves generated each second. The maximum PRF depends on the scan range (R) and the acoustic velocity (c):

$$PRF_{max} = \frac{c}{2R}$$

pulse repetition period (PRP) The time interval between successive transmit pulses. It is equal to the inverse of pulse repetition frequency.

quality control (QC) The routine testing of equipment to ensure proper function. An effective QC program is necessary to obtain high-quality images on a consistent basis.

quarter wavelength transducer A transducer that uses a one-quarter wavelength matching layer at the radiating surface of the crystal to reduce crystal–tissue impedance mismatch.

Q-value A transducer parameter that characterizes the pulse length and bandwidth of the transducer.

range ambiguity artifact The misplacement of a reflector in the B-mode image when the detected echo was not created from the most recent transmitted pulse.

range gate The selection of a time interval (time delay and time length) after pulsed wave transmission during which the detected echoes are processed for display. Since distance from the transducer is defined by the

elapsed time, analysis is restricted to echoes originating from a specific depth.

rarefaction A low-pressure region or a region of decreased density in a medium created by the action of the sound wave.

rayl The unit of acoustic impedance, which is equal to kilogram per square meter per second (kg/m^2-s).

Rayleigh scattering Scattering from small structures with dimensions very much less than the wavelength of the sound wave.

read zoom A method to magnify the image size on the monitor.

real-time scanning An automated scanning technique in which a rapid sequence of images is acquired and displayed one after the other to depict motion or changing field of view.

rectification Signal processing by which the negative components of the radiofrequency signal are converted to positive components or eliminated.

reflection An interaction that results in a fraction of the sound intensity redirected into the medium from which it came after striking an acoustic interface. The angle of incidence equals the angle of reflection. The intensity of the reflected wave depends on the composition of the interface.

reflectivity The combination of factors—including acoustic impedance mismatch, size, shape, and angle of incidence—that determine the intensity of a reflected echo from an interface.

refraction A process whereby sound enters one medium from another, resulting in a bending or deviation of a sound beam from the expected straight-line path. Refraction obeys Snell's law, which is based on the ratio of the velocity of sound in the respective media.

reject Signal processing that discards signals that are less than a selected level.

relaxation time A time indicative of the rate in which a molecule returns to its original position after being displaced by a force.

reverberation An artifact in B-mode imaging created when repeated reflections occur between two strong reflectors.

ring-down artifact An image artifact created when an object vibrates at a characteristic resonance frequency. This artifact resembles a comet tail artifact without the specific banding often seen with the comet tail.

ringing Continued expansion and contraction of a crystal after excitation by a short duration voltage pulse.

risks versus benefits An assessment of the potential harm associated with a particular agent compared with the expected medical outcome.

scan converter A device that stores scan data in the form of echo signal strengths with the corresponding locations of the interfaces.

scan line The sampling direction of the sound beam. Multiple lines of sight are necessary to compose a B-mode image. Also called *line of sight*.

scan range The maximum depth from which a returning echo can be detected with the correct assignment of reflector depth. The maximum depth of the field of view.

scattering The redirection of sound energy resulting from the sound beam striking an interface whose physical dimension is less than one wavelength. Also called *nonspecular reflection*.

sector scanner A real-time scanner that produces a pie-shaped field of view.

sensitivity The ability of the scanner to detect weak-reflecting objects at a specific distance from the transducer.

shadowing The reflectors distal to a highly attenuating object appear lower in signal strength than adjacent reflectors with similar reflectivities.

side lobes Secondary intensity lobes displaced from the main beam.

signal The voltage variation induced by a pressure wave incident on a piezoelectric crystal. The subsequent manipulation of a time-dependent voltage pattern is called *signal processing*.

signal processing The manipulation of a received echo signal to enhance the presentation of scan data.

signal-to-noise ratio (SNR) The strength of the echo signal as compared with the noise level. Contrast resolution and sensitivity improve as the signal-to-noise ratio is increased.

slice thickness The out-of-plane (elevation) thickness that contributes to the echo formation at that location in the image.

slope A time gain compensation control to adjust amplification with depth.

smoothing A spatial filtering technique for reducing noise in the image.

Snell's law A mathematic description of the principle of refraction that relates the bending of the wave with the ratio of the acoustic velocities for the media.

sound Mechanical vibrations or pressure waves that the human ear can detect. The frequency range is between 20 and 20,000 hertz (Hz). Sound waves require a medium for propagation. The term *sound* is commonly used in the broad sense to include mechanical vibrations of all frequencies, including ultrasound.

spatial average intensity Average of intensity measurements over the cross-sectional area of the beam.

spatial average, pulse average intensity (I[SAPA]) The pulse average intensity averaged over the beam cross-sectional area. May be approximated as the ratio of ultrasonic power to the product of duty factor and beam cross-sectional area.

spatial average, temporal average intensity (I[SATA]) The temporal average intensity averaged over the beam cross-sectional area. May be approximated as the ratio of ultrasonic power to the beam cross-sectional area.

spatial average, temporal peak intensity (I[SATP]) The temporal peak intensity averaged over the beam cross-sectional area.

spatial compounding A real-time imaging method in which scan lines for consecutive frames are steered at different angles and the scan data are combined to form a composite image.

spatial peak intensity Location in the ultrasonic field where intensity has the highest value.

spatial peak, pulse-averaged intensity (I[SPPA]) The maximum pulse-averaged intensity in the ultrasonic field.

spatial peak, temporal average intensity (I[SPTA]) The maximum temporal average intensity in the ultrasonic field.

spatial peak, temporal peak intensity (I[SPTP]) The maximum temporal peak intensity in the ultrasonic field.

spatial pulse length The spatial extent of the transmitted pulse. The spatial pulse length is the product of the number of cycles in the pulse and the wavelength.

speckle Interference pattern incident on a transducer produced by echoes from multiple scatterers. The signal does not exhibit a one-to-one correspondence with the scatters. The speckle pattern is frequency dependent.

spectral analysis The process of determining the individual Doppler shift frequencies that are present in the complex Doppler signal and the relative importance of each.

spectral broadening The introduction of additional frequency components in the complex Doppler signal caused by limitations in the detection technique.

spectral invert A control to alter the assigned flow direction of the Doppler spectral waveform with respect to the baseline.

specular reflector An interface much larger than the wavelength of the sound wave.

stable cavitation The expansion and contraction of pre-existing microbubbles in response to the applied pressure oscillations.

static B-mode imaging Original form of brightness mode scanning in which the brightness of a dot indicates the amplitude of the signal at the location of the interface.

subdicing The crystal element of an array is divided into several smaller subelements. These subelements are electrically wired together to act conjointly. Subdicing helps reduce the intensity of grating lobes.

synchronous scanner A type of scanner for Doppler imaging in which gray-scale and flow data are acquired simultaneously along a line of sight.

temporal average intensity The time average of intensity at a point in space.

temporal peak intensity The peak value of the intensity at a point in space.

temporal resolution The ability to depict the movement of structures accurately.

thermal index The ratio of the in situ acoustic power to the acoustic power required to raise tissue temperature by 1°C.

time gain compensation (TGC) A B-mode control to vary amplification of the signal with depth to compensate for intensity loss caused by attenuation.

tissue harmonic imaging Imaging mode that detects harmonic frequencies created by the nonlinear propagation of ultrasound through tissue.

tissue-mimicking (TM) phantom A phantom made of materials that mimic the ultrasonic properties of tissue

with respect to velocity, attenuation, and scattering. Small, strong reflectors are placed in well-defined geometric patterns within the phantom to assess axial resolution, lateral resolution, dead zone, and distance accuracy.

transducer Any device that converts one form of energy into another form. In ultrasound, a piezoelectric crystal converts an electrical stimulus into an ultrasound pulse and the returning echo into an electrical signal.

transient cavitation Short-lived bubbles undergo large variation in size before completely collapsing.

transit time broadening Introduction of frequency components above and below the actual Doppler shift because sampling is performed with a finite beam size.

transmission coefficient A coefficient that describes the fraction of intensity of a beam transmitted through an acoustic interface.

transverse wave The motion of the particles in the medium is perpendicular to the direction of wave propagation.

ultrasonic field The region over which sound energy is transmitted.

ultrasound High-frequency (>20 kilohertz [kHz]) mechanical vibrations or pressure waves that the human ear cannot detect.

uniformity Signals obtained for interfaces with similar reflective properties located at the same depth have the same amplitude.

variance map Color assignment in Doppler imaging based on the distribution of velocities within the sampling volume.

vector array A transducer with multiple crystals in a linear format that steers the beam via electronic phasing to extend the width of the field of view. Also called, "compound linear array".

velocity error The incorrect assignment of reflector size or position caused by acoustic velocity deviation from 1540 meters per second (m/s) along the beam path. Also called *propagation error*.

velocity map The assignment of various color hues or saturation based on flow velocity in Doppler imaging.

velocity scale In flow detection, the range of velocities that can be displayed without aliasing.

vertical distance Measurement of distance in the direction along the central axis of the beam.

wall filter A high-pass filter that eliminates low-frequency Doppler shift frequencies associated with slow-moving structures such as the vessel wall.

wavefront The compression zone within one wave cycle. Successive wavefronts illustrate the beam pattern generated by an ultrasound source.

wavelength A physical characteristic of a wave that is the distance for one complete wave cycle.

write zoom Magnification technique applied during data collection to improve spatial detail by mapping the detected echoes within a field of view that has reduced physical dimensions.

zone sonography A B-mode imaging method in which echo wavetrain data for each channel following a series of broad beam transmitted pulses are mathematically reconstructed to form the image.

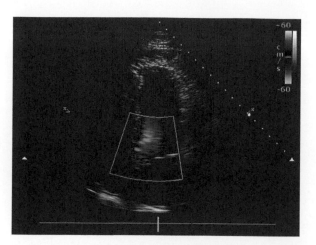

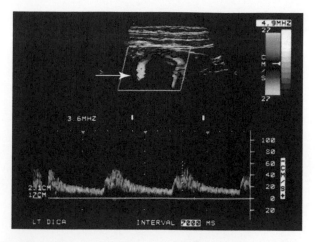

COLOR PLATE 1 Apical 4-chamber view of the heart obtained with a 3 MHz sector transducer. The color ROI box defines the portion of the 2D field of view for color display (see Fig. L15-1).

COLOR PLATE 2 Linear array image with color box showing increased brightness where the color angle to flow approaches 0° (*arrow*). Spectral Doppler with angle correction shows correct flow velocity (see Fig. L15-2).

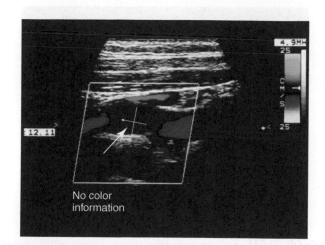

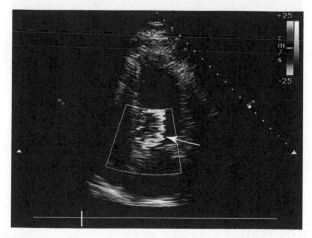

COLOR PLATE 3 Linear array color flow image with color ROI box. A perpendicular color angle to flow in the center of the box shows an area of no color (*arrow*). Color flow is observed near the box edges where an adequate angle to flow exists (see Fig. L15-4).

COLOR PLATE 4 Color aliasing creates a "mosaic pattern" (*arrow*) that helps draw the viewer's eye to high velocity flow (see Fig. L15-5).

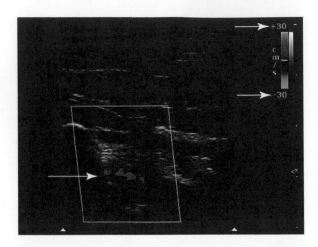

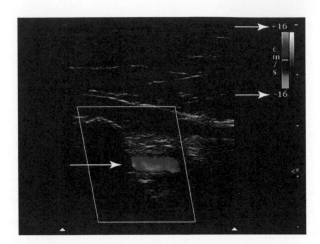

COLOR PLATE 5 Color scale set to +/− 30 cm/s (*small arrows*). Note the poorly displayed color flow within the vertebral artery (*large arrow*) (see Fig. L15-6).

COLOR PLATE 6 Color scale decreased to +/− 16 cm/s (*small arrows*). Note the color flow within the vertebral artery (*large arrow*) is more uniform than in Fig. L15-6 (see Fig. L15-7).

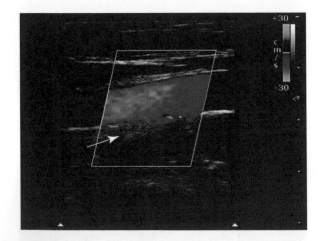

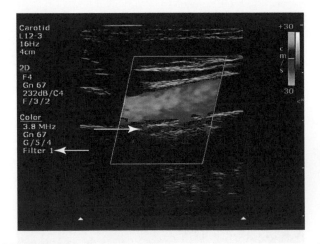

COLOR PLATE 7 Color gain set too high which causes color bleed outside the vessel walls (*arrow*) (see Fig. L15-8).

COLOR PLATE 8 Color wall filter set on lowest setting (*small arrow*) results in color wall motion artifact (*large arrow*) (see Fig. L16-2).

Printed and bound by CPI Group (UK) Ltd, Croydon, CR0 4YY

03/10/2024

01040311-0020